HIV ESSENTIALS

Eighth Edition

Paul E. Sax, MD
Clinical Director
Division of Infectious Disease and HIV Program
Brigham and Women's Hospital
Professor of Medicine
Harvard Medical School
Boston, MA

2017

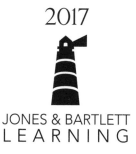

JONES & BARTLETT
LEARNING

World Headquarters
Jones & Bartlett Learning
5 Wall Street
Burlington, MA 01803
978-443-5000
info@jblearning.com
www.jblearning.com

Jones & Bartlett Learning books and products are available through most bookstores and online booksellers. To contact Jones & Bartlett Learning directly, call 800-832-0034, fax 978-443-8000, or visit our website at www.jblearning.com.

Substantial discounts on bulk quantities of Jones & Bartlett Learning publications are available to corporations, professional associations, and other qualified organizations. For details and specific discount information, contact the special sales department at Jones & Bartlett Learning via the above contact information or send an email to specialsales@jblearning.com.

Production Credits

Executive Editor: Nancy Anastasi Duffy
Senior Production Editor: Daniel Stone
Manufacturing and Inventory Control Supervisor: Amy Bacus

Composition: diacriTech, Chennai, India
Cover Design: Scott Moden
Printing and Binding: Cenveo, Inc.
Cover Printing: Cenveo, Inc.

ISBN-13: 978-1-284-12470-5

6048

Printed in the United States of America
20 19 18 17   10 9 8 7 6 5 4 3 2

EDITORIAL NOTE

The last decade of HIV treatment has seen substantial improvements in efficacy, safety, and tolerability of antiretroviral th erapy (ART). Now essentially any patient taking ART can achieve and maintain virologic suppression, all but eliminating the risk of AIDS-related complications. As such, emphasis has shifted in many patients from the sole goal of controlling viral replication to the long-term need of preventing complications of aging, in particular cardiovascular disease and malignancies.

The goal of this guide is to provide practitioners actively involved in HIV care with rapid access to practical information useful for patient management. W hen possible, we cite US national guidelines from the Department of Health and Human Services and the International AIDS Society–USA; these are available at aidsinfo.nih.gov or www.iasusa.org respectively, and readers are advised to check these sites for the most recent updates. Recommendations are also based on interpret ation of clinical trials, cohort studies, case reports, and personal experience.

While there have been several advances in the HIV field since the last edition of this guide, three in particular stand out: First, HIV treatment is now recommended for all people, regardless of clinical status or CD4 cell count; second, HIV prevention now has greatly advanced, with treatment as prevention and pre-exposure prophylaxis (PrEP) now being our primary tools; and third, HCV treatment has been completely transformed with simple and highly effective interferon-free strategies.

This volume is dedicated to people living with HIV who have partnered with us to learn how to manage this condition, and to the doctors, nurses, social workers, pharmacists,and other healthcare professionals who focus on HIV as a specialty and continue to teach all of us how to get better at what we do.

Paul E. Sax, MD

TABLES AND FIGURES

TABLE OF CONTENTS

TABLE OF CONTENTS (cont'd)

CONTRIBUTORS

Paul E. Sax, MD
Clinical Director, Division of
   Infectious Diseases and HIV Program
Brigham and Women's Hospital
Professor of Medicine
Harvard Medical School
Boston, Massachusetts

Kari Furtek
South Texas Veterans Health Care
   System (STVHCS)
San Antonio, Texas

David W. Kubiak, PharmD, BCPS
Infectious Disease Clinical Pharmacist
Brigham and Women's Hospital
Adjunct Clinical Assistant
Professor of Pharmacy
Bouvé College of Health Sciences
School of Pharmacy
Northeastern University
Boston, Massachusetts

ACKNOWLEDGMENTS

To accomplish the task of presenting the data compiled in this reference, a small, dedicated team of professionals was assembled. This team focused their energy and discipline for many months into typing, revising, designing, illustrating, and formatting the many chapters that make up this text. We wish to acknowledge Monica Crowder Kaufman for her important contribution. We would also like to thank the many contributors who graciously contributed their time and energy.

Paul E. Sax, MD

NOTICE

HIV Essentials has been developed as a concise, practical, and authoritative guide for the evaluation and treatment of HIV infection. The clinical recommendations set forth in this book are those of the authors and are offered as general guidelines, not specific instructions for individual patients. Clinical judgment should always guide the physician in the selection, dosing, and duration of antimicrobial therapy for individual patients. Not all medications have been accepted by the US Food and Drug Administration for indications cited in this book, and antimicrobial recommendations are not limited to indications in the package insert. The use of any drug should be preceded by careful review of the package insert, which provides indications and dosing approved by the US Food and Drug Administration. The information provided in this book is not exhaustive, and the reader is referred to other medical references and the manufacturer's product literature for further information. Clinical use of the information provided and any consequences that may arise from its use is the responsibility of the prescribing physician. The authors, editors, and publisher do not warrant or guarantee the information herein contained and do not assume and expressly disclaim any liability for errors or omissions or any consequences that may occur from use of this information.

ABBREVIATIONS FOR ANTIRETROVIRAL AGENTS

3TC	lamivudine	FPV	fosamprenavir
ABC	abacavir	FTC	emtricitabine
ATV	atazanavir	IDV	indinavir
ATV/c	atazanavir/cobicistat	LPV/r	lopinavir/ritonavir
d4T	stavudine	MVC	maraviroc
ddC	zalcitabine	NFV	nelfinavir
ddI	didanosine	NVP	nevirapine
DLV	delavirdine	RAL	raltegravir
DRV	darunavir	RPV	rilpivirine
DRV/c	darunavir/cobicistat	RTV	ritonavir
DTG	dolutegravir	SQV	saquinavir
EFV	efavirenz	TAF	tenofovir alafenamide
ENF	enfuvirtide	TDF	tenofovir disoproxil fumarate
ETR	etravirine	TPV	tipranavir
EVG	elvitegravir	ZDV	zidovudine
EVG/c	elvitegravir/cobicistat		

OTHER ABBREVIATIONS

AFB	acid fast bacilli	EMB	ethambutol
ALT	alanine transferase	ENT	ear, nose, throat
ANC	absolute neutrophil count	Enterobacteriaceae:	Citrobacter,
ARC	AIDS-related complex		Edwardsiella, Enterobacter, E. coli,
ARDS	adult respiratory distress syndrome		Klebsiella, Proteus, Providencia,
ART	antiretroviral therapy		Salmonella, Serratia, Shigella
AST	aspartamine transferase	ESR	erythrocyte sedimentation rate
β-lactams	penicillins, cephalosporins,	ESRD	end-stage renal disease
	cephamycins (not monobactams	ET	endotracheal
	or carbapenems)	EVR	early virologic response
BAL	bronchoalveolar lavage	FUO	fever of unknown origin
BID	twice daily	GI	gastrointestinal
ICU	intensive care unit	gm	gram
CD4	CD4 T-cell lymphocyte	GU	genitourinary
CIE	counter-immunoelectrophoresis	HSV	herpes simplex virus
CMV	cytomegalovirus	HU	hydroxyurea
CNS	central nervous system	I & D	incision and drainage
CPK	creatine phosphokinase	IFA	immunofluorescent antibody
CrCl	creatinine clearance	IgA	immunoglobulin A
CSF	cerebrospinal fluid	IgG	immunoglobulin G
CT	computerized tomography	IgM	immunoglobulin M
DFA	direct fluorescent antibody	IM	intramuscular
DIC	disseminated intravascular coagulation	INH	isoniazid
DNA	deoxyribonucleic acid	INSTI	integrase strand
DS	double strength		transfer inhibitor
e.g.	for example	IRIS	immune reconstitution
ELISA	enzyme-linked immunosorbent assay		inflammatory syndrome

IV/PO	IV or PO	PPD	purified protein derivative
IV	intravenous	PO	oral
kg	kilogram	PZA	pyrazinamide
L	liter	q__d	every__days
LFT	liver function test	q__h	every__hours
MAC	*Mycobacterium avium* complex	QD	once daily
mcg	microgram	qmonth	once a month
mcL	microliter	qweek	once a week
mg	milligram	RBC	red blood cells
mL	milliliter	RBV	ribavirin
min	minute	RNA	ribonucleic acid
MRI	magnetic resonance imaging	RT-PCR	reverse-transcriptase polymerase chain reaction
MRSA	methicillin-resistant *S. aureus*		
MSSA	methicillin-sensitive *S. aureus*	RVR	rapid virologic response
NNRTI	non-nucleoside reverse transcriptase inhibitor	SGOT/SGPT	serum transaminases
		SLE	systemic lupus erythematosus
NRTI	nucleoside reverse transcriptase inhibitor	sp.	species
		SQ	subcutaneous
NSAID	nonsteroidal anti-inflammatory drug	SS	single strength
OI	opportunistic infection	TB	tuberculosis
PBS	protected brush specimen	TID	three times per day
PCP	*Pneumocystis jirovecii* (carinii) pneumonia	TMP	trimethoprim
		TMP-SMX	trimethoprim-sulfamethoxazole
PCR	polymerase chain reaction	VCA	viral capsid antigen
PI	protease inhibitor	VZV	varicella zoster virus
PMN	polymorphonuclear leucocytes	WBC	white blood cells

Chapter 1

Overview of HIV Infection

OVERVIEW OF HIV INFECTION

Infection with human immunodeficiency virus (HIV-1) leads to a chronic and, without treatment, usually fatal infection characterized by progressive immunodeficiency, a long clinical latency period, and opportunistic infections. The hallmark of HIV disease is infection and viral replication within T-lymphocytes expressing the CD4 antigen (helper-inducer lymphocytes), a critical component of normal cell-mediated immunity. Qualitative defects in CD4 responsiveness and progressive depletion in CD4 cell counts increase the risk for opportunistic infections such as *Pneumocystis jirovecii (carinii)* pneumonia, and neoplasms such as lymphoma and Kaposi's sarcoma. HIV infection can also disrupt blood monocyte, tissue macrophage, neutrophil, and B-lymphocyte (humoral immunity) function, predisposing to infection with encapsulated and gram negative bacteria. Direct attack of CD4-positive cells in the central and peripheral nervous system can cause HIV meningitis, peripheral neuropathy, and dementia.

More than 1 million people in the United States and 30 million people worldwide are infected with HIV. Without treatment, the average time from acquisition of HIV to an acquired immunodeficiency syndrome (AIDS)-defining opportunistic infection is about 10 years; survival then averages 1–2 years. There is tremendous individual variability in these time intervals, with some patients progressing from acute HIV infection to death within 1–2 years, and others not manifesting HIV-related immunosuppression for > 20 years after HIV acquisition. Antiretroviral therapy (ART) has markedly improved the overall prognosis of HIV disease, so that patients who start ART before they have clinical or laboratory evidence of immunosuppression have estimated survival comparable to those without HIV. The approach to HIV infection is shown in Figure 1.1.

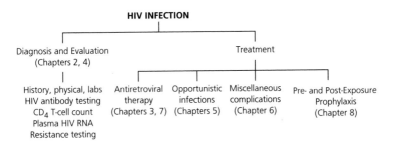

Figure 1.1. Approach to HIV Infection

STAGES OF HIV INFECTION

A. Viral Transmission. HIV infection is acquired primarily by sexual contact (anal, vaginal, infrequently oral), exposure to contaminated blood (through sharing of needles by injection drug users, less commonly transfusion of contaminated blood products), or maternal-fetal (perinatal) transmission. Sexual practices with the highest risk of transmission include unprotected receptive anal intercourse (especially with mucosal tearing), unprotected receptive vaginal intercourse (especially during menses), and unprotected rectal/vaginal intercourse in the presence of genital ulcers (e.g., primary syphilis, genital herpes, chancroid). Lower risk sexual practices include insertive anal/vaginal intercourse and oral-genital contact. The risk of transmission after a single encounter with an HIV source has been estimated to be 1 in 150 with needle sharing, 1 in 300 with occupational percutaneous exposure, 1 in 300–1000 with receptive anal intercourse, 1 in 500–1250 with receptive vaginal intercourse, 1 in 1000–3000 with insertive vaginal intercourse, and 1 in 3000 with insertive anal intercourse. Transmission risk increases with the number of encounters and when the source of infection has higher HIV RNA plasma levels (Lancet 2001;357:1149–53). Virologically suppressive ART all but eliminates the risk of HIV transmission to uninfected partners (N Engl J Med. 2011 Aug 11;365(6):493–505; N Engl J Med. 2016 September 1;375:830–839; JAMA 2016;316(2):171–181). The strategy of pre-exposure prophylaxis—taking two antiretroviral drugs, tenofovir disoproxil fumarate (TDF) and emtricitabine (FTC)—also reduces the risk of acquiring HIV (N Engl J Med. 2015, December 3;373:2237–2246; Lancet 2016 January 2;387:53–60). The mode of transmission does not affect the natural history of HIV disease, though patients with active or past injection drug use may have shortened survival due to comorbid complications (AIDS 2007;21:1185–97).

B. Acute (Primary) HIV Infection (pp. 4–5). Acute HIV occurs 1–4 weeks after transmission and is accompanied by a burst of viral replication with a decline in CD4 cell count. Many, but not all, patients manifest a symptomatic mononucleosis-like syndrome, which is often not diagnosed clinically, both because of the nonspecific nature of the symptoms and lack of clinical suspicion by clinicians.

C. Seroconversion. Development of a positive HIV antibody test usually occurs within 4 weeks of acute infection, and invariably (with few exceptions) by 6 months.

D. Asymptomatic HIV Infection. Asymptomatic HIV lasts a variable amount of time (average 8–10 years) and is accompanied by a gradual decline in CD4 cell counts and a relatively stable HIV RNA level (sometimes referred to as the viral "set point").

E. Early Symptomatic HIV Infection. Previously referred to as "AIDS-related complex (ARC)," findings include thrush or vaginal candidiasis (persistent, frequent, or poorly responsive to treatment), herpes zoster (recurrent episodes or involving multiple derma-tomes), oral hairy leukoplakia, peripheral neuropathy, diarrhea, or constitutional symp-toms (e.g., low-grade fevers, weight loss).

F. AIDS is defined by a CD4 cell count < 200/mm^3, a CD4 cell percentage of total lympho-cytes < 14%, or one of several AIDS-related opportunistic infections. Common opportunistic infections include *Pneumocystis jirovecii (carinii)* pneumonia (PCP), cryptococcal meningitis, recurrent bacterial pneumonia, *Candida esophagitis*, central nervous system (CNS) toxo-plasmosis, tuberculosis, and non-Hodgkin's lymphoma. Other AIDS indicators in HIV-infected patients include candidiasis of the bronchi, trachea, or lungs; disseminated/extrapulmonary coccidiomycosis, cryptococcosis, or histoplasmosis; chronic (> 1 month) intestinal cryptospo-ridiosis or isosporiasis; Kaposi's sarcoma; lymphoid interstitial pneumonia/pulmonary lym-phoid hyperplasia; disseminated/extrapulmonary mycobacterial (non-tuberculous) infection, in particular *Mycobacterium avium* complex (MAC); progressive multifocal leukoencepha-lopathy (PML); recurrent *Salmonella septicemia*; or HIV wasting syndrome.

G. Advanced HIV Disease is a term sometimes applied to patients who have a CD4 cell count < 50/mm^3. Most AIDS-related deaths occur with this severe degree of immuno-suppression, though rarely patients with such depleted CD4 cell counts can be stable for months or even years. Common late stage opportunistic infections are caused by cytomegalovirus (CMV) disease (retinitis, colitis) or disseminated *Mycobacterium avium* complex (MAC). Nearly all patients in this category either are newly diagnosed with HIV infection (and hence have not yet started ART) or are not adherent to prescribed therapy.

ACUTE (PRIMARY) HIV INFECTION

A. Description. Acute clinical illness associated with primary acquisition of HIV, occur-ring 1–4 weeks after viral transmission (range: 6 days to 6 weeks). Symptoms develop in 50–90%, but are often mistaken for the flu, mononucleosis, or other nonspecific viral syndrome. Approximately 25% are asymptomatic. More severe symptoms may correlate with a higher viral set point and more rapid HIV disease progression (J AIDS 2007;45:445–8). Even without therapy, most patients recover, reflecting develop-ment of a partially effective immune response and reduction in susceptible CD4 cells. Unfortunately, damage to the immune system through depletion of the gut-associ-ated lymphoid tissue occurs rapidly (AIDS 2007;21:1–11) and may not be preventable even with effective ART. The "HIV reservoir"—a term used to describe the latent form of HIV that persists even after suppressive therapy—is also seeded during this time (EBioMedicine 2016 http://www.ebiomedicine.com/article/S2352-3964(16)30330-9/fulltext).

B. Differential Diagnosis includes Epstein-Barr virus (EBV), CMV, viral hepatitis, enteroviral infection, secondary syphilis, toxoplasmosis, herpes simplex virus (HSV) with erythema multiforme, drug reaction, Behçet's disease, and acute lupus.

C. Signs and Symptoms reflect hematogenous dissemination of virus to lymphoreticular and neurologic sites (Curr Opin HIV AIDS. 2008 Jan;3(1):10–5):

- Fever (75%).
- Fatigue (68%)
- Pharyngitis (40%). Typically non-exudative (unlike EBV, which is usually exudative).
- Arthralgia/myalgia (49%)
- Rash (48%). Maculopapular viral exanthem of the face and trunk is most common, but can involve the extremities, palms, and soles.
- Diarrhea (27%).
- Neurologic symptoms (24%). Headache is most common. Neuropathy, Bell's palsy, and meningoencephalitis are rare, but may predict worse outcome.
- Weight loss (25%).
- Oral/genital ulcerations (10–20%).

D. Laboratory Findings

1. **Complete Blood Count (CBC).** Lymphopenia followed by lymphocytosis (common). Atypical lymphocytosis is variable, but usually low level (unlike EBV, where atypical lymphocytosis may be 20–30% or higher). Thrombocytopenia occurs in some.

2. **Elevated Transaminases** in some but not all patients.

3. **Depressed CD4 Cell Count.** Can rarely be low enough to induce opportunistic infections, most commonly mucosal candidiasis or PCP.

4. **Heterophile Antibody Testing** is more likely to be positive in acute EBV than acute HIV, though the latter can rarely also trigger a positive result.

5. **HIV Antibody.** Usually negative, although persons with prolonged symptoms of acute HIV may have positive antibody tests if diagnosed late during the course of illness. In general, the "fourth-generation" HIV screening tests that combine antigen with antibody detection are recommended.

6. **HIV RNA (viral load).** Generally very high (100,000 copies/mL or even 10-fold higher), in particular in patients with highly symptomatic disease. However, the viral load will spontaneously drop 100-fold or more between 2–8 weeks, reflecting partially effective immune response.

E. Confirming the Diagnosis of Acute HIV Infection

1. **Obtain Fourth Generation Antigen/Antibody Combination Assay.** Test is approximately 80% sensitive during symptomatic acute HIV infection, turning positive at an HIV RNA level of approximately 30,000 copies/mL (JAMA 2016 Feb;315(7):682–90).

2. **Order Quantitative or Qualitative Viral Load Test** (HIV RNA PCR). As noted above, most individuals will have very high HIV RNA (> 100,000 copies/mL). Quantitative HIV RNA tests are not FDA approved for HIV diagnosis, but they are more widely available than qualitative tests since they are commonly used for monitoring of the efficacy of ART.

3. **Order Other Tests/Serologies if HIV RNA Test Is Negative.** Order throat cultures for bacterial/viral respiratory pathogens, syphilis antibody, hepatitis serologies and HCV RNA, EBV VCA IgM/IgG, CMV IgM/IgG, and hepatitis serologies as appropriate to establish a diagnosis for patient's symptoms. In addition, these tests may be indicated to diagnose sexually transmitted infections that may have been acquired concurrently with HIV.

F. **Management of Acute HIV Infection**

1. **Initiate Antiretroviral Therapy.** Patients with diagnosed acute HIV infection should be treated with combination antiretroviral therapy, with recommended regimens similar to those outlined in Chapter 3. Demonstrated benefits of early therapy include preservation of immunologic status (CD4 cell count) and reducing the risk of transmission to others (N Engl J Med. 2013 Jan;368(3):218–30); in addition, treatment may hasten symptom recovery and reduce the size of the latent HIV reservoir. Because the results of resistance testing are generally not available at the time of treatment initiation, patients should start with boosted protease inhibitor (PI)-based or integrase inhibitor-based treatment given the relatively higher risk of transmitted non-nucleoside reverse transcriptase inhibitor (NNRTI) resistance.

2. **Obtain HIV Resistance Genotype** (Chapter 4) because of the possibility of transmission of antiretroviral therapy-resistant virus. Transmitted drug resistance is more easily detectable during acute HIV Infection than chronic disease, presumably because some of the transmitted drug mutations revert back to wild-type over time (J Acquir Immune Defic Syndr 2012 Oct 1; 61:258). A genotype resistance test is preferred; therapy can be started pending results of the test. Again, because transmitted NNRTI resistance completely reduces the activity of initial NNRTI-based therapy, initial treatment with two nucleoside reverse transcriptase inhibitors (NRTIs) plus a boosted PI or an integrase inhibitor is preferred in this setting.

3. **Rationale for Treatment of Acute HIV Infection.** Two randomized and one observational study strongly suggest benefits of early therapy (N Engl J Med. 2013; 368:207; N Engl J Med. 2013; 368:218; J Infect Dis. 2012 Jan 1;205(1):87). These benefits include hastening symptom resolution, reducing viral transmission, lowering virologic "set point," reduction of the viral reservoir, and preserving both absolute and virus-specific CD4 responses. Eradication of HIV is not possible with currently available agents (Nat Med 2003;9:727–8), but should HIV cure strategies one day be feasible, it is likely that those treated during acute HIV infection will be the best candidates since they have smaller latent reservoirs as measured by cell-associated DNA (EBioMedicine 2016 http://www.ebiomedicine.com/article/S2352-3964(16)30330-9/fulltext).

Chapter 2

Testing for HIV and Baseline Evaluation

HIV DIAGNOSTIC TESTING

A. **Whom to Test**

1. **All patients with signs, symptoms, or laboratory findings consistent with HIV disease.** In addition to the typical AIDS-related opportunistic infections, HIV disease may present with nonspecific symptoms such as fatigue, weight loss, low-grade fevers, or diarrhea. Signs on examination such as generalized lymphadenopathy, oral candidiasis, seborrhea, vascular skin lesions suggestive of Kaposi's sarcoma, herpes zoster, severe mucosal herpes infections, or recurrent or severe vaginal candidiasis should also be tested. Laboratory findings suggestive of HIV infection include cytopenias (all three cell lines may be involved) or polyclonal hyperglobulinemia.

2. **All patients with symptoms consistent with acute HIV infection.** The characteristic symptoms of acute HIV are covered in more detail in Chapter 1.

3. **All patients with possible exposure to HIV.** This includes both sexual and occupational exposures. Common settings in which testing is done include during evaluation for other sexually transmitted infections and prior to the initiation of pre-exposure prophylaxis (PrEP).

4. **All pregnant women.** Testing during pregnancy is recommended, and repeat testing later in pregnancy should be done to exclude HIV acquired since the first negative test.

5. **All adults and adolescents between the ages of 13 and 75.** One-time screening of sexually active individuals in this age range is recommended by guidelines issued by both the Centers for Disease Control (MMWR Recomm Rep. 2006;55(RR-14):1) and the U.S. Preventive Services Task Force (Ann Intern Med. 2013;159(1):51–60).

6. **Repeat testing is recommended in high-risk individuals.** This should be done annually or more frequently depending on the nature of the risk. In the United States, high-risk categories include: Men who have sex with men (MSM), injection drug users, people who exchange sex for money or drugs, sexual partners of people known to be HIV infected, and persons who have multiple sexual partners of unknown HIV status.

B. **Testing for HIV**

1. **Testing for HIV in most clinical settings.** The guidelines for laboratory testing for HIV were substantially revised in 2014 (http://www.cdc.gov/hiv/pdf/hivtestingalgorithmrecommendation-final.pdf). The preferred initial screening test is now a fourth-generation HIV-1 antigen/HIV 1/2 antibody test, replacing previous antibody-only tests due to its increased sensitivity in the period shortly after HIV acquisition. Reactive tests are then confirmed with an antibody assay that differentiates HIV-1 from HIV-2. This algorithm (**Figure 2-1**) is recommended for all asymptomatic individuals, patients with symptoms of established HIV infection, as well as those without recent HIV exposure.

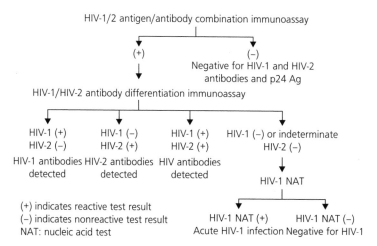

Figure 2.1. Recommended Laboratory HIV Testing Algorithm for Serum or Plasma Specimens

1. Laboratories should conduct initial testing for HIV with an FDA-approved antigen/antibody combination immunoassay[a] that detects HIV-1 and HIV-2 antibodies and HIV-1 p24 antigen to screen for established infection with HIV-1 or HIV-2 and for acute HIV-1 infection. No further testing is required for specimens that are nonreactive on the initial immunoassay.

2. Specimens with a reactive antigen/antibody combination immunoassay result (or repeatedly reactive, if repeat testing is recommended by the manufacturer or required by regulatory authorities) should be tested with an FDA-approved antibody immunoassay that differentiates HIV-1 antibodies from HIV-2 antibodies. Reactive results on the initial antigen/antibody combination immunoassay and the HIV-1/HIV-2 antibody differentiation immunoassay should be interpreted as positive for HIV-1 antibodies, HIV-2 antibodies, or HIV antibodies, undifferentiated.

3. Specimens that are reactive on the initial antigen/antibody combination immunoassay and nonreactive or indeterminate on the HIV-1/HIV-2 antibody differentiation immunoassay should be tested with an FDA-approved HIV-1 nucleic acid test (NAT).

   • A reactive HIV-1 NAT result and nonreactive HIV-1/HIV-2 antibody differentiation immunoassay result indicates laboratory evidence for acute HIV-1 infection.

   • A reactive HIV-1 NAT result and indeterminate HIV-1/HIV-2 antibody differentiation immunoassay result indicates the presence of HIV-1 infection confirmed by HIV-1 NAT.

   • A negative HIV-1 NAT result and nonreactive or indeterminate HIV-1/HIV-2 antibody differentiation immunoassay result indicates a false-positive result on the initial immunoassay.

4. Laboratories should use this same testing algorithm, beginning with an antigen/antibody combination immunoassay, with serum or plasma specimens submitted for testing after a reactive (preliminary positive) result from any rapid HIV test.

[a] Exception: As of April 2014, data are insufficient to recommend use of the FDA-approved single-use rapid HIV-1/HIV-2 antigen/antibody combination immunoassay as the initial assay in the algorithm.

The benefits of this new algorithm include: 1) greater likelihood of detecting recently acquired HIV infection; 2) rapid differentiation between HIV-1 and HIV-2, without the requirement of supplemental tests; 3) an explicit recommendation to order HIV RNA in settings where the initial screening test is positive and the differentiation assay is negative. Importantly, the new testing algorithm eliminates the need for a confirmatory western blot antibody test. While highly accurate in diagnosing established HIV infection, the western blot turned positive slowly after HIV acquisition, with a longer "window period" than more modern tests.

2. **Testing for HIV during symptomatic acute HIV or if exposure was recent.** Because the HIV-1 antigen/HIV 1/2 antibody test is less sensitive than HIV RNA for detection of recently acquired HIV, clinicians should send both tests if patients have symptoms consistent with acute HIV or if they acknowledge recent (< 2 weeks) possible HIV exposures.

3. **Indeterminate test results.** This most commonly occurs with a reactive HIV-1 antigen/HIV 1/2 antibody and a negative differentiation assay. As shown in the algorithm above, this should prompt testing with HIV RNA to exclude acute HIV infection. If the HIV RNA is negative, the interpretation is that the HIV-1 antigen/HIV 1/2 antibody was falsely positive.

C. **HIV Antibody Tests**

1. **Rapid HIV Tests (OraQuick ADVANCE Rapid HIV Test; OraQuick In-Home HIV Test; Uni-Gold Recombigen HIV).** The OraQuick was approved in 2004 and can be performed on whole blood, plasma, or oral mucosal transudate samples. The UniGold test is limited to blood samples. Results are returned in 10–20 minutes and are comparable in accuracy to a single screening test. As a result, *a reactive rapid test must be confirmed with standard two-step HIV testing*. A major advantage of this rapid test includes the ability to give patients a negative result at the time of care; there also is some evidence that individuals given a positive rapid test result are more likely to return for their confirmative serology results. Since the test can be done at the point of care (no CLIA certification is required), it is particularly useful in the evaluation of source patients of needlestick injuries and for women in labor who did not receive HIV testing during prenatal care. There have been reports of high rates of false positive rapid tests when oral samples are used in low-prevalence settings (Ann Intern Med 2008 Aug 5;149[3]:153–60); as a result, some sites have switched to using blood rapid testing, either with the OraQuick or the Uni-Gold. A version of the mouth swab rapid test from OraQuick was approved for in-home use in 2012; this does not require contact with a healthcare provider. Positive results from home tests must also be confirmed by standard HIV testing.

2. **Home Test Kit (Home Access HIV-1 Test System).** This system can be purchased over the counter at pharmacies, or ordered by phone or over the Internet (homeaccess.com). Users receive a kit that includes a stylet for obtaining a sample

of blood from the fingertip, which is then placed on filter paper and mailed to the company for testing. The standard test will return a result within 7 days and costs $44; users can purchase overnight shipping for an additional cost and a more rapid turnaround time. By using a code provided with each kit, users can call and obtain their results anonymously. Phone counseling is available to explain the results, as well as a database of local HIV providers if the test result is positive. The Home Access test employs ELISA testing, which is done in duplicate. All individuals with reactive tests on the system must have results confirmed by standard testing.

3. **OraSure.** his office-based test was approved in 1996 and uses a special swab that collects oral mucosal transudate (not saliva) when it is held between the cheek and the gum. This system obtains quantities of antibody that are comparable to or exceed those from serum samples. Once the specimen is collected, it is sent to a central laboratory for antibody testing, which can be performed on the same sample. As a result, the sensitivity and specificity of the test are comparable to standard blood HIV antibody testing (JAMA 1997;277:254).

D. **Selected Licensed HIV Diagnostic Tests**
   1. **p24 Antigen.** Approved for diagnosis of acute HIV infection. However, due to low sensitivity of this test, HIV RNA has replaced p24 antigen in clinical practice, and hence this test is rarely ordered. Testing for p24 antigen is now incorporated into the HIV-1 antigen/HIV 1/2 antibody combination assay used for standard screening.

   2. **Nucleic Acid-Based Tests.** In the United States, donated blood has been screened with nucleic acid-based tests since the late 1990s, shortening the time between infection and detectability of infection to about 12 days. As a result, the rate of acquiring HIV from a blood transfusion is now estimated at one infection per 2 million units transfused (JAMA 2003;289:959). A related test, the Aptima HIV-1 RNA Qualitative Assay, was approved for HIV diagnosis in 2006. Like quantitative HIV RNA tests, this assay can be used to diagnose acute HIV infection before antibodies develop, but results are provided only as positive or negative. Additionally, it can confirm HIV infection in a person with a positive HIV ELISA or rapid test. It is not known whether the rate of false positivity with the Aptima test is lower than the rate with RT-PCR or bDNA.

   3. **Combined HIV Antigen/Antibody Combination Assays.** These tests detect both HIV antibody and p24 antigen. As such, the test turns positive before antibody alone testing, shortening the window period between HIV acquisition and test positivity. The sensitivity of the test for acute HIV compared with HIV RNA testing is somewhat lower as p24 antigen is less likely to be positive than HIV RNA.

E. **Summary:** Timeline for HIV tests to turn positive after acquisition (**Table 2.1**) and sequence of appearance of laboratory markers for HIV-1 infection (**Figure 2.2**) follow.

Table 2.1. Timeline for HIV Tests to Turn Positive

Test	Time to Positive After HIV Acquisition and Comments
Qualitative or quantitative HIV RNA or other nucleic acid test (NAT)	10 days. Patients with negative tests fall into two categories: 1) those in the "eclipse" period just after HIV acquisition, before HIV viremia; 2) those rare patients (< 1%) with established HIV who are "HIV controllers," meaning they control HIV replication without ART. The former can only be diagnosed with f/u testing in 1–2 weeks; the latter already will have a positive HIV antibody.
p24 antigen	14–20 days; note that p24 antigen detection may be transient since as antibodies develop, they bind to the p24 antigen and form immune complexes that interfere with p24 assay detection. Also important is that p24 antigen may be negative with very recently acquired HIV infection.
IgM antibody	20–23 days; this test is incorporated into 3rd and 4th generation HIV antibody tests.
IgG antibody	28–48 days; these antibodies persist for the duration of HIV infection, and are detected using earlier generation ELISA antibody tests and the western blot.

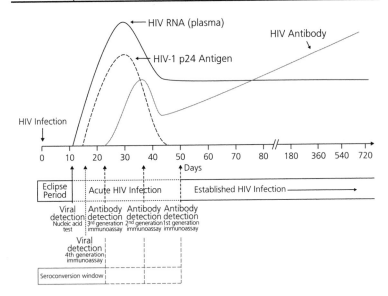

Figure 2.2. Sequence of Appearance of Laboratory Markers for HIV-1 Infection

Note. Units for vertical axis are not noted because their magnitude differs for RNA, p24 antigen, and antibody.

Reproduced from Centers for Disease Control and Prevention and Association of Public Health Laboratories. Laboratory Testing for the Diagnosis of HIV Infection: Updated Recommendations. http://www.cdc.gov/hiv/pdf/hivtestingalgorithmrecommendation-final.pdf. June 27, 2014. Modified from MP Busch, GA Satten (1997), with updated data from Fiebig (2003), Owen (2008), and Masciotra (2011, 2013).

QUANTITATIVE PLASMA HIV RNA (HIV VIRAL LOAD ASSAYS)

HIV viral load assays measure the amount of HIV RNA in plasma. The high sensitivity of these assays allows detection of virus in virtually all patients not on antiretroviral therapy. These tests are most commonly used to monitor the response to antiretroviral therapy; they can also be used to diagnose acute HIV infection.

A. Uses of HIV RNA Assay

1. **Diagnosis of Acute HIV Infection.** Except for the brief (10 days or less) "eclipse" period, this is our most sensitive test for acute HIV infection. Not FDA-approved for this indication, but widely used nonetheless given its high sensitivity and specificity and widespread availability.

2. **Helps in Initial Evaluation of HIV Infection.** Establishes baseline HIV RNA and determines (along with CD4 cell count) the urgency of starting ART, as HIV RNA correlates with rate of CD4 decline (Ann Intern Med 1997 Jun 15;126(12):946–54).

3. **Monitors Response to Antiviral Therapy.** HIV RNA rapidly declines after starting or changing effective antiretroviral therapy, with measurable decreases occurring within days. Patients who achieve virologic suppression (less than lower limit of detection of sensitive assays, typically 20–40 copies/mL) have the most durable response to antiviral therapy and the best clinical prognosis. No change in HIV RNA suggests that therapy will be ineffective or, more commonly, that the patient is noncompliant.

4. **Estimates Risk for Opportunistic Infection.** For patients with similar CD4 cell counts, the risk of opportunistic infections is higher with higher HIV RNAs. HIV RNA is not formally incorporated into opportunistic infection prevention guidelines.

B. Assays and Interpretation

1. **Tests, Sensitivities, and Dynamic Range.** Most US sites use automated RT-PCR (Roche or Abbott) assays, which have replaced the older (and less accurate) bDNA and previous less-sensitive RT-PCRs. Any assay can be used to diagnose acute HIV infection and guide/monitor therapy, but the same test should be used to follow patients longitudinally. Both currently and previously used quantitative HIV RNA tests are summarized below, the former included to provide guidance regarding test results from older medical records.

   a. **RT-PCR Amplicor** (Roche): Sensitivity = 400 copies/mL; dynamic range = 400–750,000 copies/mL. Assay discontinued, no longer used.

   b. **RT-PCR Ultrasensitive 1.5** (Roche): Sensitivity = 50 copies/mL; dynamic range = 50–75,000 copies/mL. Assay discontinued, no longer used.

   c. **bDNA Versant 3.0** (Bayer): Sensitivity = 75 copies/mL; dynamic range = 75–500,000 copies/mL. Assay discontinued, no longer used.

   d. **Nucleic acid sequence-based amplification** (NASBA), NucliSens HIV-1 QT (bioMerieux): Sensitivity = 10 copies/mL; dynamic range = 176–3.5 million copies/mL (depends on volume).

    e. **RealTime HIV-1 assay** (Abbott): PCR-based assay. Sensitivity = 40 copies/mL; dynamic range = 40–10 million copies/mL.

    f. **COBAS AmpliPrep/COBAS TaqMan HIV-1 test** (Roche): Sensitivity = 20 copies/mL; dynamic range = 20–10 million copies/mL.

2. **Correlation Between HIV RNA and CD4 Cell Count.** HIV RNA assays correlate inversely with CD4 cell counts (higher HIV RNA, lower CD4), but do so imperfectly (e.g., some patients with high CD4 counts have relatively high HIV RNA levels, and vice versa.) For any given CD4, higher HIV RNA levels correlate with more rapid CD4 decline. In response to antiretroviral therapy, changes in HIV RNA precede changes in CD4 cell count.

3. **Significant Change in HIV RNA Assay.** This is defined by at least a 2-fold (0.3 log) change in viral RNA (accounts for normal variation in clinically stable patients), or a 3-fold (0.5 log) change in response to new antiretroviral therapy (accounts for intra-laboratory and patient variability). For example, if an HIV RNA result = 50,000 copies/mL, then the range of possible actual values = 25,000–100,000 copies/mL, and the value needed to demonstrate antiretroviral activity is ≤ 17,000 copies/mL. In clinical practice, adherent patients will frequently have at least a 100-fold (2-log) decrease to ART at 4 weeks; as a result, determining whether a given individual is adherent based on HIV RNA response is usually quite accurate.

C. **Indications for HIV RNA Testing.** This test is indicated for the diagnosis of acute HIV infection and for initial evaluation of newly diagnosed HIV. It is the single most important monitoring test for HIV treatment efficacy; it should be performed 2–8 weeks after starting a new antiretroviral regimen. If HIV RNA is detectable at 2–8 weeks, repeat every 4–8 weeks until suppression to < 200 copies/mL, then every 3–6 months. Clinically stable patients with long-term virologic suppression may reduce the frequency of HIV RNA testing to 1–2 times yearly.

INITIAL ASSESSMENT OF HIV-INFECTED PATIENTS

A. **Clinical Evaluation.** The history and physical examination should focus on diagnoses associated with HIV infection. Compared to patients without HIV, the severity, frequency, and duration of these conditions are usually increased in HIV disease; many are also common in non-HIV infected patients, so their presence is consistent with but not diagnostic of HIV.

    1. **Dermatologic:** Herpes simplex (oral/anogenital); herpes zoster (especially recurrent, cranial nerve, or disseminated); molluscum contagiosum; staphylococcal abscesses; tinea nail infections; Kaposi's sarcoma (from human herpesvirus-8 [HHV-8] infection); petechiae (from immune thrombocytopenic purpura [ITP]); seborrheic dermatitis; new or worsening psoriasis; eosinophilic pustular folliculitis; severe cutaneous drug eruptions (especially sulfonamides)

    2. **Oropharyngeal:** Oral candidiasis; oral hairy leukoplakia (from EBV); Kaposi's sarcoma (most commonly on palate or gums); gingivitis/periodontitis; warts; aphthous ulcers (especially esophageal/perianal)

3. **Constitutional Symptoms:** Fatigue, fevers, chronic diarrhea, weight loss
4. **Lymphatic:** Persistent, generalized lymphadenopathy
5. **Others:** Active tuberculosis (TB) (especially extrapulmonary); non-Hodgkin's lymphoma (especially CNS); unexplained leukopenia, anemia, thrombocytopenia (especially ITP); myopathy; miscellaneous neurologic conditions (cranial/peripheral neuropathies, Guillain-Barre syndrome, mononeuritis multiplex, aseptic meningitis, cognitive impairment)

B. **Baseline Laboratory Testing (Table 2.2).** See also Clin Infect Dis. Jan 2014;58(1):e1–34.

Table 2.2. Baseline Laboratory Testing for HIV-Infected Patients*

Test	Rationale
Repeat HIV test	Indicated for patients unable to document a prior positive test or detectable HIV RNA in their medical records, and for "low-risk" individuals with a positive test (to detect computer/clerical error). A detectable HIV RNA testing provides an additional means of confirming HIV infection, so repeating HIV testing is rarely required. Critical in ruling out cases of suspected factitious HIV.
CBC with differential, platelets	Detects cytopenias (e.g., ITP) seen in HIV. Needed to calculate CD4 cell count.
Chemistry panel ("SMA 20")	Detects renal dysfunction and electrolyte/liver function test (LFT)/ glucose abnormalities, which may accompany HIV and associated infections (e.g., HIV nephropathy, HCV).
Fasting lipid profile	Since HIV and many antiretroviral agents influence lipid levels, a lipid profile before treatment provides a useful baseline.
CD4 cell count	Determines the urgency of antiretroviral therapy and need for opportunistic infection (OI) prophylaxis. Best test for defining risk of OIs and prognosis.
HIV RNA assay ("viral load")	Provides a marker for the pace of HIV disease progression. Provides a second test confirming HIV diagnosis. Determines response to antiretroviral therapy.
HIV resistance genotype	Identifies patients infected with a resistant virus, hence may guide selection of initial ART regimen.
Tuberculin skin test (standard 5 TU of purified protein derivative, PPD) or interferon gamma release assay (IGRA)	Detects latent TB infection and targets patients for preventive therapy. Anergy skin tests are not recommended due to poor predictive value.

Table 2.2. Baseline Laboratory Testing for HIV-Infected Patients* (cont'd)

Test	Rationale
PAP smear	Risk of cervical cancer is nearly twice as high in HIV-positive women vs. uninfected controls; some advocate anal pap smears for men who have sex with men.
Toxoplasmosis serology (IgG)	Identifies patients at risk for subsequent cerebral/systemic toxo-plasmosis and the need for prophylaxis if severely immunosuppressed. Those with negative tests should be counseled on how to avoid infection
Syphilis serology (RPR or VDRL or syphilis EIA)	Identifies co-infection with syphilis, which is epidemiologically linked to HIV. Disease may have accelerated course in HIV patients.
Hepatitis C serology (anti-HCV)	Identifies HCV infection and usually chronic carriage. If positive, follow with HCV genotype and HCV viral load assay. If patient is antibody-negative but at high risk for hepatitis or has unexplained abnormal liver function tests, order HCV RNA to exclude a false-negative result.
Hepatitis B serologies (HBsAb, HBcAb, HBsAg)	Identifies patients who are immune to hepatitis B (HBsAb) or chronic carriers (HBsAg). If all three are negative, hepatitis B vaccine is indicated.
Hepatitis A serology (anti-HAV)	Identifies candidates for hepatitis A vaccine; if anti-HAV positive, already immune.
G6PD screen	Identifies patients at risk for dapsone or primaquine-associated hemolysis.
CMV serology (IgG)	Identifies patients who should receive CMV-negative or leukocyte-depleted blood if transfused.
VZV serology (IgG)	Identifies patients at risk for varicella (chickenpox), and those who should avoid contact with active varicella or herpes zoster patients. Serology-negative patients exposed to chickenpox should receive varicella-zoster immune globulin (VZIG); varicella vaccine if CD4 > 350/ mm^3.
Chest x-ray	Sometimes ordered as a baseline test for future comparisons. May detect healed granulomatous diseases/other processes. Indicated in all tuberculin skin test or IGRA-positive patients.
HLA-B*5701	Needed if therapy with abacavir is planned. Patients negative for HLA-B*5701 have almost no risk of severe hypersensitivity reaction to abacavir.

*   See also Clin Infect Disease Clin Infect Dis. 2013 Nov 13.

Table 2.3. Laboratory Testing Schedule for Monitoring HIV-Infected Patients Before and After Initiation of Antiretroviral Therapy[a]

Laboratory Test	Entry into Care	ART Initiation[b] or Modification	2 to 8 Weeks After ART Initiation or Modification	Every 3 to 6 Months	Every 6 Months	Every 12 Months	Treatment Failure	Clinically Indicated	If ART Initiation Is Delayed[c]
				Timepoint/Frequency of Testing					
HIV Serology	√ If HIV diagnosis has not been confirmed								
CD4 Count	√	√		√ During first 2 years of ART or if viremia develops while patient on ART or CD4 count <300 cells/mm³		√ After 2 years on ART with consistently suppressed viral load: CD4 count 300–500 cells/mm³: • Every 12 months CD4 count >500 cells/mm³: • CD4 monitoring is optional	√	√	√ Every 3–6 months

Table 2.3. Laboratory Testing Schedule for Monitoring HIV-Infected Patients Before and After Initiation of Antiretroviral Therapy[a] (cont'd)

Laboratory Test	Entry into Care	ART Initiation[b] or Modification	2 to 8 Weeks After ART Initiation or Modification	Every 3 to 6 Months	Every 6 Months	Every 12 Months	Treatment Failure	Clinically Indicated	If ART Initiation Is Delayed[c]
				Timepoint/Frequency of Testing					
HIV Viral Load	✓	✓	✓[d]	✓[e]	✓[e]		✓	✓	Repeat testing is optional
Resistance Testing	✓	✓[f]					✓	✓	✓[f]
HLA-B*5701 Testing		✓ If considering ABC							
Tropism Testing		✓ If considering a CCR5 antagonist					✓ If considering a CCR5 antagonist or for failure of CCR5 antagonist-based regimen	✓	

Hepatitis B Serology[a,h]	✓	✓ May repeat if patient is nonimmune and not chronically infected with HBV[h]			✓ May repeat if patient is nonimmune and not chronically infected with HBV[h]			✓
Hepatitis C Antibody Test (if positive, confirm with HCV RNA test)	✓	✓ May repeat for at-risk patients if negative result at baseline			✓ May repeat for at-risk patients if negative result at baseline			✓
Basic Chemistry[i,j]	✓	✓	✓				✓	✓ Every 6–12 months
ALT, AST, T. bilirubin	✓	✓	✓				✓	✓ Every 6–12 months
CBC with Differential	✓	✓ If on ZDV	✓ If on ZDV or if CD4 testing is done	✓			✓	✓ Every 3–6 months

Table 2.3. Laboratory Testing Schedule for Monitoring HIV-Infected Patients Before and After Initiation of Antiretroviral Therapy[a] (cont'd)

Laboratory Test	Entry into Care	ART Initiation[b] or Modification	2 to 8 Weeks After ART Initiation or Modification	Timepoint/Frequency of Testing						
				Every 3 to 6 Months	Every 6 Months	Every 12 Months	Treatment Failure	Clinically Indicated	If ART Initiation Is Delayed[c]	
Fasting Lipid Profile[k]	✓	✓			✓ If abnormal at last measurement	✓ If normal at last measurement		✓	✓ If normal at baseline, annually	
Fasting Glucose or Hemoglobin A1C	✓	✓		✓ If abnormal at last measurement		✓ If normal at last measurement		✓	✓ If normal at baseline, annually	
Urinalysis[i,j]	✓	✓			✓ If on TAF or TDF[i]	✓		✓		
Pregnancy Test		✓ In women with childbearing potential						✓		

Guidelines for the Use of Antiretroviral Agents in HIV-1-Infected Adults and Adolescents

a   This table pertains to laboratory tests done to select an antiretroviral (ARV) regimen and monitor for treatment responses or ART toxicities. Please refer to the HIV Primary Care guidelines for guidance on other laboratory tests generally recommended for primary healthcare maintenance of HIV patients.[1]

b   If ART initiation occurs soon after HIV diagnosis and entry into care, repeat baseline laboratory testing is not necessary.

c   ART is indicated for all HIV-infected individuals and should be started as soon as possible. However, if ART initiation is delayed, patients should be retained in care, with periodic monitoring as noted above.

d If HIV RNA is detectable at 2 to 8 weeks, repeat every 4 to 8 weeks until viral load is suppressed to <200 copies/mL, and thereafter, every 3 to 6 months.

e In patients on ART, viral load typically is measured every 3 to 4 months. However, for adherent patients with consistently suppressed viral load and stable immunologic status for more than 2 years, monitoring can be extended to 6-month intervals.

f Based on current rates of transmitted drug resistance to different ARV medications, standard genotypic drug-resistance testing in ARV-naive persons should focus on testing for mutations in the reverse transcriptase (RT) and protease (PR) genes. If transmitted integrase strand transfer inhibitor (INSTI) resistance is a concern, providers should also test for resistance mutations to this class of drugs. In ART-naive patients who do not immediately begin ART, repeat testing before initiation of ART is optional if resistance testing was performed at entry into care. In virologically suppressed patients who are switching therapy because of toxicity or for convenience, viral amplification will not be possible; therefore, resistance testing should not be performed. Results from prior resistance testing can be helpful in constructing a new regimen.

g If HBsAg is positive, TDF or TAF plus either FTC or 3TC should be used as part of the ARV regimen to treat both HBV and HIV infections. Preliminary data from clinical trials have demonstrated TAF activity against HBV. Final results from ongoing clinical trials will help to define the role of TAF in the treatment of HBV/HIV coinfection.

h If HBsAg, HBsAb, and anti-HBc are negative, hepatitis B vaccine series should be administered. Refer to HIV Primary Care and Opportunistic Infections guidelines for more detailed recommendations.[1,2]

i Serum Na, K, HCO_3, Cl, BUN, creatinine, glucose (preferably fasting), and creatinine-based estimated glomerular filtration rate. Serum phosphorus should be monitored in patients with chronic kidney disease who are on TAF- or TDF-containing regimens.[3]

j Consult the Guidelines for the Management of Chronic Kidney Disease in HIV-Infected Patients: Recommendations of the HIV Medicine Association of the Infectious Diseases Society of America for recommendations on managing patients with renal disease.[3] More frequent monitoring may be indicated for patients with evidence of kidney disease (e.g., proteinuria, decreased glomerular dysfunction) or increased risk of renal insufficiency (e.g., patients with diabetes, hypertension).

k Consult the National Lipid Association's recommendations for management of patients with dyslipidemia.[4]

Urine glucose and protein should be assessed before initiating TAF- or TDF-containing regimens, and monitored during treatment with these regimens.

Key to Acronyms: 3TC = lamivudine; ABC = abacavir; ALT = alanine aminotransferase; ART = antiretroviral therapy; AST = aspartate aminotransferase; BUN = blood urea nitrogen; CBC = complete blood count; Cl = chloride; CrCl = creatinine clearance; EFV = efavirenz; FTC = emtricitabine; HBsAb = hepatitis B surface antibody; HBsAg = hepatitis B surface antigen; HBV = hepatitis B virus; HCO_3 = bicarbonate; K = potassium; NA = sodium; TAF = tenofovir alafenamide; TDF = tenofovir disoproxil fumarate; ZDV = zidovudine.

References

1. Aberg JA, Gallant JE, Ghanem KG, Emmanuel P, Zingman BS, Horberg MA. Primary care guidelines for the management of persons infected with HIV: 2013 update by the HIV Medicine Association of the Infectious Diseases Society of America. *Clin Infect Dis.* Jan 2014;58(1):e1–34. Available at http://www.ncbi.nlm.nih.gov/pubmed/24235263.

2. Panel on Opportunistic Infections in HIV-Infected Adults and Adolescents. *Guidelines for the prevention and treatment of opportunistic infections in HIV-infected adults and adolescents: recommendations from the Centers for Disease Control and Prevention, the National Institutes of Health, and the HIV Medicine Association of the Infectious Diseases Society of America.* Available at http://aidsinfo.nih.gov/contentfiles/lvguidelines/adult_oi.pdf. Accessed June 6, 2016.

3. Lucas GM, Ross MJ, Stock PG, et al. Clinical practice guideline for the management of chronic kidney disease in patients infected with HIV: 2014 update by the HIV Medicine Association of the Infectious Diseases Society of America. *Clin Infect Dis.* Nov 1 2014;59(9):e96–138. Available at http://www.ncbi.nlm.nih.gov/pubmed/2534519.

4. Jacobson TA, Ito MK, Maki KC, et al. National lipid association recommendations for patient-centered management of dyslipidemia: part 1—full report. *J Clin Lipidol.* Mar-Apr 2015;9(2):129–169. Available at http://www.ncbi.nlm.nih.gov/pubmed/25911072.

Reproduced from Panel on Antiretroviral Guidelines for Adults and Adolescents. Guidelines for the use of antiretroviral agents in HIV-1-infected adults and adolescents. AIDSinfo. https://aidsinfo.nih.gov/contentfiles/lvguidelines/adultandadolescentgl.pdf. July 14, 2016.

Table 2.4. Use of CD4 Cell Count for Interpretation of Patient Signs and Symptoms in HIV Infection

CD4 (cells/mm³)	Associated Conditions
> 500	Most illnesses are similar to those in HIV-negative patients. Some increased risk of bacterial infections (pneumococcal pneumonia, sinusitis), herpes zoster, tuberculosis, skin conditions.
200–500*	Generalized lymphadenopathy, bacterial infections (especially pneumococcal pneumonia, sinusitis), cutaneous Kaposi's sarcoma, vaginal candidiasis, ITP.
50–200*	Thrush, oral hairy leukoplakia, several HIV-associated opportunistic infections (e.g., *P. jirovecii [carinii]* pneumonia, cryptococcal meningitis, toxoplasmosis). Most opportunistic infection do not occur until CD4 cell counts < 100/mm³ (Ann Intern Med 1996;124:633–42).
< 50*	Disseminated *Mycobacterium avium* complex, CMV retinitis, HIV-associated wasting, neurologic disease (neuropathy, encephalopathy)

*   Patients remain at risk for all processes noted in earlier stages. Once patients are receiving suppressive antiretroviral therapy for > 6 months, all opportunistic infections become rare even if CD4 cell counts remain low.

C. **CD4 Cell Count (Lymphocyte Subset Analysis)**

1. **Overview.** Acute HIV infection is characterized by a decline in CD4 cell count, followed by a gradual rise associated with clinical recovery. Without ART, chronic HIV infection shows progressive declines (~ 50–80 cells/year, but with wide interpatient variability) in CD4 cell count followed by more rapid decline 1–2 years prior to opportunistic infection (AIDS-defining diagnosis). Cell counts remain stable over 5–10 years in most patients, while others may show rapid declines (> 300 cells/year). Since variability exists within individual patients and between laboratories, it is useful to repeat any value that is clinically unexpected.

2. **Uses of CD4 Cell Count**

    a. **Gives context of degree of immunosuppression** for interpretation of symptoms/signs (**Table 2.4**).

    b. **Helpful in determining how urgently to start ART.** HIV treatment is now recommended for all patients regardless of CD4 cell count; however, the urgency of starting therapy is much greater with counts < 200 even without symptoms. For prophylaxis against PCP, toxoplasmosis, and MAC/CMV infection, CD4 cell counts of 200/mm³, < 100/mm³, and < 50/mm³ are used as threshold levels, respectively, though the last of these is of questionable benefit if patients start ART promptly (JAMA 2016;316(2):191–210).

c. **Provides estimate of risk of opportunistic infection or death.** Patients with CD4 cell counts < 50/mm³ (almost all of whom are not taking ART) are at markedly increased risk of death from AIDS complications. In the pre-ART era, the median survival was approximately 1–2 years without treatment, though rarely some patients with these low counts survived > 3 years (J Infect Dis. 1995;171(4):829–836). Today, prognosis is influenced by HIV RNA, presence/history of opportunistic infections or neoplasms, performance status, concomitant illnesses and, most importantly, by the proportion of time these individuals are taking ART.

Chapter 3

Treatment of HIV Infection

INITIATION OF ANTIRETROVIRAL THERAPY (Table 3.2)

Combination antiretroviral therapy (ART) improves clinical outcomes across the entire spectrum of HIV disease, including those with a prior AIDS-defining illness (N Engl J Med. 1997 Sep 11;337(11):725–33), asymptomatic individuals with moderate immunosuppression (CD4 200–350) (N Engl J Med. 2011;365:1471–81), and even in those with normal CD4 cell counts (N Engl J Med. 2015 Aug 27;373(9):795–807). In addition, suppressive ART virtually eliminates the risk of HIV transmission (N Engl J Med. 2011;365(6):493–505). Although there are potential disadvantages of antiretroviral therapy for those with asymptomatic HIV disease and high CD4 cell counts (medication side effects, cost, and development of resistance), these risks are outweighed by the clinical and public health benefits.

The primary goals of therapy are prolonged suppression of viral replication to undetectable levels (HIV RNA < 20–40 copies/mL depending on assay), restoration/preservation of immune function, and improved clinical outcome. Once initiated, antiretroviral therapy should be continued indefinitely, as intermittent treatment has been associated with increased risk of HIV-related and non-HIV-related complications (N Engl J Med. 2006 Nov 30;355(22):2283–69).

Table 3.1. Antiretroviral Agents Used for HIV Infection

Drug (abbreviation; trade name, manufacturer)	Formulations	Usual Adult Dosing[§]
NUCLEOSIDE (AND NUCLEOTIDE) REVERSE TRANSCRIPTASE INHIBITORS (NRTIs)		
Abacavir sulfate (ABC; Ziagen, ViiV; also available generically)	300-mg tablets; 20-mg/mL oral solution	300 mg BID or 600 mg QD
Abacavir sulfate/lamivudine (Epzicom, ViiV)	600-/300-mg tablet	One 600-/300-mg tablet QD
Abacavir sulfate/lamivudine/ zidovudine (Trizivir, ViiV)	300-/150-/300-mg tablet	One 300-/150-/300-mg tablet BID
Didanosine (ddI; Videx/Videx EC, Bristol-Myers Squibb; Oncology/Immunology; also available generically)	125-, 200-, 250-, 400-mg delayed-release enteric-coated capsules; 100-, 167-, 250-mg powder	Capsule: < 60 kg: 250 mg QD ≥ 60 kg: 400 mg QD 250 mg QD with tenofovir (best avoided) Powder: < 60 kg: 167 mg BID ≥ 60 kg: 250 mg BID probably Administration: Take on empty stomach at least 30 minutes before or 2 hours after meal

Table 3.1. Antiretroviral Agents Used for HIV Infection (cont'd)

Drug (abbreviation; trade name, manufacturer)	Formulations	Usual Adult Dosing§
NUCLEOSIDE (AND NUCLEOTIDE) REVERSE TRANSCRIPTASE INHIBITORS (NRTIs) (cont'd)		
Emtricitabine (FTC; Emtriva, Gilead Sciences)	200-mg capsule	200 mg QD
Lamivudine (3TC; Epivir, ViiV)	150-, 300-mg tablets; 10-mg/mL oral solution	150 mg BID or 300 mg QD
Lamivudine/zidovudine (Combivir, ViiV; also available generically)	150-/300-mg tablet	One 150-/300-mg tablet BID
Stavudine (d4T; Zerit, Bristol-Myers Squibb Virology)	15-, 20-, 30-, 40-mg capsules; 1-mg/mL oral solution	< 60 kg: 30 mg BID ≥ 60 kg: 40 mg BID
Tenofovir disoproxil fumarate (TDF; Viread, Gilead Sciences)	300-mg tablet	One 300-mg tablet QD
Tenofovir disoproxil fumarate/emtricitabine (TDF/FTC, Truvada, Gilead Sciences)	300-/200-mg tablet	One 300-/200-mg tablet QD
Tenofovir alafenamide emtricitabine (TAF/FTC, Descovy, Gilead Sciences)	25-/200-mg tablet	One 25-/200 mg tabled QD
Zidovudine (ZDV; Retrovir, ViiV; also available generically)	100-mg capsule; 300-mg tablet; 10-mg/5-mL oral solution; 10-mg/mL IV solution	200 mg TID or 300 mg BID (or with 3TC as Combivir or with abacavir and 3TC as Trizivir) 5–6 mg/kg daily
NON-NUCLEOSIDE REVERSE TRANSCRIPTASE INHIBITORS (NNRTIs)*		
Delavirdine mesylate (DLV; Rescriptor, ViiV)‡	100-, 200-mg tablets	400 mg TID (100-mg tablets can be dispersed in water; 200-mg tablet should be taken intact). Separate dosing from ddI or antacids by 1 hour, with or without food
Efavirenz (EFV; Sustiva, Bristol-Myers Squibb Oncology/Immunology; outside USA known as Stocrin)‡	50-, 100-, 200-mg capsules; 600-mg tablet	600 mg QD; best taken prior to bed to reduce incidence of CNS side effects
Etravirine (ETR; Intelence, Janssen Therapeutics)	100-mg tablets; 200-mg tablets	Two 100-mg tablets twice daily after a meal or one 200-mg tablet twice daily after a meal

Table 3.1. Antiretroviral Agents Used for HIV Infection (cont'd)

Drug (abbreviation; trade name, manufacturer)	Formulations	Usual Adult Dosing§
NON-NUCLEOSIDE REVERSE TRANSCRIPTASE INHIBITORS (NNRTIs)* (cont'd)		
Nevirapine (NVP; Viramune, Boehringer Ingelheim; also available generically)‡	200-mg tablet; 50-mg/5-mL oral suspension (pediatric)	200 mg QD × 2 weeks, then 200 mg BID
Nevirapine Extended Release (NVP XR, Viramune XR, Boehringer Ingelheim)	400-mg tablet	200 mg immediate release QD x 14 days then 400 mg XR QD thereafter
Rilpivirine (RPV, Edurant, Janssen Therapeutics)	25-mg tablet	1 tablet daily with a meal
COMBINATION NRTI/NNRTI		
Tenofovir disoproxil fumarate/ efavirenz/emtricitabine/ (TDF/ FTC/EFV, Atripla, Bristol-Myers Squibb, and Gilead)	One 600-,/200-,/300-mg tablet daily on an empty stomach, generally given before bed	One 600-/200-/300-mg tablet daily
Tenofovir disoproxil fumarate/ emtricitabine/rilpivirine (Complera, Gilead, and Janssen)	300-,/200-,/25-mg tablet	One tablet daily with a meal
Tenofovir alafenamide/ emtricitabine/rilpivirine (TAF/FTC/ RPV, Odefsey, Gilead, and Janssen)	25-,/200-,/25-mg tablet	One tablet daily with a meal
PROTEASE INHIBITORS (PIs)†		
Atazanavir sulfate (ATV; Reyataz, Bristol-Myers Squibb Virology)‡	100-, 150-, 200-, 300-mg capsules	400 mg QD, or 300 mg QD in combination with ritonavir 100 mg QD. For treatment-experienced patients, or when used with tenofovir or efavirenz or nevirapine use: 300 mg in combination with 100 mg of ritonavir. Take with food
Darunavir (DRV; Prezista, Janssen Therapeutics)	400-, 600-mg, 800-mg tablets	600 mg BID with ritonavir 100 mg BID (treatment experienced); 800 mg QD with ritonavir 100 mg QD (treatment naïve)

Table 3.1. Antiretroviral Agents Used for HIV Infection (cont'd)

Drug (abbreviation; trade name, manufacturer)	Formulations	Usual Adult Dosing§
PROTEASE INHIBITORS (PIs)† (cont'd)		
Fosamprenavir (FPV; Lexiva, ViiV)‡	700-mg tablet	PI-naïve patients: 1400 mg BID, or 700 mg BID in combination with ritonavir 100 mg BID, or 1400 mg QD in combination with ritonavir 200 mg QD or 100 mg QD PI-experienced patients: 700 mg BID in combination with ritonavir 100 mg BID
Indinavir sulfate (IDV; Crixivan, Merck)‡	200-, 333-, 400-mg capsules	800 mg TID, or 800 mg BID in combination with ritonavir 100 mg or 200 mg BID Administration: Unboosted: Take 1 hour before or 2 hours after meals; may take with skim milk/low-fat meal Boosted: Take with or without food. Separate dosing from ddI by 1 hour
Lopinavir/ritonavir (LPV/r; Kaletra, Abbott)‡	200-/50-mg tablet; 80-/20-mg/mL oral solution	Two tablets (400/100 mg) BID; 5-mL oral solution BID. Four tablets (800/200 mg) QD an option for treatment-naïve patients With EFV or NVP: 3 tablets (600/150 mg) BID or 6.7 mL BID
Nelfinavir mesylate (NFV; Viracept, ViiV)	250-, 625-mg tablets; 50-mg/gm oral powder	750 mg TID or 1250 mg BID. Take with food
Ritonavir (RTV; Norvir, Abbott)‡	100-mg tablet or capsule; 600-mg/7.5-mL solution; 80-mg/mL oral solution	600 mg BID as sole PI; 100–400 mg daily in 1–2 divided doses as pharmacokinetic booster for other PIs Administration: Take with food or up to 2 hours after a meal to improve tolerability

Table 3.1. Antiretroviral Agents Used for HIV Infection (cont'd)

Drug (abbreviation; trade name, manufacturer)	Formulations	Usual Adult Dosing§
PROTEASE INHIBITORS (PIs)† (cont'd)		
Saquinavir (SQV; Invirase, Roche)‡	200-, 500-mg hard-gel capsules	1000 mg BID in combination with ritonavir 100 mg BID. Take with food
Tipranavir (TPV; Aptivus, Boehringer Ingelheim)‡	250-mg soft-gel capsule	500 mg BID in combination with ritonavir 200 mg BID. Take with food
PROTEASE INHIBITORS/PHARMOCOKINETIC BOOSTER COMBINATIONS		
Atazanavir/cobicistat (ATV/c; Avataz, Bristol-Myers Squibb Virology)	300-mg/150-mg tablet	1 tablet QD. Take with food
Darunavir/cobicistat (DRV/c; Prezcobix, Janssen Therapeutics)	800-mg/150-mg tablet	1 tablet QD. Take with food
FUSION INHIBITORS		
Enfuvirtide (T-20; Fuzeon, Roche)‡	Injectable (lyophilized powder). Each single-use vial contains 108 mg of enfuvirtide to be reconstituted with 1.1 mL of sterile water for injection for delivery of approximately 90 mg/mL	90 mg BID IV. Administered subcutaneously into upper arm, anterior thigh, or abdomen
CCR5 ANTAGONIST		
Maraviroc (MVC; Selzentry, ViiV)	150-, 300-mg tablets	150 mg, 300 mg or 600 BID depending on concomitant drugs (see p. 205 for details); may be taken with or without food
INTEGRASE INHIBITORS		
Raltegravir (RAL; Isentress, Merck)	400-mg tablet	One 400-mg tablet BID
Dolutegravir (DTG; Tivicay, ViiV)	50-mg tablet	No integrase inhibitor resistance: one 50-mg tablet QD; with integrase inhibitor resistance: one 50-mg tablet BID

Table 3.1. Antiretroviral Agents Used for HIV Infection (cont'd)

Drug (abbreviation; trade name, manufacturer)	Formulations	Usual Adult Dosing[§]
COMBINATION NRTI/INTEGRASE INHIBITOR		
Abacavir sulfate/lamivudine/ dolutegravir (ABC/3TC/DTG, Triumeq, ViiV)	600-mg/300-mg/50-mg tablet	One tablet QD.
Tenofovir disoproxil fumarate/ emtricitabine/elvitegravir/ cobicistat (TDF/FTC/EVG/c; Stribild, Gilead-Sciences)	300-mg/200-mg/150-mg/ 150-mg tablet	One tablet QD with food
Tenofovir alafenamide/ emtricitabine/elvitegravir/ cobicistat (TAF/FTC/ EVG/c; Genvoya, Gilead Sciences)	25-mg/200-mg/150-mg/ 150-mg tablet	One tablet QD with food.

*   Nevirapine and efavirenz are cytochrome p450 cyp3A4 inducers; delavirdine is an inhibitor; etravirine has mixed effects. Consult package insert for full drug interaction profile.

†   All protease inhibitors are hepatically metabolized by the cytochrome p450 system; they also are specific inhibitors of cyp3A4 and have induction effects on other enzymes. Consult package insert for full drug-drug interaction profile.

‡   Consult package insert for full drug interaction profile.

§   See Chapter 9 for dosing adjustments in renal or hepatic insufficiency. Unless otherwise stated, medication may be taken with or without food.

SELECTION OF AN OPTIMAL INITIAL ANTIRETROVIRAL REGIMEN (Tables 3.2–3.7)

Selection of the optimal initial antiretroviral regimen must take into consideration antiviral potency, tolerability, and safety. In the DHHS and IAS-USA Guidelines (Tables 3.3 and 3.4), all recommended regimens consist of three active agents: an NRTI pair (containing 3TC or FTC as one of the drugs) plus an integrase inhibitor; the DHHS Guidelines also includes ritonavir-boosted darunavir as an option. As such, choosing a specific regimen therefore can be reduced to four major decisions (see Table 3.2).

Table 3.2. Major Decisions in Selecting the Initial Antiretroviral Regimen

Decision	Comment
What is the optimal NRTI pair?	Because of the availability of once-daily, fixed-dose formulations and a low risk of toxicity, most patients should start a regimen with tenofovir alafenamide-emtricitabine (TAF/FTC). Abacavir/lamivudine (ABC/3TC) may also be used if the integrase inhibitor is dolutegravir. TAF-based options are generally preferable to TDF due to a safer renal and bone profile of TAF; the only exceptions are when HIV treatment is given with rifamycin drugs and during pregnancy; pre-exposure prophylaxis (PrEP, see Chapter 8) is another setting where TDF is preferred over TAF. ABC therapy must be preceded by testing for HLA-B*5701 to reduce the risk of ABC hypersensitivity. Several (but not all) studies have found an association between ABC treatment and an increased risk of myocardial infarction.
Should the third drug be an integrase inhibitor or ritonavir-boosted darunavir?	Most comparative clinical trials have demonstrated the superiority of integrase inhibitor-based treatment over ritonavir-boosted PIs (Lancet 2014;383(9936):2222–2231; Ann Intern Med. 2014 Oct 7; 161(7):461-471; Lancet HIV 2016 May 27;3(9):e410–e420); as a result, the IAS-USA Guidelines list only integrase-based options as recommended first-line regimens. The only advantage of DRV/r-based initial therapy is that intermittent treatment very rarely leads to PI resistance, and hence some might choose this option for individuals with uncertain adherence. Note that the integrase inhibitor DTG has similarly not selected for integrase resistance when given as initial therapy.
Which integrase inhibitor should be selected?	Each of the three available integrase inhibitors has advantages and disadvantages. RAL has the fewest drug interactions, but must be taken twice daily and is not available as coformulated full regimen. EVG/c is coformulated with the optimal NRTI pair (TAF/FTC), but has the most drug interactions due to the requirement for cobicistat for once-daily dosing. DTG is once daily and has the highest resistance barrier, but is only coformulated with ABC/3TC. Based on these factors, for patients not requiring a single tablet for treatment, the two-pill regimen of TAF/FTC plus DTG provides the best combination of efficacy and safety. For those wanting a single pill option, and who do not have significant drug interactions, TAF/FTC/EVG/c is preferred.
Should a single-tablet regimen be used?	Some data suggest that adherence and clinical outcomes are improved with regimens that consist of one tablet daily compared with those that are multiple pills (AIDS 2010 Nov 27;24(18):2835–40. PLoS One 2012;7(2):e31591; Medicine 2015;94:e1677). Among recommended first-line regimens, there are three that are single tablets once daily: TAF (and TDF)/FTC/EVG/c and ABC/3TC/DTG. Alternative options include TAF (and TDF)/FTC/RPV and TDF/FTC/EFV. For the RPV options, TAF/FTC/RPV should be used only when the pre-treatment HIV RNA is < 100,000 copies/mL and the CD4 cell count > 200 to reduce the risk of virologic failure. TDF/FTC/EFV is highly effective virologically, but EFV leads to a high rate of neuropsychiatric side effects; one study found a more than 2-fold increased risk of suicidal ideation in those randomized to EFV-based regimens (Ann Intern Med. 2014 July 1;161(1):1–10).

Table 3.3. DHHS Guidelines: What to Start: Initial Combination Regimens for the Antiretroviral-Naive Patient (Last updated July 14, 2016)

An antiretroviral (ARV) regimen for a treatment-naive patient generally consists of two nucleoside reverse transcriptase inhibitors (NRTIs) in combination with a third active ARV drug from one of three drug classes: an integrase strand transfer inhibitor (INSTI), a non-nucleoside reverse transcriptase inhibitor (NNRTI), or a protease inhibitor (PI) with a pharmacokinetic (PK) enhancer (booster) (cobicistat or ritonavir).

Recommended Regimen Options
Recommended regimens are those with demonstrated durable virologic efficacy, favorable tolerability and toxicity profiles, and ease of use.

INSTI plus Two-NRTI Regimen:
- DTG/ABC/3TC[a] **(AI)**—if **HLA-B*5701 negative**
- DTG plus either TDF/FTC[a] **(AI)** or TAF/FTC[b] **(AII)**
- EVG/c/TAF/FTC **(AI)** or EVG/c/TDF/FTC **(AI)**
- RAL plus either TDF/FTC[a] **(AI)** or TAF/FTC[b] **(AII)**

Boosted PI plus Two NRTIs:
- DRV/r plus either TDF/FTC[a] **(AI)** or TAF/FTC[b] **(AII)**

Alternative Regimen Options
Alternative regimens are effective and tolerable, but have potential disadvantages when compared with the recommended regimens, have limitations for use in certain patient populations, or have less supporting data from randomized clinical trials. **However, an alternative regimen may be the preferred regimen for some patients.**

NNRTI plus Two NRTIs:
- EFV/TDF/FTC[a] **(BI)**
- EFV plus TAF/FTC[b] **(BII)**
- RPV/TDF/FTC[a] **(BI)** or RPV/TAF/FTC[b] **(BII)**—if HIV RNA < 100,000 copies/mL and CD4 > 200 cells/mm³

Boosted PI plus Two NRTIs:
- (ATV/c orATV/r) plus either TDF/FTC[a] **(BI)** or TAF/FTC[b] **(BII)**
- DRV/c **(BIII)** or DRV/r **(BII)** plus ABC/3TC[a]—if HLA-B*5701 negative
- DRV/c plus either TDF/FTC[a] **(BII)** or TAF/FTC[b] **(BII)**

---

[a] 3TC may be substituted for FTC, or vice versa, if a non-fixed dose NRTI combination is desired.

[b] The evidence supporting this regimen is based on relative bioavailability data coupled with data from randomized, controlled switch trials demonstrating the safety and efficacy of TAF-containing regimens.

Rating of Recommendations: *A = Strong; B = Moderate; C = Optional.*

Rating of Evidence: *I = Data from randomized controlled trials; II = Data from well-designed nonrandomized trials, observational cohort studies with long-term clinical outcomes, relative bioavailability/bioequivalence studies, or regimen comparisons from randomized switch studies; III = Expert opinion*

Key to Abbreviations: 3TC = lamivudine, ABC = abacavir, ART = antiretroviral therapy, ARV = antiretroviral, ATV/r = atazanavir/ritonavir, COBI = cobicistat, CrCl = creatinine clearance, CVD = cardiovascular disease, DRV/r = darunavir/ritonavir, DTV = dolutegravir, EFV = efavirenz, EVG = elvitegravir, FDA = Food and Drug Administration, FPV/r = fosamprenavir/ritonavir, FTC = emtricitabine, INSTI = integrase strand transfer inhibitor, LPV/r = lopinavir/ritonavir, NNRTI = nonnucleoside reverse transcriptase inhibitor, NRTI = nucleos(t)ide reverse transcriptase inhibitor, PI = protease inhibitor, PPI = proton pump inhibitor, RAL = raltegravir, RPV = rilpivirine, RTV = ritonavir, TDF = tenofovir, ZDV = zidovudine

Table 3.4. IAS-USA Guidelines: Recommended Initial Antiretroviral Therapy Regimens[a]

Regimen	Rating
Dolutegravir/abacavir/lamivudine	AIa
Dolutegravir plus tenofovir alafenamide/emtricitabine[b]	AIa
Elvitegravir/cobicistat/tenofovir alafenamide/emtricitabine[b]	AIa
Raltegravir plus tenofovir alafenamide/emtricitabine[b]	AIII

[a] Regimens are listed in alphabetic order by integrase strand transfer inhibitor component. Components separated with a slash (/) indicate that they are available as coformulations.

[b] In settings in which tenofovir alafenamide/emtricitabine is not available, tenofovir disoproxil fumarate (with emtricitabine or lamivudine) remains an effective and generally well-tolerated option. Given the limited long-term experience with tenofovir alafenamide, some clinicians may prefer to continue using tenofovir disoproxil fumarate pending broader experience with tenofovir alafenamide in clinical practice.

Table 3.5. IAS-USA Guidelines: Strength of Recommendation and Quality of Evidence Rating Scale[a]

Rating	Definition
Strength of recommendation	
A	Strong support for the recommendation
B	Moderate support for the recommendation
C	Limited support for the recommendation
Quality of evidence	
Ia	Evidence from ≥ one randomized clinical trials published in the peer-reviewed literature
Ib	Evidence from ≥ one randomized clinical trials presented in abstract form at peer-reviewed scientific meetings
IIa	Evidence from nonrandomized clinical trials or cohort or case-control studies published in the peer-reviewed literature
IIb	Evidence from nonrandomized clinical trials or cohort or case-control studies presented in abstract form at peer-reviewed scientific meetings
III	Recommendation based on the panel's analysis of the accumulated available evidence

[a] Adapted in part from the Canadian Task Force on Periodic Health Examination.

Table 3.6. IAS-USA Guidelines: Advantages and Disadvantages of Currently Available Integrase Strand Transfer Inhibitors

	Dolutegravir	Elvitegravir	Raltegravir
Year of US Food and Drug Administration approval	2013	2012	2007
Advantages	Superior to efavirenz and ritonavir-boosted darunavir in comparative clinical trials. Once-daily dosing. Coformulated with abacavir/lamivudine as part of a complete initial regimen. Dolutegravir (not coformulated) pill size is small. Lowest risk of resistance with virologic failure. Relatively few drug interactions. Can be taken with or without food. Superior to raltegravir in treatment-experienced patients.	Superior to ritonavir-boosted atazanavir in comparative clinical trial in HIV-infected women. Once-daily dosing. Coformulated with cobicistat, tenofovir disoproxil fumarate/ emtricitabine or tenofovir alafenamide/emtricitabine as a complete regimen.	Superior to ritonavir-boosted atazanavir and ritonavir-boosted darunavir in comparative clinical trial. Longest safety record. Fewest drug interactions. Can be taken with or without food.
Disadvantages	Only available coformulation is with abacavir/lamivudine. Raises serum creatinine owing to inhibition of tubular secretion of creatinine. Higher rates of insomnia and headache than comparators in some studies. Largest tablet among coformulated single-pill regimens.	Requires pharmacokinetic boosting with cobicistat or ritonavir for once-daily dosing. Most drug interactions. Cobicistat raises serum creatinine owing to inhibition of tubular secretion of creatinine. Should be taken with food.	Currently must be taken twice daily (formulation consisting of two pills given once daily in development). Not coformulated as part of a complete regimen.

Table 3.7. IAS-USA Guideiines Initial Antiretroviral Treatment Options for Those Who Cannot Take Integrase Inhibitors: Advantages and Disadvantages[a]

	Darunavir (Boosted with Cobicistat or Ritonavir) plus TAF/ Emtricitabine, TDF/ Emtricitabine, or Abacavir/Lamivudine[b]	Efavirenz/TDF/ Emtricitabine	Rilpivirine/TAF (or TDF)/Emtricitabine
Advantages	Low risk of resistance with virologic failure, even with intermittent adherence.	High efficacy in patients with baseline HIV RNA >100,000 copies/mL. Extensive experience in patients with concomitant tuberculosis. Widely available globally.	Lowest risk of rash among NNRTI-based therapies. Low risk of metabolic adverse effects. Smallest tablet among single-pill regimens.
Disadvantages	Requires pharmacokinetic boosting; many drug interactions. Ritonavir-boosted darunavir inferior to raltegravir and dolutegravir in separate comparative clinical trials. Results of comparative, fully powered studies of cobicistat-boosted darunavir as initial therapy are not yet available.	Relatively high rate of rash. No single-tablet form available with TAF. High rates of neuropsychiatric adverse effects. Increased risk of suicidality in 1 study; avoid in patients with history of depression.	Not recommended for patients with HIV RNA > 100,000 copies/mL or CD4 cell count < 200/μL owing to increased risk of virologic failure. Must be taken with a meal to optimize absorption. Should not be administered with proton pump inhibitors; stagger dosing if given with an H_2 blocker.

Abbreviations: InSTI, integrase strand transfer inhibitor; NNRTI, nonnucleoside reverse transcriptase inhibitor; TAF, tenofovir alafenamide; TDF, tenofovir disoproxil fumarate.

[a] Nonnucleoside reverse transcriptase inhibitor–based regimens should not be used without baseline resistance data because of the possible presence of transmitted NNRTI-resistant virus. In the rare circumstance in which maraviroc might be included in initial therapy, initiation should not occur before confirmation of CC chemokine receptor 5 tropism.

[b] Cautions on the use of abacavir and TAF or TDF are described in the text.

Special considerations when selecting initial ART (adapted from IAS USA 2016 guidelines):

1. **Pregnancy** (see Chapter 7). NRTI options include (in order of author's preference) TDF/FTC, ABC/3TC, and ZDV/3TC. Raltegravir is currently the recommended integrase inhibitor; DRV/r or ATV/r may be used if a boosted PI is the best option. For women who become pregnant while receiving TDF/FTC/EFV or ABC/3TC plus EFV and have virologic suppression, this regimen should be continued.

2. **Hepatitis B Coinfection** (see Chapter 5). All patients with chronic hepatitis B should be treated with a regimen containing either TAF or TDF with either FTC or 3TC (in addition to a third active HIV agent) as TAF and TDF have the greatest activity against hepatitis B. Use of FTC or 3TC without TAF or TDF risks development of HBV resistance to FTC.

3. **Hepatitis C Coinfection** (see Chapter 5). Many antiretroviral agents have significant drug interactions with some anti-HCV drugs. Among the currently recommended first-line regimens, TAF/FTC plus DTG or RAL, or ABC/3TC/DTG have the fewest drug interactions, and hence are the preferred options. In general, HIV treatment should be started before HCV therapy, with the latter undertaken once a patient has HIV virologic suppression and is tolerating the ART regimen well. If one of the above regimens cannot be used for HIV, close attention to HIV and HCV drug interactions is essential. Good online resources include www.hep-druginteractions.org and hcvguidelines.org.

4. **Osteoporosis.** Patients who start regimens containing TDF have significantly greater declines in bone density than non-TDF-containing treatments. As such, for patients with osteoporosis, TAF/FTC or ABC/3TC should be selected as the NRTI pair.

5. **Cardiovascular Disease.** Concerns over an association between ABC and an increased risk of myocardial infarction were first raised in an observational study reported in 2008 (Lancet 2008 April 2; 371(9622):1417–1426). Since that time, several but not all studies evaluating this risk have found the same association, with an important exception a meta-analysis of randomized clinical trials comparing ABC to alternative treatments (J Acquir Immune Defic Syndr. 2012 Dec 1;61(4):441–7). Although there is no proven single mechanism for the association between ABC and MI, current theories include increased inflammation, increased leucocyte adhesion, altered endothelial function, and increased platelet activation. Despite the fact that the data from these studies are not conclusive, they argue for avoidance of ABC in patients who have or who are at risk of cardiovascular disease. As a result, the NRTI combination of choice in this setting is either TAF/FTC or TDF/FTC.

6. **Kidney Disease.** TDF-based treatments are more likely to cause renal injury and chronic renal disease than regimens that do not include TDF; this difference is more pronounced when TDF is given with a ritonavir-boosted PI. Atazanavir has also been implicated in causing renal disease. TDF should be avoided in those with renal impairment (estimated GFR < 60 mL/min), with preferential use of TAF (if eGFR is greater than 30 mL/min) or ABC. For patients with moderate-severe renal impairment who cannot take either TAF or ABC, the two-drug regimens DRV/r plus DTG, or plus 3TC can be considered.

ANTIRETROVIRAL THERAPY ADVERSE EFFECTS

Although the tolerability and safety of antiretroviral therapy has improved substantially, adverse events have been reported with all the available agents. In addition, subjective side effects remain one of the most common causes of medication non-compliance and treatment failure. Certain drugs — such as d4T, ddI, and indinavir — are now rarely used in developed countries due to their relatively poor adverse event profile, but may still be used in resource-limited settings that do not have access to the newest agents.

Clinicians should be particularly alert to potential side effects that may occur in patients who already have underlying disease processes, or who are taking concomitant medications with overlapping toxicities. For example, individuals co-infected with hepatitis B and C generally have higher rates of hepatotoxicity; those with psychiatric disease are more prone to the adverse CNS effects of efavirenz; and patients with pre-existing renal disease may be more likely to experience tenofovir DF nephrotoxicity. Table 3.8 was adapted from DHHS Guidelines for the Use of Antiretroviral Agents in HIV-1-Infected Adults and Adolescents, last updated July 14, 2016.

Table 3.8. Antiretroviral Therapy-Associated Common and/or Severe Adverse Effects: Last Updated on July 14, 2016

N/A indicates either that there are no reported cases for the particular side effect or that data for the specific ARV drug class are not available.

Adverse Effect	NRTIs	NNRTIs	PIs	INSTI	EI
Bleeding Events	N/A	N/A	Spontaneous bleeding, hematuria in hemophilia. **TPV:** Intracranial hemorrhage associated with CNS lesions, trauma, alcohol abuse, hypertension, coagulopathy, anticoagulant or antiplatelet agents, vitamin E.	N/A	N/A
Bone Density Effects	**TDF:** Associated with greater loss of BMD than other NRTIs; osteomalacia may be associated with renal tubulopathy and urine phosphate wasting. **TAF:** Smaller declines in BMD than with TDF.	Decreases in BMD observed after the initiation of any ART regimen.			N/A
Bone Marrow Suppression	**ZDV:** Anemia, neutropenia	N/A	N/A	N/A	N/A

Table 3.8. Antiretroviral Therapy-Associated Common and/or Severe Adverse Effects: Last Updated on July 14, 2016 (cont'd)

Adverse Effect	NRTIs	NNRTIs	PIs	INSTI	EI
Cardiovascular Disease	**ABC and ddI:** Associated with an increased risk of MI in some cohort studies. Absolute risk greatest in patients with traditional CVD risk factors.	**RPV:** QTc prolongation.	Associated with MI and stroke in some cohorts. **SQV/r, ATV/r, and LPV/r:** PR prolongation (risks include pre-existing heart disease, other medications). **SQV/r:** QT prolongation. Obtain ECG before administering SQV.	N/A	N/A
Cholelithiasis	N/A	N/A	**ATV:** Cholelithiasis and kidney stones may present concurrently. Median onset is 42 months.	N/A	N/A
Diabetes Mellitus/Insulin Resistance	ZDV, d4T, and ddI	N/A	Reported for some (**IDV, LPV/r**), but not all PIs.	N/A	N/A
Dyslipidemia	d4T > ZDV > ABC: TG and LDL **Tenofovir lowers plasma lipids; TDF lowers them more than TAF due to higher systemic tenofovir levels.**	**EFV:** TG, LDL, HDL	**All RTV- or COBI-boosted PIs:** TG, LDL, HDL **LPV/r = FPV/r and LPV/r > DRV/r and ATV/r:** →TG	**EVG/c:** TG, LDL, HDL	N/A

Adverse Effect	NRTIs	NNRTIs	PIs	INSTI	EI
Gastrointestinal Effects	**ddI and ZDV > other NRTIs:** Nausea and vomiting **ddI:** Pancreatitis	N/A	GI intolerance (e.g. diarrhea, nausea, vomiting) Common with **LPV/r** and more frequent than with **DRV/r** and **ATV/r:** Diarrhea	**EVG/c:** Nausea and diarrhea	N/A
Hepatic Effects	Reported with most NRTIs. **ZDV, d4T, or ddI:** Steatosis most common. **ddI:** Prolonged exposure linked to noncirrhotic portal hypertension, esophageal varices. When **TAF, TDF, 3TC,** and **FTC** are withdrawn or when HBV resistance develops; HIV/HBV coinfected patients may develop severe hepatic flares.	**NVP > other NNRTIs** **NVP:** Severe hepatotoxicity associated with skin rash or hypersensitivity. Two-week NVP dose escalation may reduce risk. Risk is greater for women with pre-NVP CD4 count >250 cells/mm^3 and men with pre-NVP CD4 count >400 cells/mm^3. NVP should **never** be used for postexposure prophylaxis, or in patients with hepatic insufficiency (Child-Pugh B or C).	**All PIs:** Drug-induced hepatitis and hepatic decompensation have been reported; greatest frequency with TPV/r. **IDV, ATV:** Jaundice due to indirect hyperbilirubinemia. **TPV/r:** **Contraindicated** in patients with hepatic insufficiency (Child-Pugh B or C).	N/A	**MVC:** Hepatotoxicity with or without rash or HSRs reported.

Table 3.8. Antiretroviral Therapy-Associated Common and/or Severe Adverse Effects: Last Updated on July 14, 2016 (cont'd)

Adverse Effect	NRTIs	NNRTIs	PIs	INSTI	EI
Hypersensitivity Reaction Excluding rash alone or Stevens-Johnson syndrome	**ABC: <u>Contraindicated</u>** if HLA-B*5701 positive. Median onset 9 days; 90% of reactions occur within first 6 weeks of treatment. HSR symptoms (in order of descending frequency): Fever, rash, malaise, nausea, headache, myalgia, chills, diarrhea, vomiting, abdominal pain, dyspnea, arthralgia, and respiratory symptoms. Symptoms worsen with continuation of ABC. Patients, regardless of HLA-B*5701 status, should not be rechallenged with ABC if HSR is suspected.	**NVP:** Hypersensitivity syndrome of hepatotoxicity and rash that may be accompanied by fever, general malaise, fatigue, myalgias, arthralgias, blisters, oral lesions, conjunctivitis, facial edema, eosinophilia, renal dysfunction, granulocytopenia, or lymphadenopathy. Risk is greater for ARV-naïve women with pre-NVP CD4 count > 250 cells/mm³ and men with pre-NVP CD4 count > 400 cells/mm³. Overall, risk is higher for women than men. Two-week dose escalation of NVP reduces risk.	N/A	**RAL:** HSR reported when RAL given in combination with other drugs known to cause HSR. All ARVs should be stopped if HSR occurs. **DTG:** Reported in < 1% of patients in clinical development program.	**MVC:** Reported as part of a syndrome related to hepatotoxicity.

Adverse Effect	NRTIs	NNRTIs	PIs	INSTI	EI
Lactic Acidosis	Reported with **NRTIs,** especially **d4T, ZDV,** and **ddi:** Insidious onset with GI prodrome, weight loss, and fatigue. May rapidly progress with tachycardia, tachypnea, jaundice, weakness, mental status changes, pancreatitis, and organ failure. Mortality high if serum lactate >10 mmol/L. Women and obese patients at increased risk.	N/A	N/A	N/A	N/A
Lipodystrophy	Lipoatrophy: **d4T > ZDV**. May be more likely when **NRTIs** combined with **EFV** than with an **RTV-boosted PI**.	Lipohypertophy: Trunk fat increase observed with EFV., PI, and RAL-containing regimens; however, causal relationship has not been established.			N/A
Myopathy/ Elevated Creatine Phosphokinase	**ZDV:** Myopathy	N/A	N/A	**RAL:** CPK, weakness, and rhabdomyolysis	N/A

Table 3.8. Antiretroviral Therapy-Associated Common and/or Severe Adverse Effects: Last Updated on July 14, 2016 (cont'd)

Adverse Effect	NRTIs	NNRTIs	PIs	INSTIs	EI
Nervous System/ Psychiatric Effects	**d4T > ddI** and **ddC:** Peripheral neuropathy: (can be irreversible). **d4T:** Associated with rapidly progressive, ascending neuromuscular weakness resembling Guillain-Barré syndrome (rare).	**EFV:** Somnolence, insomnia, abnormal dreams, dizziness, impaired concentration, depression, psychosis, and suicidal ideation. Symptoms usually subside or diminish after 2 to 4 weeks. Bedtime dosing may reduce symptoms. Risks include psychiatric illness, concomitant use of agents with neuropsychiatric effects, and increased EFV concentrations because of genetic factors or increased absorption with food. An association between EFV and suicidal ideation, suicide, and attempted suicide (especially among younger patients and those with history of mental illness or substance abuse) was found in a retrospective analysis of comparative trials. **RPV:** Depression, suicidality, sleep disturbances.	N/A	**All INSTIs:** Insomnia, depression, and suicidality have been infrequently reported with INSTI use, primarily in patients with preexisting psychiatric conditions.	N/A

Adverse Effect	NRTIs	NNRTIs	PIs	INSTI	EI
		All NNRTIs	ATV, DRV, FPV, LPV/r, TPV	RAL, EVG	MVC
Rash	FTC: Hyperpigmentation	N/A			N/A
Renal Effects/ Urolithiasis	TDF: SCr, proteinuria, hypophosphatemia, urinary phosphate wasting, glycosuria, hypokalemia, non-anion gap metabolic acidosis. Concurrent use of TDF with COBI or RTV-containing regimens appears to increase risk. TAF: Less impact on renal biomarkers and lower rates of proteinuria than TDF.	N/A	ATV and LPV/r: Increased risk of chronic kidney disease in a large cohort study. IDV: SCr, pyuria, renal atrophy or hydronephrosis. IDV, ATV: Stone, crystal formation; adequate hydration may reduce risk.	COBI and DTG: Inhibits Cr secretion without reducing renal glomerular function.	
Stevens-Johnson Syndrome/ Toxic Epidermal Necrosis	ddl, ZDV: Reported cases.	NVP > DLV, EFV, ETR, RPV	FPV, DRV, IDV, LPV/r, ATV: Reported cases.	RAL	N/A

Reproduced from Panel on Antiretroviral Guidelines for Adults and Adolescents. Guidelines for the use of antiretroviral agents in HIV-1-infected adults and adolescents. AIDSinfo. https://aidsinfo.nih.gov/contentfiles/lvguidelines/adultandadolescentgl.pdf. July 14, 2016.

Key to Abbreviations: 3TC = lamivudine; ABC = abacavir; ART= antiretroviral therapy; ARV = antiretroviral; ATV = atazanavir; ATV/r = atazanavir/ritonavir; BMD = bone mineral density; CD4 = CD4 T lymphocyte; CNS = central nervous system; COBI = cobicistat; CPK = creatine phosphokinase; Cr = creatinine; CrCl = creatinine clearance; CVD = cardiovascular disease; d4T = stavudine; ddC = zalcitabine; ddI = didanosine; DLV = delavirdine; DRV = darunavir; DRV/r = darunavir/ritonavir; DTG = dolutegravir; ECG = electrocardiogram; EFV = efavirenz; EI = entry inhibitor; ETR = etravirine; EVG = elvitegravir; FPV = fosamprenavir; FPV/r = fosamprenavir/ritonavir; FTC = emtricitabine; GI = gastrointestinal; HBV = hepatitis B virus; HDL = high-density lipoprotein; HSR = hypersensitivity reaction; IDV = indinavir; INSTI = integrase strand transfer inhibitor; LDL = low-density lipoprotein; LPV/r = lopinavir/ritonavir; MI = myocardial infarction; MVC = maraviroc; NFV = nelfinavir; NNRTI = non-nucleoside reverse transcriptase inhibitor; NRTI = nucleoside reverse transcriptase inhibitor; NVP = nevirapine; PI = protease inhibitor; RAL = raltegravir; RPV = rilpivirine; RTV = ritonavir; SCr = serum creatinine; SQV = saquinavir; SQV/r = saquinavir/ritonavir; TAF = tenofovir alafenamide; TDF = tenofovir disoproxil fumarate; TG = triglyceride; TPV = tipranavir; TPV/r = tipranavir/ritonavir; ZDV = zidovudine.

Chapter 4

Management of the Treatment-Experienced Patient

ANTIRETROVIRAL TREATMENT FAILURE

Antiretroviral treatment failure can be defined in various ways. These include virologic failure (inability to achieve virologic suppression, or occurrence of virologic rebound), immunologic failure (also referred to as poor CD4 recovery), and clinical failure (HIV disease progression). Immunologic and clinical failure rarely occur in patients who are taking their antiretrovirals faithfully and are virologically suppressed. The bulk of clinical decisions, therefore, depend on diagnosis, evaluation, and management of virologic failure.

A. Virologic Response Definitions (Adapted from DHHS Guidelines for the Use of Antiretroviral Agents in HIV-1-Infected Adults and Adolescents: Management of the Treatment-Experienced Patient—Virologic Failure, last updated April 8, 2015

1. **Virologic Suppression:** A confirmed HIV RNA level below the lower level of detection of available assays. Generally this is 20 copies/mL (Roche) or 40 copies/mL (Abbott).

2. **Virologic Failure:** The inability to achieve or maintain suppression of viral replication to an HIV RNA level < 200 copies/mL. The use of 200 copies/mL allows for intermittent detection of low-level viremia ("blip," see below) without prompting resistance testing or changing of the regimen. Once virologic failure is confirmed, blood should be sent for genotypic resistance testing.

3. **Incomplete Virologic Response:** Two consecutive plasma HIV RNA levels ≥ 200 copies/ mL after 24 weeks on an ART regimen in a patient who has not yet had documented virologic suppression on this regimen. A patient's baseline HIV RNA level may affect the time course of response, and some regimens will take longer than others to suppress HIV RNA levels. Integrase-inhibitor-based therapy usually achieve virologic suppression by 8 weeks of treatment.

4. **Virologic Rebound:** Confirmed HIV RNA ≥ 200 copies/mL after virologic suppression.

5. **Virologic Blip:** After virologic suppression, an isolated detectable HIV RNA level that is followed by a return to virologic suppression. Usually these are between 20–200 copies/mL. There is an increased frequency of detecting low-level HIV RNA (20–200 copies/mL) with the current more sensitive HIV RNA assays (J Acquir Immune Defic Syndr. 2009 May 1;51(1):3–6). While some studies indicate an increased risk of eventual virologic failure in those who have HIV RNA repeatedly detected between 20–200 copies/mL, the optimal strategy for managing these patients is not known. For now, our practice is not to switch treatments in patients who have newly detectable HIV RNA < 200 copies/mL, especially if not confirmed with a second value.

Most patients with virologic failure fall into one of the following categories based on results of genotype testing.

1. **Failure with No Resistance.** This is predominantly due to poor adherence, either from never taking prescribed ART or taking it successfully and then abruptly stopping.

2. **Failure with One or Two Class Resistance.** This is most commonly seen in patients who fail their first treatment regimen with intermittent adherence.

3. **Failure with Extensive Multi-Class Resistance.** The cause of this treatment failure is sequential treatment with less potent drugs, often given as "sequential monotherapy" — meaning a single drug was added to a failing regimen. Such patients often were fully adherent, but the regimen was not sufficiently potent or active to achieve suppression. Almost all of these patients have lengthy treatment histories, including the period from 1996–2000 during the early introduction of combination ART.

B. Evaluation of Virologic Failure

1. **Determine the Etiology.** Since poor adherence is by far the most common cause of treatment failure, it is critical to assess whether they are taking ART as directed. Patients may not admit to poor adherence, and hence they should be queried in a non-judgmental way — for example, "Many patients have difficulty taking their medications regularly. Has this been a challenge for you?" or, "Can you let me know how often you missed your medications in the last week? The last month?" Ask them to bring in their actual pill bottles to confirm that they are taking the right medications, and that food requirements are understood and unanticipated drug interactions can be resolved. Pharmacy refill records are extremely useful, as patients rarely refill prescriptions of medications that they are not taking. Finally, query for underlying causes of poor adherence, including side effects, insurance issues, pill burden, substance abuse, and mental illness.

2. **Evaluate for Resistance.** Resistance testing is a highly complex diagnostic strategy that for optimal effect requires both a thorough review of the patient treatment history and an understanding of the strengths and limitations of the resistance assays. Criteria for resistance are under continuous evaluation and evolution. It is therefore important to consult with updated guidelines, such as those published by the International AIDS Society. (https://www.iasusa.org/content/drug-resistance-mutations-in-HIV, see Appendix 1).

    Types of resistance tests:

   a. **Genotype testing.** In most settings where resistance testing is indicated, genotype testing is preferred over phenotype testing. Not only have a large number of studies validated the predictive value of genotype testing to help enhance treatment response, but genotype testing is also more easily standardized from lab to lab, less expensive, and has faster turnaround time than phenotype. Standard genotype resistance tests offer results for NRTIs, NNRTIs, and PIs; testing for genotypic resistance to integrase inhibitors usually must be ordered separately. Laboratories will typically require an HIV RNA level of > 500 copies to perform a genotype test. The GenoSure Archive test can extract HIV DNA from patients with lower viral loads (or even undetectable viral loads), and then perform sequencing to detect if there is "archived" resistance to all the major HIV drug classes. This test should not generally be used in patients with virologic failure, but may be helpful when for technical reasons or very low level HIV RNA, standard genotyping is not successful.

   b. **Phenotype testing.** Phenotype testing, usually in conjunction with a genotype test, may rarely be done as an adjunct to genotype tests. Situations might include: (1) occurrence of certain viral strains that make sequencing difficult for the laboratory;

(2) highly complex or contradictory genotype results, especially in multiple PI-resistant cases; and (3) when used in conjunction with therapeutic drug monitoring of protease inhibitors (rarely done in the United States currently). Phenotype testing may be useful in patients with high-level PI resistance, where activity of darunavir (generally the recommended PI) is uncertain, and tipranavir may rarely be a better option. In such a setting, the clinical cutoffs provided by phenotype testing detail whether these drugs are fully active, partially active, or unlikely to be active virologically.

c. **Co-receptor tropism assay.** HIV enters the CD4 cell using both the CD4 receptor and either a CCR5 receptor (R5-tropic viruses) or a CXCR4 receptor (X4-tropic viruses). R5-tropic viruses are commonly transmitted and predominate in early infection. Over time, there is a shift in virus population to those that use both receptors (dual tropic) or to a mixture of R5 and X4 viruses. The CCR5 antagonist drug maraviroc is only active against R5-tropic viruses. As a result, when considering use of this agent, a co-receptor tropism assay should be ordered. It is reasonable to consider repeating this test for patients who experience virologic failure on maraviroc.

One available tropism assay currently is a modification of the Monogram phenotype; results return in 3–4 weeks, and indicate whether the viral population is R5 tropic, of dual or mixed tropism (D/M), or X4 tropic. The report also provides a summary statement about whether CCR5 antagonist drugs will be active. A second version of this assay is available for patients who have virologic suppression; it is potentially useful for those who may need to switch to a maraviroc-containing regimen due to toxicity, but no prior tropism test is available. Importantly, there has not yet been clinical validation of this second assay. Finally, a genotypic tropism assay is also available from Quest Laboratories. It provides similar information to the phenotypic assay, with results returning in 1–3 weeks and at much lower cost than the phenotype.

3. **Select the optimal Next Regimen.** In all patients with virologic failure, clinicians should devise a treatment strategy that will again lead to virologic suppression. With very few exceptions, this should be achievable even in patients with extensive drug resistance given the high potency of currently available agents. The specific regimen employed will depend on the cause of the treatment failure and the results of resistance testing.

a. **Virologic failure with no resistance detected.** Although resistance mutations are rare in these non-adherent patients, the testing is still of value since a negative genotype prevents unnecessary switching to potentially more expensive, toxic, or complex regimens. As noted above, most of these patients are experiencing virologic failure due to poor adherence. Many times, they will be taking none of the prescribed medications, and this can be confirmed using pharmacy refill data.

Adherence can be affected by a multitude of factors, including but not limited to drug side effects, cost, medication access, housing, food security, patient safety, healthy literacy, mental illness, and substance abuse. Ideally all involved factors should be addressed with the assistance of a multidisciplinary team including social workers, case managers, pharmacists, and psychiatrists. If available, the use of community health workers for directly observed therapy can increase adherence in certain patient populations.

The best characteristics for a new regimen in such a setting take into account potential side effects, regimen complexity, and likelihood of resistance with intermittent therapy. Single pill options from the recommended regimens, such as abacavir/lamivudine/dolutegravir or elvitegravir/cobicistat/tenofovir AF/emtricitabine, should be considered. The two-pill option of tenofovir alafenamide/emtricitabine plus dolutegravir is particularly attractive (albeit slightly more complex), as the pill sizes are small, and the regimen has a relatively high barrier to resistance should virologic failure occur again. Some clinicians may select darunavir-based treatment, as resistance is exceedingly rare when virologic failure occurs on these regimens. However, the side effect profile and virologic efficacy are not as favorable as with the integrase inhibitor-based regimens.

After selecting a new regimen—or, alternatively, continuing the same regimen with enhanced adherence support—clinicians should follow these patients closely with both clinical and laboratory evaluations. HIV RNA should decline at least one log (and usually more) 2–4 weeks after starting treatment, and relatively frequent virologic monitoring (for example every 4–8 weeks) should be done until the HIV RNA is suppressed.

b. **Virologic failure with single or dual class resistance.** Intermittent adherence to first-line regimens that are based on NNRTIs and the integrase inhibitors raltegravir and elvitegravir may select for single or dual class resistance. Errors in medication prescribing or dispensing, drug interactions, and patient's misunderstanding of dosing strategies (for example, taking rilpivirine-based therapies without food) may all be responsible.

Clinical trials have evaluated treatment strategies in patients after failure of first-line dual-NRTI plus NNRTI-based therapy, most of whom had single or dual class resistance (Lancet 2013;381:2091–2099; NEJM 2014;371: 234–247). In these studies, the subsequent regimens included lopinavir/ritonavir with randomization to add the integrase inhibitor raltegravir, or to add nucleoside analogs chosen at the discretion of the study investigators. The studies demonstrated high levels of virologic suppression regardless of which strategy was chosen, indicating that when using a boosted protease inhibitor for second-line therapy, both a fully active drug (such as an integrase inhibitor) or recycled nucleoside analogs (which continue to exert partial antiviral activity) will suffice. While studies of second line-treatment after failure of an integrase inhibitor have not been done, one can extrapolate from these studies that a similar approach (boosted PI plus NRTIs or fully active integrase inhibitor) would be successful, especially if using a more active and better tolerated PI such as darunavir. In addition, the SAILING study demonstrated that dolutegravir was more active than raltegravir in treatment- experienced patients with virologic failure and resistance (Lancet. 2013 Aug 24;382(9893):700–8). As a result, dolutegravir is the integrase inhibitor of choice for this population.

c. **Virologic failure with extensive multi-class resistance (See Table 4-1).** Patients treated in the 1990s often received antiretroviral regimens that were inadequately potent to suppress viral replication despite excellent medication adherence. In addition, the practice of adding a new class of drugs to an existing regimen—so-called "serial monotherapy"—would only transiently reduce HIV RNA. Both of these situations led to selection of extensive multi-class drug resistance involving NRTI, NNRTI, and the protease inhibitor classes.

Table 4.1. Categories of Virologic Failure Based on Resistance Pattern

Resistance Pattern	Cause of Virologic Failure	Management
No mutations	Non-adherence *or* Adherence then abrupt stop of medications	Assess for adherence and tolerability. Resume regimen unless the cause of poor adherence was drug toxicity; consider treatment simplification if possible.
1 or 2 class resistance	Intermittent adherence *or* Administration/absorption errors (drug-drug interactions, incorrect dosing, dietary effects)	Assess for adherence and inquire about pharmacokinetic factors. Change to boosted PI regimen plus either NRTIs or (if no integrase resistance), an integrase inhibitor.
Multi-class resistance	Treated previously with suboptimal regimens *or* History of intermittent adherence to multiple regimens	Review all previous resistance testing. Obtain supplemental testing if warranted and not yet available, such as integrase resistance genotype, resistance phenotype, or viral tropism assay. Goal is to find regimen with 2–3 active drugs.

Virologic failure in this patient population requires meticulous attention to current and past resistance testing. Supplemental assessments, including a resistance phenotype (especially in those with complex PI resistance), integrase genotype, and a viral tropism assay may be required. Once this information is obtained, the goal is to find a regimen that has at least two fully active drugs.

Certain drugs in each drug class deserve special mention for management in this patient population. These include the following: (1) **NRTIs:** 3TC and FTC appear to offer ongoing virologic activity even in the presence of the signature M184V mutation. (2) **NNRTIs:** Etravirine often retains viral activity even in those with prior resistance to NRTIs, and is fully active against the K103N mutation, most commonly selected by efavirenz. Rilpivirine also is active against K103N-containing viruses, but it less potent than etravirine and hence less commonly used in this setting. (3) **PIs:** In treatment-experienced patients, darunavir is generally the protease inhibitor of choice, as it is active against most viruses with protease inhibitor mutations. The drug can be used once daily if there are no darunavir-associated mutations (see Appendix 1), but twice daily if these are present. In rare situations, the protease inhibitor tipranavir retains activity against viruses resistant to darunavir. The disadvantages of tipranavir include a higher pill burden, more side effects, and more drug interactions, hence it only should be used in this circumstance where darunavir is not active. (4) **Integrase inhibitors:** Dolutegravir is generally preferred in this setting, as it was demonstrated superior to raltegravir in treatment-experienced patients with virologic failure and drug resistance (Lancet 2013 Aug 24;382(9893):700–708). The coformalation ECF-TAF can be used with darunavir as a two-pill option for salvage therapy provided there are no darunavir-associated mutations, there are three or fewer thymidine-associated mutations, and no evidence of integrase inhibitor resistance. (5) **Maraviroc:** The only CCR5 antagonist, maraviroc provides an additional antiviral option only for patients whose viral tropism test indicates that they have R5-using virus. It is not active against CXCR4 or dual-tropic virus.

Once information from various resistance tests and complete treatment history has been obtained, a regimen consisting of a boosted protease inhibitor (typically darunavir, given once or twice daily), the integrase inhibitor dolutegravir, and a third active agent will lead to virologic suppression even in patients of extensive multi-class resistance. In the TRIO study, the combination of raltegravir, etravirine, and darunavir/ritonavir (often with inclusion of NRTIs at the discretion of the investigators) yielded virologic suppression in 90% of study subjects at 24 weeks (Clin Infect Dis 2009;49:1441–1449), a rate comparable to that seen in treatment-naïve patients.

In rare situations, antiretroviral drug resistance is so extensive that a suppressive regimen cannot be constructed. In this context, continued antiretroviral therapy may nonetheless maintain immunologic stability and prevent clinical events, likely because treatment is selecting for less fit virus, and in particular NRTIs retain antiviral activity even in the presence of extensive resistance. Though the optimal regimen for patients in this setting has not been determined, a combination of nontoxic NRTIs (such as TAF/FTC) plus a ritonavir-boosted protease inhibitor is a reasonable option. Continued therapy with drug classes with relatively low resistance barriers such as NNRTIs and integrase inhibitors should be avoided.

IMPORTANT GENOTYPIC RESISTANCE PATTERNS

(see also Appendix 1: Drug Resistance Mutations in HIV-1)

A. Nucleoside Reverse Transcriptase Inhibitors (NRTIs)

1. 3TC/FTC: M184V

- M184V emerges rapidly (days-weeks) in non-suppressive treatment regimens. This leads to a large reproducible increase in resistance of the virus to 3TC and FTC. On its own, M184V reduces the susceptibility of viruses to abacavir and ddI; however, these drugs do retain clinically significant antiviral activity even with M184V. Some studies (e.g., NEJM 2006;43:535–40) have indicated that the incidence of M184V on treatment failure is lower in patients treated with FTC than 3TC, possibly due to FTC's longer half-life and greater potency.

- Despite this resistance, significant antiviral activity of 3TC/FTC-containing regimens is often maintained for a prolonged period of time. Common explanations include: (1) M184V increases viral susceptibility to certain other NRTIs, notably ZDV, d4T, and tenofovir; (2) viruses with M184V have a lower replication capacity in vitro than wild-type viruses; and (3) 3TC/FTC exert an antiviral effect despite the presence of high-level phenotypic resistance.

- The combination of rapid development of resistance to 3TC/FTC, the potential benefits of the M184V mutation otherwise, and the excellent tolerability of these drugs leads to a clinical dilemma: should the drug be continued even in the face of resistance? Our practice is typically to continue the 3TC/FTC in patients who otherwise have extensive resistance and may benefit from the reduced viral fitness imparted by the M184V mutation. Supportive data for this approach is derived from studies in which patients receiving 3TC and having M184V experienced significant increases in HIV RNA after 3TC was discontinued (Clin Infect Dis 2005;41:236–42; AIDS 2006;20:795–803).

2. **ZDV/d4T: Thymidine-Associated Mutations (TAMs)**

- The thymidine-associated mutations are M41L, D67N, K70R, L210W, T215Y, and K219Q.
- TAMs emerge slowly and sequentially with ZDV and d4T-containing regimens. As ZDV and d4T are combined with 3TC or FTC for initial therapy, the M184V mutation generally evolves before the occurrence of TAMs.
- As with other non-suppressive regimens, in general the longer a patient is on an ZDV or d4T-containing regimen with a detectable HIV RNA, the greater the number of TAMs the patient will accumulate.
- The degree of resistance to ZDV and d4T as well as other NRTIs correlates with the total number of TAMs. Only one or two TAMs may reduce susceptibility to ZDV or d4T, whereas three or more TAMs are required to reduced susceptibility (and virologic response) to ABC, ddI, and TDF. (Note that M184V plus only one TAM will reduce viral susceptibility to ABC.)
- Often patients will evolve along one of two different TAM pathways: (1) M41L, L210W, T215Y: this occurs more commonly and is associated with broader resistance, including all other NRTIs as well as tenofovir; or (2) D67N, K70R, and K219Q: this induces a lower level of resistance, and tenofovir treatment retains significant activity.

3. **Tenofovir: K65R**

- K65R reduces in vitro susceptibility to tenofovir, 3TC, ddI, and abacavir. In patients with prior ZDV or d4T treatment and associated TAMs, selection of K65R rarely occurs.
- As with the TAMs described above, in a typical combination regimen using TDF, 3TC or FTC, and EFV, the first mutations to appear are M184V (selected by 3TC and FTC) and NNRTI-associated mutations. In patients with continued non-suppressive therapy, K65R may also develop.
- The consequence of M184V and K65R is broad NRTI resistance (analogous to multiple TAMs). Viruses harboring the K65R mutation remain susceptible to ZDV, and are sometimes "hypersusceptible," indicating that ZDV is more active vs. K65R mutants than against wild-type virus.

- Rates of K65R development are substantially higher in HIV subtype C than B. Subtype C is more common in Africa, B in North America and Western Europe.
- As with M184V, in vitro data suggest that K65R reduces replication capacity, and that both together reduce replication capacity more than either one alone.
- K65R also may develop in treatment-naïve patients placed on abacavir, ddI, or d4T-containing initial regimens. More commonly, however, d4T will select for TAMs, and ddI and abacavir for L74V.

4. **Abacavir, ddI: L74V**

- Virologic failure of initial therapy with abacavir or ddI (plus 3TC or FTC) most commonly selects initially for the M184V mutation, followed by L74V.
- L74V reduces susceptibility to ABC and ddI; ZDV remains fully active. The data on TDF activity are conflicting.

5. **Multinucleoside Resistance Patterns: Q151M and T69ins**

- Before the triple-therapy era, Q151M and T69 insertion mutation pattern (T69ins) developed in patients who were on prolonged ZDV/ddI or d4T/ddI-containing regimens with virologic failure.
- The occurrence of these mutational patterns is rare today.
- Q151M reduces susceptibility to all NRTIs except tenofovir.
- If the T69ins is accompanied by one or more TAMs, all NRTIs (including tenofovir) show reduced susceptibility.

B. **Non-Nucleoside Reverse Transcriptase Inhibitors (NNRTIs).**

1. **Nevirapine and Efavirenz.** Unsuccessful treatment with these NNRTIs leads rapidly to selection of NNRTI-associated resistance mutations. These mutations generally share two important properties: (1) a nearly complete loss of antiviral activity of the agent being used (contrast 3TC or FTC resistance); and (2) a high degree of cross-resistance between nevirapine, delavirdine, and efavirenz. As a result, sequencing of these older NNRTIs after resistance develops is not possible. The most common resistance mutation selected by efavirenz is K103N, and nevirapine often selects for Y181C, except when given with ZDV. Less common mutational patterns seen with NNRTIs are L100I, V106A/M, Y181C/I, Y188L, G190S/A, and M230L.

2. **Etravirine** was the first NNRTI with documented clinical activity against some NNRTI-resistant viruses. In the DUET studies, treatment-experienced patients with documented NNRTI resistance received either etravirine or placebo; they also received an optimized background regimen containing at least DRV + RTV, plus other agents selected by the investigators. At 24 weeks, viral load and CD4 cell count data significantly favored etravirine over placebo (Lancet 2007;370:39–48). In this study, response to etravirine was diminished only when patients had at least three of the following mutations (which are also included in the IAS–USA

set): V90I, A98G, L100I, K101E/P, V106I, V179D/F, Y181C/I/V, and G190A/S. Importantly, baseline presence of the K103N mutation—the most common mutation seen in patients with treatment failure on efavirenz—does not reduce response to etravirine.

3. **Rilpivirine** most commonly selects for the resistance mutation E138K. This mutation reduces susceptibility to all other NNRTIs, including etravirine. Subsequent treatment strategies for patients with the E138K mutation would therefore include at least two active agents outside the NNRTI drug class. Rilpivirine is also active against K103N mutations.

C. Protease Inhibitors (PIs)

1. Nelfinavir: D30N

Virologic failure on a nelfinavir-containing regimen is most commonly associated with the D30N mutation, sometimes with N88D. While conferring high-level resistance to NFV, other PIs retain activity against these viruses.

- Clinical studies have confirmed that second PIs–especially when "boosted" with ritonavir–can be used to salvage virologic failures with D30N mutations. A potential disadvantage of this strategy is that 3TC and sometimes other NRTI-based mutations are often present as well.
- A minority of treatment failures with nelfinavir will select for the L90M mutation, which is associated with broader resistance to PIs than D30N. The L90M pathway is more common in non-subtype B viruses, which are considerably more prevalent outside of the United States and Western Europe.

2. Atazanavir: I50L

- In patients without prior PI treatment, unboosted atazanavir selects for the I50L mutation, usually after selection of 3TC or other NRTI resistance. As with D30N and nelfinavir, I50L reduces susceptibility to ATV but not to other PIs.
- On phenotype testing, viruses with I50L alone often demonstrate hypersusceptibility to other PIs–that is, non-ATV PIs appear to be more active against these viruses than against wild-type strains. The clinical significance of this phenomenon is unknown, as there are no controlled studies evaluating sequencing of PIs after ATV failure.
- PI-experienced patients treated with ATV rarely select for I50L, and more typical PI mutations emerge.
- As with other boosted PIs, resistance to atazanavir rarely if ever develops when the drug is used in treatment-naive patients.

3. Fosamprenavir: I50V

- Use of unboosted FPV may select for the I50V mutation, generally occurring (as with NFV and ATV) along with some degree of NRTI resistance.
- I50V reduces susceptibility to lopinavir, ritonavir, and darunavir; other PIs retain activity, at least as measured by phenotype testing.
- Sequencing of PIs after development of I50V or other patterns of FPV failure has not been studied in controlled trials.

- Since unboosted fosamprenavir may select for mutations that confer cross-resistance to darunavir (the most important PI in treatment-experienced patients), it should be avoided.

4. **Darunavir:**

   - The darunavir-related resistance mutations are V11I, V32I, L33F, I47V, I50V, I54L/M, T74P, L76V, I84V, and L89V. If patients have none of these mutations, they may be treated with once-daily darunavir/ritonavir or darunavir/cobicistat (800/100 mg daily; AIDS 2011;25:929–39). If they have one or more of these mutations and still retain full or partial susceptibility to darunavir based on phenotype testing, they should receive twice-daily darunavir/ritonavir (600/100 mg twice daily).

   - In patients with extensive darunavir resistance based on genotype, a resistance phenotype can provide information about whether tipranavir retains activity. However, darunavir is generally preferred due to favorable tolerability, safety, profile, lower pill burden, and fewer drug-drug interactions.

D. **Integrase Inhibitors**

   1. **Raltegravir and Elvitegravir.** As with other antiretroviral drug classes, treatment failure with raltegravir or elvitegravir may select for mutations that confer resistance to these agents. Because the use of integrase inhibitors both in clinical trials and clinical practice occurred after there was a more complete understanding of optimal antiretroviral strategies, in particular the need to include multiple active agents, resistance to integrase inhibitors is relatively rare.

   2. The resistance pattern for raltegravir generally involves a major mutation at one of Q148H/K/R, N155H, or Y143R/H/C, with addition of one or more minor mutations that decrease susceptibility further. The most common inital mutation with elvitegravir failure is E92Q. Cross-resistance between raltegravir and elvitegravir can be assumed; that is, no significant antiviral effect can be expected by switching from one drug to the other once resistance has developed.

   3. **Dolutegravir** retains activity against many raltegravir and elvitegravir-resistant viruses, especially if treatment failure with RAL and EVG is not prolonged. Dolutegravir has a higher barrier to resistance then raltegravir and elvitegravir, and resistance to the drug in treatment-naïve patients with virologic failure has thus far not been reported. Resistance to dolutegravir, however, is possible, especially when previous treatment selected for mutations at position 148. While a 148 mutation alone does not lead to high-level dolutegravir resistance, additional mutations added to 148 will reduce viral susceptibility. Dolutegravir should be given twice daily in patients with documented integrase inhibitor resistance.

POOR CD4 RECOVERY DESPITE VIROLOGIC SUPPRESSION

After starting ART, CD4 recovery is fastest in the first 3 months, with a more gradual increase thereafter and continuing for a least a decade. Most patients with virologic suppression will eventually achieve a CD4 cell count > 500 cells/mm³; starting ART prior to significant CD4 decline is the best strategy for maintaining normal counts. However, approximately 15–20% of those who start ART with significantly depleted counts will plateau at a level substantially below normal, with extreme cases being < 200. While the occurrence of AIDS-related complications is rare in these patients, they do appear to be at higher risk of non-AIDS related complications such as cardiovascular, renal, and bone disease.

A modifiable cause will be identified in rare cases of poor CD4 recovery. These include use of certain older antivirals (zidovudine, the combination of tenofovir and didanosine, interferon), or untreated infections (HCV or HIV-2) and/or malignancies. However, in the vast majority of individuals, no reversible cause of the immunologic failure can be found. Modification or intensification of the ART regimen has been evaluated in prospective clinical studies, with no consistently beneficial effect. As a result, changing ART is generally not recommended. As noted above, the best way to prevent immunologic failure is to start ART before significant CD4 decline.

A. Regimen Switching in the Setting of Virologic Suppression

Although it may seem counterintuitive to switch ART regimens when patients are virologically suppressed, this strategy may be indicated for several reasons. These are listed below (adapted from DHHS Guidelines for the Use of Antiretroviral Agents in HIV-1-Infected Adults and Adolescents: Management of the Treatment-Experienced Patient):

1. **To Simplify the Regimen by Reducing Pill Burden and Dosing Frequency.** There are several one-pill daily regimens now available; patients on multi-pill treatments may wish to switch, especially if they are taking pills twice daily.

2. **To Enhance Tolerability and Decrease Short- or Long-Term Toxicity.** This is particularly important if patients are receiving older agents no longer recommended due to toxicity. For example, patients receiving any of the following drugs should have their regimens scrutinized carefully to allow for a safer treatment: NRTIs: stavudine, didanosine, zidovudine; NNRTIs: delavirdine, nevirapine, efavirenz (especially with neuropsychiatric side effects); PIs: saquinavir, indinavir, nelfinavir, lopinavir/ritonavir.

3. **To Prevent or Mitigate Drug-Drug Interactions.** For example, a patient receiving a ritonavir-boosted PI or elvitegravir/cobicistat may require intermittent inhalational or intra-articular corticosteroids. The ritonavir and/or cobicistat could increase concentrations of these drugs to dangerous levels, leading to hypercortisolism.

4. **To Eliminate Food or Fluid Requirements.** Rilpivirine is very dependent on food for optimal absorption; individual patients may have difficulty remembering to take the medication with a meal.

5. **To Allow for Optimal Use of ART during Pregnancy or Should Pregnancy Occur.**

6. **To Reduce Costs.** Although generic ART may reduce costs of HIV treatment in the future, as of late 2016 in the US, the cost of ART is roughly similar between recommended regimens.

B. General Principles of Regimen Switching

1. **Maintain Virologic Suppression without Jeopardizing Future Options.** In order to maximize the chances of a safe switch virologically, the patient's treatment history and prior resistance testing should be meticulously reviewed.

Table 4.2. Specific Regimen Switching Strategies

Good Supporting Evidence	Selected Strategies Under Evaluation	Strategies Not Recommended
• *Within class switches.* Examples include EFV to RPV, TDF or ABC to TAF, RAL to EVG/c or DTG. These switches generally can be made without considering resistance issues. • *Between class switches.* Examples include boosted PI to RPV or INSTI. These switches can only be made if activity of the other agents in the regimen is known. • *RTV-boosted PI plus 3TC or FTC.* Several studies have demonstrated that in patients receiving boosted PI plus 2 NRTIs, switching to boosted PI plus 3TC or FTC maintains virologic suppression. This should only be undertaken if there is no history of resistance to 3TC or FTC.	• *ECF/TAF + DRV.* In patients with prior treatment failure and resistance to 2 or more drug classes, switch to this two-pill regimen maintained virologic suppression. This strategy should not be used in those with prior INSTI or DRV resistance, or more than 3 thymidine-associated mutations. • *DTG + 3TC or DTG + RPV.* Several studies are evaluating these two-agent regimens. Pending the results of these studies, these strategies should be used only in rare circumstances.	*In clinical trials of various sizes and study designs, each of the following strategies demonstrated suboptimal virologic suppression:* • RTV-boosted monotherapy • DTG monotherapy • ATV/r plus RAL • Switches to maraviroc using proviral DNA to assess tropism status

2. **Assume "Once Resistant, Always Resistant."** Resistance mutations that are detected on genotype at the time of failure may not be detected on later tests once the selective pressure of that particular medication or drug class is removed. However, there is good evidence that this resistance is "archived," and will emerge if the same drug is used again. Clinicians should therefore presume that this treatment is not a fully active option for future regimens. A resistance assay using proviral DNA (GenoSure Archive) may be useful in this setting, though the sensitivity of this assay for archived mutations is not 100%. As a result, detection of resistance can be trusted more than absence of resistance.

3. **Switching from a Regimen with a High Resistance Barrier to a Low Resistance Barrier Should Be Undertaken Cautiously.** Patients virologically suppressed on boosted PI-containing regimens may experience virologic failure if an NNRTI or integrase inhibitor replaces the boosted PI if the other components of the regimen are not fully active. This was best demonstrated in a study of patients on regimens containing LPV/r + NRTIs who were randomized to switch to RAL or remain on LPV/r; those with a prior history of multiple regimens and prior treatment failure experienced more virologic failure

when switching to RAL (Lancet 2010 Jan 13; 375(9712):396–407). It is not known whether dolutegravir (with its higher barrier to resistance than EVG and RAL) will have this same risk.

4. **Consider Other Medical Issues Prior to the Switch.** Patients with chronic hepatitis B (HBSAg positive) should in general not switch off TDF or TAF; if such a switch is mandatory due to progressive renal disease, entecavir should be added. Patients receiving multiple other medications should have this list screened carefully for drug interactions prior to switching to any regimen containing ritonavir or cobicistat.

5. **After Switching Therapy, Patients Should Be Monitored Closely.** A clinic visit or phone call is recommended 1–2 weeks after the change, and HIV RNA along with safety labs (renal and liver function tests) 4–8 weeks and 12–16 weeks later. Correct dosing of the regimen should not be assumed, but confirmed with the patient. Once virologic suppression and stable safety labs are documented 12–16 weeks after the switch, a twice-yearly monitoring plan can be resumed.

C. Regimen Switch Strategies in the Setting of Drug Toxicity

Patients experiencing drug-related adverse effects should have their regimens scrutinized for potential switch options (**Table 4.3**). Utilizing the principles described above, clinicians can generally make these switches safely and with a low risk of virologic failure. Acute adverse events, especially those that are potentially life threatening, should prompt cessation of all antiretroviral agents. Examples include severe cutaneous drug reactions (most commonly seen with NNRTIs) and marked hepatotoxicity. In the setting of less urgent issues such as jaundice or urolithiasis from atazanavir, hyperlipidemia from a ritonavir-boosted PI, or proteinuria with TDF, the offending agent can be stopped with substitution of an alternative drug provided virologic suppression can be ensured.

Table 4.3. Antiretroviral Therapy-Associated Adverse Events that Can Be Managed with Substitution of Alternative Antiretroviral Agent

| Adverse Event | ARV Agent(s) or Drug Class | | Comments |
	Switch from	Switch to	
Bone Density Effects	TDF[a]	ABC[b] or TAF NRTI sparing regimens or regimens using only 3TC or FTC as NRTI may be considered if appropriate.	Declines in BMD have been observed upon initiation of most ART regimens. Switching from TDF to alternative ARV agents has been shown to increase bone density, but the clinical significance of this increase remains uncertain. TAF is associated with smaller declines in BMD than TDF, and with improvement in BMD upon switching from TDF. The long-term impact of TAF on patients with osteopenia or osteoporosis is unknown; close clinical monitoring is recommended in this setting.

Table 4.3. Antiretroviral Therapy-Associated Adverse Events that Can Be Managed with Substitution of Alternative Antiretroviral Agent (cont'd)

| Adverse Event | ARV Agent(s) or Drug Class | | Comments |
	Switch from	Switch to	
Bone Marrow Suppression	ZDV	TDF, TAF, or ABC[b]	ZDV has been associated with neutropenia and macrocytic anemia.
Central Nervous System, Neuropsychiatric Side Effects Dizziness, suicidal ideation, abnormal dreams, depression	EFV, RPV	ETR or a PI/c or PI/r INSTI may be considered (see Comments column).	In most patients, EFV-related CNS effects subside within 4 weeks after initiation of the drug. Persistent or intolerable effects should prompt substitution of EFV. INSTIs are associated with insomnia. Depression and suicidality have been infrequently reported with INSTI use, primarily in patients with pre-existing psychiatric conditions.
Dyslipidemia Hypertriglyceridemia (with or without elevated LDL level)	RTV- or COBI-boosted regimens; EFV; EVG/c	RAL, DTG, RPV	Elevated TG and LDL levels are more common with LPV/r and FPV/r than with other RTV-boosted PIs. Improvements in TG and LDL levels have been observed with switch from LPV/r to ATV or ATV/r.[c]
Gastrointestinal Effects Nausea, diarrhea	LPV/r	ATV/c, ATV/r, DRV/c, DRV/r, RAL, DTG, EVG/c	GI intolerance is common with boosted PIs and is linked to the total dose of RTV. More GI toxicity is seen with LPV/r than with ATV/r or DRV/r. GI effects are often transient, and do not warrant substitution unless persistent and intolerable.
	Other RTV- or COBI-boosted regimens	RAL, DTG, NNRTIs	In a trial of treatment-naive patients, rates of diarrhea and nausea were similar for EVG/c/TDF/FTC and ATV/r plus TDF/FTC.
Hypersensitivity Reaction	ABC	TDF or TAF	Never rechallenge with ABC following a suspected HSR, regardless of the patient's HLA-B*5701 status.
	NVP, EFV, ETR, RPV	Non-NNRTI ART	Risk of HSR with NVP is higher for women and those with high CD4 cell counts.

Table 4.3. Antiretroviral Therapy-Associated Adverse Events that Can Be Managed with Substitution of Alternative Antiretroviral Agent (cont'd)

Adverse Event	ARV Agent(s) or Drug Class		Comments
	Switch from	Switch to	
	DTG, RAL MVC	Non-INSTI ART Suitable alternative ART	Reactions to NVP, ETR, RAL, DTG, and MVC may be accompanied by elevated liver transaminases.
Insulin Resistance	LPV/r, FPV/r	INSTI, RPV	Results of switch studies have been inconsistent. Studies in HIV-negative patients suggest a direct causal effect of LPV/r (and IDV) on insulin resistance. However, traditional risk factors may be stronger risk factors for insulin resistance than use of any PI.
Jaundice and Icterus	ATV, ATV/c, ATV/r	DRV/c, DRV/r, INSTI, or NNRTI	Increases in unconjugated bilirubin are common with ATV and generally do not require modification of therapy unless resultant symptoms are distressing to the patient.
Lipoatrophy Subcutaneous fat, wasting of limbs, face, buttocks	d4T, ZDV	TDF, TAF, or ABC[b]	Peripheral lipoatrophy is a legacy of prior thymidine analog (d4T and ZDV) use. Switching from these ARVs prevents worsening lipoatrophy, but fat recovery is typically slow (may take years) and incomplete.
Lipohypertrophy	Accumulation of visceral, truncal, dorso-cervical, and breast fat has been observed during ART, particularly during use of older PI-based regimens (e.g., IDV), but whether ART directly causes fat accumulation remains unclear. There is no clinical evidence that switching to another first-line regimen will reverse weight or visceral fat gain.		
Rash	NNRTIs (especially NVP and EFV)	PI- or INSTI-based regimen	Mild rashes developing after initiation of NNRTIs other than NVP rarely require treatment switch. When serious rash develops due to any NNRTI, switch to another drug class.
	DRV/c, DRV/r	ATV/c, ATV/r, or another drug class (e.g., INSTI)	Mild rashes following DRV/r use may resolve with close follow-up only. For more severe reactions, change to an alternative boosted PI or an agent from another drug class.

Table 4.3. Antiretroviral Therapy-Associated Adverse Events that Can Be Managed with Substitution of Alternative Antiretroviral Agent (cont'd)

| Adverse Event | ARV Agent(s) or Drug Class | | Comments |
	Switch from	Switch to	
Renal Effects Including proximal renal tubulopathy, elevated creatinine	TDF[a]	ABC[b] or TAF (for patients with CrCl > 30 mL/min) or NRTI-sparing regimens, or regimens using only 3TC or FTC as NRTI may be considered if appropriate.	TDF may cause tubulopathy. Switching from TDF to TAF is associated with improvement in proteinuria and renal biomarkers. The long-term impact of TAF on patients with pre-existing renal disease, including overt proximal tubulopathy, is unknown, and close clinical monitoring is recommended in this setting.
	ATV/c, ATV/r, LPV/r	DTG, RAL, or NNRTI	COBI and DTG, and to a lesser extent RPV, can increase SCr through inhibition of creatinine secretion. This effect does not affect glomerular filtration. However, assess for renal dysfunction if SCr increases by > 0.4 mg/dL.
Stones Nephrolithiasis and cholelithiasis	ATV, ATV/c, ATV/r	DRV/c, DRV/r, INSTI, or NNRTI	Assuming that ATV is believed to be causing the stones.

Reproduced from DHHS Guidelines for the Use of Antiretroviral Agents in HIV-1-Infected Adults and Adolescents: Recommendations of the Panel on Clinical Practices for Treatment of HIV Infection, last updated July 14, 2016; http://aidsinfo.nih.gov/guidelines/html/1/adult-and-adolescent-arv-guidelines/31/adverse-effects-of-arv.

[a] In patients with chronic active HBV infection, another agent active against HBV should be substituted for TDF.

[b] ABC should be used only in patients known to be HLA-B*5701 negative.

[c] TDF reduces ATV levels; therefore, unboosted ATV should not be co-administered with TDF. Long-term data for unboosted ATV are unavailable.

Key to Abbreviations: ABC = abacavir; ART = antiretroviral therapy; ARV = antiretroviral; ATV = atazanavir; ATV/c = atazanavir/cobicistat; ATV/r = atazanavir/ritonavir; BMD = bone mineral density; CNS = central nervous system; COBI or c = cobicistat; d4T = stavudine; DRV/c = darunavir/cobicistat; DRV/r = darunavir/ritonavir; DTG = dolutegravir; EFV = efavirenz; ETR = etravirine; EVG = elvitegravir; FPV/r = fosamprenavir/ritonavir; FTC = emtricitabine; GI = gastrointestinal; HBV = hepatitis B virus; HSR = hypersensitivity reaction; IDV = indinavir; INSTI = integrase strand transfer inhibitor; LDL = low-density lipoprotein; LPV/r = lopinavir/ritonavir; MVC = maraviroc; NNRTI = non-nucleoside reverse transcriptase inhibitor; NVP = nevirapine; PI = protease inhibitor; PI/c = protease inhibitor/cobicistat; PI/r = protease inhibitor/ritonavir; RAL = raltegravir; RPV = rilpivirine; RTV = ritonavir; SCr = serum creatinine; TAF = tenofovir alafenamide; TDF = tenofovir disoproxil fumarate; TG = triglycerides; ZDV = zidovudine.

Chapter 5

Prophylaxis and Treatment of Opportunistic Infections

PROPHYLAXIS OF OPPORTUNISTIC INFECTIONS

Patients with HIV disease are at risk for infectious complications not otherwise seen in immunocompetent patients. Such opportunistic infections occur in proportion to the severity of immune system dysfunction (reflected by CD4 cell count depletion). While community-acquired infections (e.g., pneumococcal pneumonia) can occur at any CD4 cell count, the "classic" HIV-related opportunistic infections (PCP, toxoplasmosis, cryptococcus, disseminated *Mycobacterium avium* complex [MAC], CMV) generally do not occur until CD4 cell counts are dramatically reduced. Specifically, it is rare to encounter PCP in HIV patients with CD4 > 200/mm^3, and CMV and disseminated MAC typically occur at median CD4 < 50/mm^3. Furthermore, for patients receiving suppressive antiretroviral therapy, opportunistic infections occur very infrequently, regardless of the CD4 cell count. Indications for prophylaxis and specific prophylaxis regimens are summarized in Table 5.1 and detailed in Table 5.2. The US Public Health Service/Infectious Diseases Society of America guidelines for the prevention and treatment of opportunistic infections in persons infected with HIV can be found at aidsinfo.nih.gov, and are updated regularly (see http://aidsinfo.nih.gov/guidelines/html/4/adult-and-adolescent-oi-prevention-and-treatment-guidelines/318/introduction).

Table 5.1. Overview of Prophylaxis of Selected Opportunistic Infections (see Table 5.2 for details)

Infection	Indication for Prophylaxis	Intervention
PCP	CD4 < 200/mm^3	TMP-SMX
TB (*M. tuberculosis*)	PPD > 5 mm (current or past) or contact with active case	INH
Toxoplasma	IgG Ab (+) and CD4 < 100/mm^3	TMP-SMX
MAC	CD4 < 50/mm^3	Azithromycin (not recommended in all guidelines for patients about to start ART)
Streptococcus pneumoniae	CD4 > 200/mm^3	Pneumococcal polysaccharide and conjugate vaccines
Hepatitis B	Susceptible patients	Hepatitis B vaccine
Hepatitis A	Susceptible patients	Hepatitis A vaccine
Influenza	All patients	Annual flu vaccine
VZV	CD4 > 200/mm^3, VZV antibody negative	Varicella vaccine

Ab = antibody; TB = tuberculosis; VZV = varicella-zoster virus; other abbreviations (p. ix)

Table 5.2. Prophylaxis to Prevent First Episode of Opportunistic Disease

Pathogen	Indication	First choice	Alternative
Pneumocystis pneumonia (PCP)	CD4+ count < 200 cells/μL or oropharyngeal candidiasis CD4+ < 14% or history of AIDS-defining illness CD4+ count > 200 but < 250 cells/μL if monitoring CD4+ count every 1–3 months is not possible Note: Patients who are receiving pyrimethamine/sulfadiazine for treatment or suppression of toxoplasmosis do not require additional PCP prophylaxis.	Trimethoprim-sulfamethoxazole (TMP-SMX), 1 DS PO daily; or 1 SS daily	TMP-SMX 1 DS PO tiw **or** Dapsone 100 mg PO daily or 50 mg PO bid **or** Dapsone 50 mg PO daily + pyrimethamine 50 mg PO weekly + leucovorin 25 mg PO weekly **or** Dapsone 200 mg PO weekly + pyrimethamine 75 mg PO weekly + leucovorin 25 mg PO weekly **or** Aerosolized pentamidine 300 mg via Respigard II™ nebulizer every month **or** Atovaquone 1500 mg PO daily **or** Atovaquone 1500 mg PO daily + pyrimethamine 25 mg PO daily + leucovorin 10 mg PO daily
Toxoplasma gondii encephalitis	Toxoplasma IgG – positive patients with CD4+ count < 100 cells/μL	TMP-SMX, 1 DS PO daily	TMP-SMX 1 DS PO tiw **or** TMP-SMX 1 SS PO daily

Table 5.2. Prophylaxis to Prevent First Episode of Opportunistic Disease (cont'd)

Pathogen	Indication	First choice	Alternative
	Seronegative patients receiving PCP prophylaxis not active against toxoplasmosis should have toxoplasma serology retested if CD4+ count decline to < 100 cells/µL. Prophylaxis should be initiated if seroconversion occurred.		**or** Dapsone 50 mg PO daily + pyrimethamine 50 mg PO weekly + leucovorin 25 mg PO weekly **or** Dapsone 200 mg PO weekly + pyrimethamine 75 mg PO weekly + leucovorin 25 mg PO weekly **or** Atovaquone 1500 mg PO daily + pyrimethamine 25 mg PO daily + leucovorin 10 mg PO daily
Mycobacterium tuberculosis infection (TB) (treatment of latent TB infection or LTBI)	(+) diagnostic test for LTBI, no evidence of active TB, and no prior history of treatment for active or latent TB **or** Close contact with a person with infectious TB, with no evidence of active TB, regardless of screening test results	Isoniazid (INH) 300 mg PO daily or 900 mg PO/DOT biw for 9 months–both plus pyridoxine 25 mg PO daily **or** For persons exposed to drug-resistant TB, selection of drugs after consultation with public health authorities	Rifampin (RIF) 600 mg PO daily × 4 months **or** Rifabutin (RFB) (dose adjusted based on concomitant ART) 4 months

Table 5.2. Prophylaxis to Prevent First Episode of Opportunistic Disease (cont'd)

Pathogen	Indication	First choice	Alternative
Disseminated *Mycobacterium avium* complex (MAC) disease	CD4+ count < 50 cells/μL—after ruling out active MAC infection Note: IAS-USA Guidelines do not recommend MAC prophylaxis if patients are starting ART promptly.	Azithromycin 1200 mg PO once weekly **or** Clarithromycin 500 mg PO bid **or** Azithromycin 600 mg PO twice weekly	RFB (dosage adjustment based on concomitant ART); rule out active TB before starting RFB
Streptococcus pneumoniae infection	For individuals who have not received any pneumococcal vaccine, regardless of CD4 count, followed by: • if CD4 count ≥200 cells/μL • if CD4 count <200 cells/μL	PCV13 0.5 mL IM × 1 PPV23 0.5 mL IM at least 8 weeks after the PCV13 vaccine PPV23 can be offered at least 8 weeks after receiving PCV13 or can wait until CD4 count increased to >200 cells/μL	PPV23 0.5 mL IM × 1
	In patients who received polysaccharide pneumococcal vaccination (PPV)	One dose of PCV13 should be given at least 1 year after the last receipt of PPV23	
	Revaccination • If age 19–64 years and ≥ 5 years since the first PPV23 dose • If age ≥ 65 years, and if ≥ 5 years since the previous PPV23 dose	• PPV23 0.5 mL IM × 1 • PPV23 0.5 mL IM × 1	
Influenza A and B virus infection	All HIV-infected patients	Inactivated influenza vaccine 0.5 mL IM annually	

Table 5.2. Prophylaxis to Prevent First Episode of Opportunistic Disease (cont'd)

Pathogen	Indication	First choice	Alternative
		Live-attenuated influenza vaccine is **contraindicated** in HIV-infected patients	
Syphilis	• For individuals exposed to a sex partner with a diagnosis of primary, secondary, or early latent syphilis within past 90 days **or** • For individuals exposed to a sex partner > 90 days before syphilis diagnosis in the partner, if serologic test results are not available immediately, and the opportunity for follow-up is uncertain	Benzathine penicillin G 2.4 million units IM for 1 dose	For penicillin-allergic patients: • Doxycycline 100 mg PO bid × 14 days **or** • Ceftriaxone 1 g IM or IV daily for 8–10 days **or** • Azithromycin 2 g PO for 1 dose—not recommended for MSM or pregnant women
Histoplasma capsulatum infection	CD4+ count ≤ 150 cells/µL and at high risk because of occupational exposure or live in a community with a hyperendemic rate of histoplasmosis (> 10 cases/100 patient-years)	Itraconazole 200 mg PO daily	
Coccidioidomycosis	Positive IgM or IgG serologic test in a patient from a disease-endemic area; and CD4+ count < 250 cells/µL	Fluconazole 400 mg PO daily	

Table 5.2. Prophylaxis to Prevent First Episode of Opportunistic Disease (cont'd)

Pathogen	Indication	First choice	Alternative
Varicella-zoster virus (VZV) infection	<u>Pre-exposure prevention:</u> Patients with CD4+ count ≥ 200 cells/µL who have not been vaccinated, have no history of varicella or herpes zoster, or who are seronegative for VZV Note: routine VZV serologic testing in HIV-infected adults is not recommended. <u>Post-exposure prevention:</u> Close contact with a person with chickenpox or herpes zoster, and is susceptible (i.e., no history of vaccination or of either condition, or known to be VZV seronegative)	<u>Pre-exposure prevention:</u> Primary varicella vaccination (Varivax™), 2 doses (0.5 mL SQ each) administered 3 months apart If vaccination results in disease because of vaccine virus, treatment with acyclovir is recommended. <u>Post-exposure therapy:</u> Varicella-zoster immune globulin (VariZIG™) 125 IU per 10 kg (maximum of 625 IU) IM, administered as soon as possible and within 10 days after exposure Note: VariZIG can be obtained only under a treatment IND (800-843-7477, FFF Enterprises). Individuals receiving monthly high-dose IVIG (> 400 mg/kg) are likely to be protected if the last dose of IVIG was administered < 3 weeks before exposure.	VZV-susceptible household contacts of susceptible HIV-infected persons should be vaccinated to prevent potential transmission of VZV to their HIV-infected contacts. <u>Alternative post-exposure therapy:</u> • Acyclovir 800 mg PO 5×/day for 5–7 dys **or** • Valacyclovir 1 g PO tid for 5–7 days These alternatives have not been studied in the HIV population. If antiviral therapy is used, varicella vaccines should not be given until at least 72 hours after the last dose of the antiviral drug.

Table 5.2. Prophylaxis to Prevent First Episode of Opportunistic Disease (cont'd)

Pathogen	Indication	First choice	Alternative
Human papillomavirus (HPV) infection	Females aged 13–26 years	HPV quadravalent vaccine 0.5 mL IM months 0, 1–2, and 6 **or** HPV bivalent vaccine 0.5 mL IM at months 0, 1–2, and 6	
	Males aged 13–26 years	HPV quadravalent vaccine 0.5 mL IM at months 0, 1–2, and 6	
Hepatitis A virus (HAV) infection	HAV-susceptible patients with chronic liver disease, or who are injection-drug users, or men who have sex with men. Certain specialists might delay vaccination until CD4+ count > 200 cells/µL.	Hepatitis A vaccine 1 mL IM × 2 doses at 0 and 6–12 months IgG antibody response should be assessed 1 month after vaccination; non-responders should be revaccinated when CD4+ count > 200 cells/µL	For patients susceptible to both HAV and hepatitis B virus (HBV) infection (see below): Combined HAV and HBV vaccine (Twinrix®), 1 mL IM as a 3-dose (0, 1, and 6 months) or 4-dose series (days 0, 7, 21 to 30, and 12 months)
Hepatitis B virus (HBV) infection	Patients without chronic HBV or without immunity to HBV (i.e., anti-HBs < 10 international units/mL)	Hepatitis B vaccine IM (Engerix-B® 20 µg/mL or Recombivax HB® 10 µg/mL) at 0, 1, and 6 months **or**	
	Patients with isolated anti-HBc and negative HBV DNA	Combined HAV and HBV vaccine (Twinrix®), 1 mL IM as a 3-dose (0, 1, and 6 months) or 4-dose series (days 0, 7, 21 to 30, and 12 months)	Some experts recommend vaccinating with 40 µg doses of either HBV vaccine.

Table 5.2. Prophylaxis to Prevent First Episode of Opportunistic Disease (cont'd)

Pathogen	Indication	First choice	Alternative
	Early vaccination is recommended before CD4 count falls below 350 cells/µL. However, in patients with low CD4 cell counts, vaccination should not be deferred until CD4 count reaches > 350 cells/µL, because some patients with CD4 counts < 200 cells/µL do respond to vaccination. In general, patients should be vaccinated, regardless of CD4 cell counts.	Anti-HBs should be obtained 1 month after completion of the vaccine series.	
	Vaccine non-responders: Defined as anti-HBs < 10 IU/mL 1 month after a vaccination series. For patients with low CD4+ count at the time of first vaccination series, certain specialists might delay revaccination until after a sustained increase in CD4+ count with ART.	Revaccinate with a second vaccine series.	Some experts recommend revaccinating with 40 µg doses of either HBV vaccine.

Table 5.2. Prophylaxis to Prevent First Episode of Opportunistic Disease (cont'd)

Pathogen	Indication	First choice	Alternative
Malaria	Travel to disease-endemic area	Recommendations are the same for HIV-infected and uninfected patients. Recommendations are based on region of travel, malaria risks, and drug susceptibility in the region. Refer to the following website for the most recent recommendations based on region and drug susceptibility: http://www.cdc.gov/malaria/.	
Penicilliosis	Patients with CD4 cell counts < 100 cells/μL who live or stay for a long period in rural areas in northern Thailand, Vietnam, or Southern China	Itraconazole 200 mg once daily	Fluconazole 400 mg PO once weekly

Definitions of abbreviations: anti-HBc = hepatitis B core antibody; anti-HBs = hepatitis B surface antibody; ART = antiretroviral therapy; bid = twice daily; biw = twice a week; CD4 = CD4 T lymphocyte cell; DOT = directly observed therapy; DS = double strength; HAV = hepatitis A virus; HBV = hepatitis B virus; HPV = human papillomavirus; IgG = immunoglobulin G; IgM = immunoglobulin M; IM = intramuscular; IND = investigational new drug; INH = isoniazid; IV= intravenously; IVIG = intravenous immunoglobulin; LTBI = latent tuberculosis infection; MAC = *Mycobacterium avium* complex; MSM = men who have sex with men; PCP = *Pneumocystis* pneumonia; PCV13 = 13-valent pneumococcal conjugate vaccine; PO = orally; PPV23 = 23-valent pneumococcal polysaccharides vaccine; SQ = subcutaneous; SS = single strength; TB = tuberculosis; TIW = thrice weekly; TMP-SMX = trimethoprim-sulfamethoxazole; VZV = varicella zoster virus

Modified from Panel on Antiretroviral Guidelines for Adults and Adolescents. Guidelines for the use of antiretroviral agents in HIV-1-infected adults and adolescents. AIDSinfo. https://aidsinfo.nih.gov/contentfiles/lvguidelines/adultandadolescentgl.pdf. July 14, 2016.

Pneumocystis jirovecii (carinii) pneumonia (PCP)

Without prophylaxis, 80% of AIDS patients develop PCP, and 60–70% relapse within 1 year after the first episode. Prophylaxis with TMP-SMX also reduces the risk for toxoplasmosis and possibly bacterial infections. Among patients with prior non-life-threatening reactions to TMP-SMX, 55% can be successfully rechallenged with 1 SS tablet daily, and 80% can be rechallenged with gradual dose escalation using TMP-SMX elixir (8 mg TMP + 40 mg SMX/mL) given as 1 mL × 3 days, then 2 mL × 3 days, then 5 mL × 3 days, then 1 SS tablet (PO) QD. Primary and secondary prophylaxis may be discontinued if CD4 cell counts increase to > 200/mm^3 for 3 months or longer in response to antiretroviral therapy. Prophylaxis should be resumed if the CD4 cell count decreases to < 200/mm^3. One study found the incidence of PCP to be 0% if patients were virologically suppressed and had CD4 counts between 100–200 (Clin Infect Dis. (2010); 51(5):611–9). As a result, some clinicians elect to discontinue PCP prophylaxis in this setting.

Toxoplasmosis

Incidence of toxoplasmosis in seronegative patients is too low to warrant chemoprophylaxis. Primary prophylaxis can be discontinued if CD4 cell counts increase to > 200/mm^3 for at least 3 months in response to antiretroviral therapy. Secondary prophylaxis (chronic maintenance therapy) may be discontinued in patients who responded to initial therapy, remain asymptomatic, and whose CD4 counts increase to > 200/mm^3 for 6 months or longer in response to antiretroviral therapy. Prophylaxis should be restarted if the CD4 count decreases to < 200/mm^3. Some experts would obtain an MRI of the brain as part of the evaluation prior to stopping secondary prophylaxis.

Tuberculosis (*Mycobacterium tuberculosis*)

Indicated for skin-test or interferon gamma release assay (IGRA)-positive patients, whether current or historical. Also indicated for close (e.g., household) contacts of active cases. Consider prophylaxis for skin test-negative patients when the probability of prior TB exposure is > 10% (e.g., patients from developing countries, IV drug abusers in some cities, prisoners). However, a trial testing this strategy in the United States did not find a benefit for empiric prophylaxis. Rifamycins interact with PIs, NNRTIs, integrase inhibitors, and maraviroc—use with caution.

M. avium complex (MAC)

Macrolide options (azithromycin, clarithromycin) preferable to rifabutin given greater efficacy, better tolerability, and protection against other respiratory tract disease. Among macolide options, azithromycin is preferred over clarithromycin (fewer pills, fewer drug-drug interactions, better tolerated). Primary prophylaxis may be discontinued if CD4 cell counts increase to > 100/mm^3 and HIV RNA suppresses for 3 months or longer in response to antiretroviral therapy. Resume MAC prophylaxis for CD4 < 100/mm^3. The IAS-USA Guidelines no longer recommend MAC prophylaxis for patients with CD4 < 50 if they are to start ART promptly (JAMA. 2016;316(2):191–210). As starting ART urgently in such severely immunosuppressed patients is standard of care, we no longer give primary prophylaxis for MAC, even though it is still recommended in the DHHS Guidelines.

Pneumococcus (*Streptococcus pneumoniae*)

Incidence of invasive pneumococcal disease is > 100-fold higher in HIV patients. Efficacy of vaccine seen in multiple observational studies, though not all prospective randomized studies show protection. Vaccine may be offered to HIV patients with CD4 > 200/mm^3. Both the 23-valent pneumococcal polysaccharide vaccine and the 13-valent pneumococcal conjugate vaccine are recommended.

Influenza
Give annually (optimally between October and January). Intranasal live attenuated virus vaccine is contraindicated in immunosuppressed patients.

Hepatitis B
Check antibody response 1–3 months after completion of series. Response rate is lower than in HIV-negative controls. Repeat series if no response, especially if CD4 was low during initial series and has increased due to ART.

Vaccine non responders: Defined as anti-HBs < 10 IU/mL 1 month after a vaccination series. For patients with low CD4+ count at the time of first vaccination series, some experts might delay revaccination until after a sustained increase in CD4+ count with ART.

Management of patients with isolated antibody to hepatitis B core (i.e., "core alone") is not well defined—screen for HBV DNA to rule out occult chronic HBV prior to vaccination.

Hepatitis A
Response rate is lower than in HIV-negative controls; assess antibody response 1–3 months after vaccination. Some clinicians delay vaccination until CD4 is > 200 cells/mm³.

Measles, mumps, rubella
Single case of vaccine-strain measles pneumonia reported in a severely immunocompromised adult who received MMR; vaccine is therefore contraindicated in patients with severe immunodeficiency (CD4 < 200/mm³).

Haemophilus influenzae
Incidence of *H. influenzae* disease is increased in HIV patients, but 65% are caused by non-type B strains. Unclear whether vaccine offers protection; not generally recommended.

Neisseria meningitidis
In July 2016, the ACIP recommended that all HIV infected patients receive the meningococcal conjugate vaccine (serogroups A, C, W, and Y). There are two such vaccines available; either product can be chosen. The recommendation is for two doses, 8-12 weeks apart, with a follow-up booster dose every 5 years thereafter.

Travel vaccines
All considered safe except oral polio, yellow fever, and live oral typhoid—each a live vaccine. Most could probably be given safely to patients with high CD4 cell counts (> 350/mm³), but data are limited.

Varicella zoster virus (VZV)
If vaccination results in disease due to vaccine virus, treatment with acyclovir is recommended.

If exposure occurs and patient is nonimmune, consider administration of varicella vaccine and pre-emptive acyclovir, 800 mg 5×/day for 5 days, or valacyclovir 1 g TID × 5d or famciclovir 500 g TID × 5d.

Live attenuated zoster vaccine was found to be safe in HIV patients in one prospective study. Our practice is to give this vaccine to stable patients (on ART, CD4 > 200) if older than 60.

TREATMENT OF OPPORTUNISTIC INFECTIONS

Antiretroviral therapy (ART) and specific antimicrobial prophylaxis regimens have led to a dramatic decline in HIV-related opportunistic infections. Today, opportunistic infections occur predominantly in patients not receiving ART (due to undiagnosed HIV infection or nonacceptance of therapy), or in the period soon after starting ART (due to eliciting a previously absent inflammatory host response, called immune reconstitution inflammatory syndrome (IRIS)). Even when virologic failure occurs in clinical practice, the rate of opportunistic infections in patients compliant with ART remains low, presumably due to continued immunologic response despite virologic failure, a phenomenon that may be linked to impaired "fitness" (virulence) of resistant HIV strains. For patients on or off ART, the absolute CD4 cell count provides the best marker of risk for opportunistic infections (OIs).

The precise timing of ART in patients with acute HIV-related OIs has been debated, and hence studied in several clinical trials. Favoring early starting of ART is the critical need to improve immune status, especially in conditions with either no highly effective direct therapy (e.g., progressive multifocal leukoencephalopathy (PML) or cryptosporidiosis) or resulting from HIV itself (e.g., dementia or wasting). Concerns about about drug-drug interactions, pill burden, and the immune reconstitution inflammatory syndrome (IRIS) favor deferring treatment until the OI is stabilized. In a randomized clinical trial of patients with opportunistic infections other than TB, the strategy of starting antiretroviral therapy within 2 weeks of the OI diagnosis was compared with deferring therapy until 6–8 weeks later. The results of the study demonstrated a significant reduction in the risk of further AIDS complications or death for the early therapy arm (PLoS One. 2009;4:e5575). In addition, 3 additional studies in HIV-related TB demonstrated clinical benefit for early ART, especially when the CD4 cell count was < 50 cells/mm^3. Early ART may not be beneficial with certain central nervous system (CNS) infection such as cryptococcal meningitis or tuberculosis meningitis (Clin Infect Dis. 2010;50:1532–1538; N Engl J Med. 2014 June 26;370:2487–98); one possible explanation is that IRIS in the CNS has more ominous consequences.

Based on the above clinical trials, it is recommended that treatment in patients with acute HIV-related opportunistic infections typically start within 2 weeks of the OI diagnosis. For patients with central nervous system infections, such as cryptococcal or tuberculous meningitis, deferring treatment until 4–6 weeks of anti-infective therapy has been received is recommended. Deferring ART until clinical improvement is also justified for patients with relatively preserved CD4 cell counts who have pulmonary TB or bacterial pneumonia.

Guidelines for treatment of OIs were last updated August 17, 2016, and are available here: https://aidsinfo.nih.gov/guidelines/html/4/adult-and-adolescent-oi-prevention-and-treatment-guidelines/0.

Specific OIs are listed below in alphabetical order.

Aspergillosis, Invasive

Preferred Therapy, Duration of Therapy, Chronic Maintenance	Alternate Therapy	Other Options/Issues
Preferred therapy Voriconazole 6 mg/kg q12h IV × 1 day, then 4 mg/kg q12h IV, followed by voriconazole PO 200 mg PO q12h after clinical improvement Duration of therapy: until CD4+ count > 200 cells/µL and with evidence of clinical response	Alternative therapy Amphotericin B deoxycholate 1 mg/kg IV daily **or** Lipid formulation of amphotericin B 5 mg/kg IV daily Caspofungin 70 mg IV × 1, then 50 mg IV daily **or** Anidulafungin 200 mg IV × 1, then 100 mg IV daily **or** Posaconazole 200 mg PO qid, then, after condition improved, 400 mg bid PO	Potential for significant pharmacokinetic interactions between certain ARV agents and voriconazole; they should be used cautiously in these situations. Consider therapeutic drug monitoring and dosage adjustment if necessary.

Clinical Presentation: Pleuritic chest pain, hemoptysis, cough in a patient with advanced HIV disease. Additional risk factors include neutropenia and use of corticosteroids.

Diagnostic Considerations: Diagnosis by bronchoscopy with biopsy/culture. Open lung biopsy (usually video-assisted thoracopic surgery) is sometimes required. Radiographic appearance includes cavitation (sometimes with a characteristic "halo" around a nodule, called the air crescent sign), nodules, sometimes focal consolidation. Dissemination to CNS may occur and manifests as focal neurological deficits. As with HIV-negative patients, elevation in serum galactomannan generally occurs with invasive disease.

Pitfalls: Positive sputum culture for *Aspergillus* in advanced HIV disease should heighten awareness of possible infection. Watch for drug-drug interactions between voriconazole and antiretrovirals metabolized via the cytochrome p450 system (PIs, NNRTIs).

Therapeutic Considerations: Decrease/discontinue corticosteroids, if possible. If present, treat neutropenia with granulocyte-colony stimulating factor (G-CSF) to achieve absolute neutrophil count > 1000/mm³. There are insufficient data to recommend chronic suppressive or maintenance therapy.

Prognosis: Poor unless immune deficits can be corrected.

Bacterial Respiratory Diseases

Preferred Therapy, Duration of Therapy, Chronic Maintenance	Alternate Therapy	Other Options/Issues
Preferred empiric outpatient therapy (oral) A beta-lactam plus a macrolide (azithromycin or clarithromycin) *Preferred beta-lactams*: high-dose amoxicillin or amoxicillin/clavulanate *Alternative beta-lactams*: cefpodoxime or cefuroxime, or *For penicillin-allergic patients*: levofloxacin 750 mg PO once daily or moxifloxacin 400 mg PO once daily Duration: 7–10 days (minimum 5 days). Patients should be afebrile for 48–72 h and clinically stable before stopping antibiotics. Preferred empiric therapy for non-ICU inpatient A beta-lactam (IV) plus a macrolide (azithromycin or clarithromycin) *Preferred beta-lactams*: cefotaxime, ceftriaxone, or ampicillin-sulbactam *For penicillin-allergic patients*: levofloxacin 750 mg PO once daily or moxifloxacin 400 mg PO once daily	Alternative empiric outpatient therapy (oral) A beta-lactam plus doxycycline *Preferred beta-lactams*: high-dose amoxicillin or amoxicillin/clavulanate *Alternative beta-lactams*: cefpodoxime or cefuroxime Alternative empiric therapy for non-ICU inpatient A beta-lactam (IV) plus doxycycline Alternative empiric ICU therapy *For penicillin-allergic patients*: Aztreonam IV + (levofloxacin 750 mg IV once daily or moxifloxacin 400 mg IV once daily)	Fluoroquinolones should be used with caution in patients where TB is suspected but is not being treated. Empiric therapy with a macrolide alone is not routinely recommended, because of increasing pneumococcal resistance. Patients receiving macrolide for MAC prophylaxis should not receive macrolide monotherapy for empiric treatment of bacterial pneumonia. Chemoprophylaxis may be considered for patients with frequent recurrences of serious bacterial respiratory infections. Clinicians should be cautious of using antibiotics to prevent recurrences, because of the potential for developing drug resistance and drug toxicities.

Bacterial Respiratory Diseases (cont'd)

Preferred Therapy, Duration of Therapy, Chronic Maintenance	Alternate Therapy	Other Options/Issues
<u>Preferred empiric ICU inpatient therapy</u> A beta-lactam (IV) plus azithromycin IV or an IV respiratory fluoroquinolone (levofloxacin 750 mg once daily or moxifloxacin 400 mg, once daily) *Preferred beta-lactams*: cefotaxime, ceftriaxone, or ampicillin-sulbactam <u>Preferred empiric *Pseudomonas* therapy (if risks present)</u> An IV antipneumococcal, antipseudomonal beta-lactam plus either ciprofloxacin 400 mg IV q8–12h or levofloxacin 750 mg/day IV once daily *Preferred beta-lactams*: piperacillin-tazobactam, cefepime, imipenem, or meropenem <u>Preferred empiric methicillin-resistant *Staphylococcus aureus* (if risks present)</u> Add vancomycin IV (possibly plus clindamycin) or linezolid alone to above.	<u>Alternative empiric Pseudomonas therapy</u> An IV antipneumococcal, antipseudomonal beta-lactam plus an aminoglyscoside plus azithromycin **or** Above beta-lactam plus an aminoglycoside plus (levofloxacin 750 mg IV once daily or moxifloxacin 400 mg IV once daily) *For penicillin-allergic patients:* Replace the beta-lactam with aztreonam.	

Clinical Presentation: HIV-infected patients with bacterial pneumonia present similar to those without HIV, with a relatively acute illness (over days) that is often associated with chills, rigors, pleuritic chest pain, and purulent sputum. Patients who have been ill over weeks to months are more likely have PCP, tuberculosis, or a fungal infection. Since bacterial pneumonia can occur at any CD4 cell count, this infection is frequently the presenting symptom of HIV disease, prompting initial HIV testing and diagnosis.

Diagnostic Considerations: The most common pathogens are *Streptococcus pneumoniae*, followed by *Haemophilus influenzae*, *Pseudomonas aeruginosa*, and *Staphylococcus aureus*. The pathogens of atypical pneumonia (*Legionella pneumophila*, *Mycoplasma pneumoniae*, and *Chlamydia pneumoniae*) are rarely encountered, even with extensive laboratory investigation; nonetheless, as with HIV-negative patients, these pathogens should be covered empirically unless a specific alternative diagnosis is made. A lobar infiltrate on chest radiography is a further predictor of bacterial pneumonia. Blood cultures should be obtained preferably before starting antibiotics, as HIV patients have an increased rate of bacteremia compared to those without HIV.

Pitfalls: Sputum Gram stain and culture are generally only helpful if collected prior to starting antibiotics, and only if a single organism predominates. HIV patients with bacterial pneumonia may rarely have a more subacute opportunistic infection concurrently, such as PCP or TB. Fluoroquinolones should be used with caution for treatment of suspected bacterial pneumonia if TB is a diagnostic consideration, as they may inadvertently select for quinolone-resistant TB.

Therapeutic Considerations: Once improvement has occurred, a switch to oral therapy is generally safe. Patients with advanced HIV disease are at greater risk of bacteremic pneumonia due to gram-negative bacilli, and should be covered empirically for this condition. Preventive therapy (for example daily trimethoprim-sulfa) may be considered for patients with frequent recurrent bacterial respiratory infections.

Prognosis: Response to therapy is generally prompt and overall prognosis is good.

Bartonella Infections

Preferred Therapy, Duration of Therapy, Chronic Maintenance	Alternate Therapy	Other Options/Issues
Preferred therapy for bacillary angiomatosis, peliosis hepatis, bacteremia, and osteomyelitis Erythromycin 500 mg PO or IV q6h **or** Doxycycline 100 mg PO or IV q12h Duration of therapy: at least 3 months CNS infections and severe infections Doxycycline 100 mg PO or IV q12h +/− rifampin 300 mg PO or IV q12h **or** Erythromycin 500 mg PO or IV q6h) +/− RIF 300 mg PO or IV q12h Duration of therapy: at least 3 months Confirmed *Bartonella* endocarditis (Doxycycline 100 mg IV q12h + gentamicin 1 mg/kg IV q8h) for 2 weeks, then continue with doxycycline 100 mg IV or PO q12h Duration of therapy: at least 3 months	Alternative therapy for bacillary angiomatosis infections, peliosis hepatis, bacteremia, and osteomyelitis Azithromycin 500 mg PO daily Clarithromycin 500 mg PO bid	Severe Jarisch-Herxheimer-like reaction can occur in the first 48 hours of treatment.

Clinical Presentation: Skin lesions resemble Kaposi's sarcoma. CT of liver shows hepatomegaly and hypodense lesions. Bartonella can rarely present as a CNS mass lesion, similar to toxoplasmosis.

Diagnostic Considerations: Diagnosis by demonstrating organism by stain/culture of skin lesions or by blood culture after lysis-centrifugation.

Pitfalls: Requires lifelong suppressive therapy unless CD4 > 200 with ART. Does not grow in routine cultures.

Therapeutic Considerations: Fluoroquinolones have variable activity in case reports and in vitro; may be considered as alternative therapy. Azithromycin likely to be better tolerated than erythromycin with fewer drug-drug interactions. Long-term suppressive therapy should be given for patients with relapse or reinfection, especially if CD4 cell count remains < 200 cells/mm3.

Prognosis: Related to extent of infection/degree of immunosuppression.

Campylobacteriosis

Preferred Therapy, Duration of Therapy, Chronic Maintenance	Alternate Therapy	Other Options/Issues
For mild disease Might withhold therapy unless symptoms persist for several days. For mild-to-moderate disease Ciprofloxacin 500–750 mg PO (or 400 mg IV) q12h **or** Azithromycin 500 mg PO daily (Note: Not for patients with bacteremia) For *Campylobacter* bacteremia: Ciprofloxacin 500–750 mg PO (or 400 mg IV) q12h + an aminoglycoside Duration of therapy: Gastroenteritis: 7–10 days (5 days with azithromycin) Bacteremia: ≥14 days Recurrent bacteremia: 2–6 weeks	For mild-to-moderate disease (if susceptible): Levofloxacin 750 mg (PO or IV) q24h **or** Moxifloxacin 400 mg (PO or IV) q24h Add an aminoglycoside to fluoroquinolone in bacteremic patients.	Oral or IV rehydration if indicated. Antimotility agents should be avoided. If no clinical response after 5–7 days, consider follow-up stool culture, alternative diagnosis, or antibiotic resistance. There is an increasing rate of fluoroquinolone resistance in the United States (22% resistance in 2009). Antimicrobial therapy should be modified based on susceptibility reports. Effective ART may reduce the frequency, severity, and recurrence of campylobacter infections.

Clinical Presentation: Acute onset of diarrhea, sometimes bloody; constitutional symptoms may be prominent.

Diagnostic Considerations: Diagnosis by stool culture; bacteremia may rarely occur, so blood cultures also indicated. Suspect *Campylobacter* in AIDS patient with diarrhea and curved gram-negative rods in blood culture. Non-C. *jejuni* species may be more strongly correlated with bacteremia.

Therapeutic Considerations: Optimal therapy not well defined. Treat with quinolone or azithromycin; modify therapy based on susceptibility testing. Quinolone resistance is common and correlates with treatment failure. Imipenem is sometimes used for bacteremia.

Prognosis: Depends on underlying immune status; prognosis is generally good.

Candidiasis (Mucosal)

Preferred Therapy, Duration of Therapy, Chronic Maintenance	Alternate Therapy	Other Options/Issues
<u>Preferred therapy</u> <u>oropharyngeal candidiasis: initial episodes (7–14 day treatment)</u> Fluconazole 100 mg PO daily **or** Clotrimazole troches 10 mg PO 5 times daily **or** Miconazole mucoadhesive buccal 50-mg tablet—apply to mucosal surface over the canine fossa once daily (do not swallow, chew, or crush)	<u>Alternative therapy</u> <u>oropharyngeal candidiasis: initial episodes (7–14 day treatment)</u> Itraconazole oral solution 200 mg PO daily **or** Posaconazole oral solution 400 mg PO bid × 1, then 400 mg daily **or** Nystatin suspension 4–6 mL qid or 1–2 flavored pastilles 4–5 times daily	Chronic or prolonged use of azoles might promote development of resistance. Higher relapse rate of esophageal candidiasis seen with echinocandins than with fluconazole use.
<u>Preferred therapy esophageal candidiasis (14–21 days)</u> Fluconazole 100 mg (up to 400 mg) PO or IV daily **or** Itraconazole oral solution 200 mg PO daily	<u>Alternative therapy</u> <u>esophageal candidiasis (14–21 days)</u> Voriconazole 200 mg PO or IV bid Posaconazole 400 mg PO bid Caspofungin 50 mg IV daily Micafungin 150 mg IV daily Anidulafungin 100 mg IV × 1, then 50 mg IV daily **or** Micafungin 150 mg IV daily **or** Amphotericin B deoxycholate 0.6 mg/kg IV daily **or** Lipid formulation of amphotericin B 3–4 mg/kg IV daily	Suppressive therapy is usually not recommended unless patients have frequent or severe recurrences. If decision is to use suppressive therapy:

Candidiasis (Mucosal) (cont'd)

Preferred Therapy, Duration of Therapy, Chronic Maintenance	Alternate Therapy	Other Options/Issues
Preferred therapy uncomplicated vulvovaginal candidiasis	Alternative therapy uncomplicated vulvovaginal candidiasis Itraconazole oral solution 200 mg PO daily for 3–7 days	Oropharyngeal candidiasis Fluconazole 100 mg PO daily or tiw
Oral fluconazole 150 mg for 1 dose **or** Topical azoles (clotrimazole, butoconazole, miconazole, tioconazole, or terconazole) for 3–7 days		Itraconazole oral solution 200 mg PO daily Fluconazole 100–200 mg PO daily Esophageal candidiasis Fluconazole 100–200 mg PO daily Posaconazole 400 mg PO bid
Preferred therapy severe or recurrent vulvovaginal candidiasis Fluconazole 100–200 mg PO daily for ≥ 7 days **or** Topical antifungal ≥ 7 days	Alternative therapy fluconazole-refractory oropharyngeal candidiasis or esophageal candidiasis Amphotericin B deoxycholate 0.3 mg/kg IV daily Lipid formulation of amphotericin B 3–5 mg/kg IV daily Anidulafungin 100 mg IV × 1, then 50 mg IV daily Caspofungin 50 mg IV daily Micafungin 150 mg IV daily Voriconazole 200 mg PO or IV BID	Vulvovaginal candidiasis Fluconazole 150 mg PO once weekly
Preferred therapy complicated (severe or recurrent) vulvovaginal candidiasis Fluconazole 150 mg q72h × 2–3 doses Topical antifungal ≥ 7 days	*Fluconazole-refractory oropharyngeal candidiasis (not esophageal)* Amphotericin B oral suspension 100 mg/mL (not available in U.S.) 1 mL PO QID	

Oral Thrush (*Candida*)

Clinical Presentation: Dysphagia/odynophagia. More common/severe in advanced HIV disease.

Diagnostic Considerations: Pseudomembranous (most common), erythematous, and hyperplastic (leukoplakia) forms. Pseudomembranes (white plaques on inflamed base) on buccal muscosa/tongue/gingiva/palate scrape off easily, hyperplastic lesions do not. Diagnosis of oral thrush most commonly by clinical appearance. KOH/Gram stain of scraping showing yeast/pseudomycelia. Other oral lesions in AIDS patients include herpes simplex, aphthous ulcers, Kaposi's sarcoma, oral hairy leukoplakia.

Pitfalls: Patients may be asymptomatic.

Therapeutic Considerations: Fluconazole is superior to topical therapy in preventing relapses of thrush and treating *Candida* esophagitis. Continuous treatment with fluconazole may lead to fluconazole resistance, which is best treated initially with itraconazole suspension and, if no response, with IV echinocandin or amphotericin. Chronic suppressive therapy is usually only considered for severely immunosuppressed patients.

Prognosis: Improvement in symptoms are usually seen within 24–48 hours.

Candida Esophagitis

Clinical Presentation: Dysphagia/odynophagia, almost always in the setting of oropharyngeal thrush. Fever is uncommon.

Diagnostic Considerations: Most common cause of esophagitis in HIV disease. For persistent symptoms despite therapy, endoscopy with biopsy/culture is recommended to confirm diagnosis and assess azole resistance.

Pitfalls: May extend into stomach. Other common causes of esophagitis include CMV, herpes simplex, and aphthous ulcers. Rarely, Kaposi's sarcoma, non-Hodgkin's lymphoma, zidovudine, dideoxycytidine, and other infections may cause esophageal symptoms.

Therapeutic Considerations: Systemic therapy is preferred over topical therapy. Failure to improve rapidly (24–48 hours) on empiric therapy mandates endoscopy to look for other causes, especially herpes viruses/aphthous ulcers. Consider maintenance therapy with fluconazole for frequent relapses, although the risk of fluconazole resistance is increased. Fluconazole resistance is best treated initially with itraconazole suspension and, if no response, with IV echinocandin (caspofungin, micafungin, anidulafungin) or amphotericin. Patients with fluconazole-refractory oropharyngeal or esophageal candidiasis who responded to echinocandin should be started on voriconazole or posaconazole for secondary prophylaxis until ART produces immune reconstitution.

Prognosis: Relapse rate is related to degree of immunosuppresion. Failure to improve promptly suggests either an alternative diagnosis or azole-resistant candida.

Chagas Disease (American Trypanosomiasis)

Preferred Therapy, Duration of Therapy, Chronic Maintenance	Alternate Therapy	Other Options/Issues
Preferred therapy for acute, early chronic, and reactivated disease Benznidazole 5–8 mg/kg/day PO in 2 divided doses for 30–60 days (not commercially available in the US, contact the CDC Drug Service at drugservice@cdc.gov or (404) 639–3670, or the CDC emergency operations center at (770) 488–7100)	Alternative therapy Nifurtimox 8–10 mg/kg/day PO for 90–120 days (Contact the CDC Drug Service at drugservice@cdc.gov or (404) 639–3670, or the CDC emergency operations center at (770) 488–7100)	Treatment is effective in reducing parasitemia and preventing clinical symptoms or slowing disease progression. It is ineffective in achieving parasitological cure. Duration of therapy has not been studied in HIV-infected patients. Initiation or optimization of ART in patients undergoing treatment for Chagas disease, once the patient is clinically stable.

Clostridium difficile Diarrhea/Colitis

Preferred Therapy	Alternate Therapy	Other Options/Issues
Preferred therapy for mild disease Metronidazole 500 mg (PO) q8h–10–14 days. Avoid use of other antibactericals if possible. Preferred therapy for moderate-severe disease (fever, WBC, colitis) Vancomycin 125 mg (PO) q6h–10–14 days. Avoid use of other antibacterials if possible.	Nitazoxanide 500 mg BID × 7–10 days	Severe disease with illeus/toxic mega-colon IV metronidazole Vancomycin per rectum Surgical consultation for possible colectomy

Clinical Presentation: Diarrhea and abdominal pain following antibiotic therapy. Diarrhea may be watery or bloody. Proton pump inhibitors increase the risk. Among antibiotics, clindamycin, quinolones, and beta-lactams are most frequent. Rarely occurs after aminoglycosides, linezolid, doxycycline, TMP-SMX, daptomycin, vancomycin.

Diagnostic Considerations: Most common cause of bacterial diarrhea in United States among HIV patients (Clin Infect Dis. 2005;41:1620-7), and increased in those with low CD4 cell counts (AIDS 2013 July 19). Many different approaches to diagnosis—most commonly labs will screen with *C. difficile* toxin and antigen test; if both are positive, no further testing is done. If results are toxin negative and antigen positive, then PCR for toxin (which is more sensitive than initial screen) is done to resolve conflict. Some sites only do PCR testing (Open Forum Infect Dis. 2014 Mar; 1(1): ofu007). After therapy completed, no indication for retesting if the patient is doing well clinically.

Pitfalls: *C. difficile* toxin may remain positive in stools for weeks following treatment; do not treat positive stool toxin test unless patient has symptoms.

Therapeutic Considerations: For all disease severity, vancomycin has become the preferred agent due to concern for the more virulent strain, and based on the results of some studies suggesting vancomycin is more effective. For moderate or severe disease, or with evidence of colitis clinically (leukocytosis, fever, colonic thickening on CT scan), surgical consultation should be obtained; if ileus and/or systemic toxicity occur, then colectomy may be indicated. The duration of therapy should be extended beyond 14 days if other systemic antibiotics must be continued. Relapse occurs in 10–25% of patients, and rates may be higher in patients with HIV due to the frequent need for other antimicrobial therapy. First relapses can be treated with a repeat of the initial regimen vancomycin. For multiple relapses, a long-term taper of vancomycin is appropriate: week 1, give 125 mg 4×/day; week 2, give 125 mg 2×/day; week 3, give 125 mg once daily; week 4, give 125 mg every other day; weeks 5 and 6, give 125 mg every 3 days. Fidaxomicin, a nonabsorbed macrocyclic antibiotic, was as effective as vancomycin for *C. diff.* and associated with fewer relapses; experience in HIV-infected patients is limited. Every effort should be made to resume a normal diet and to avoid other antibacterial therapies. Probiotic treatments (such as *Lactobacillus* or *Saccharomyces boulardii*) have not yet been shown to reduce the risk of relapse in controlled clinical trials. Fecal microbiota therapy (stool transplant) should be performed for multiple relapses (Annals Int Med. 2013;158:779–80).

Prognosis: Prognosis with *C. difficile* colitis is related to severity of the colitis.

Coccidioidomycosis

Preferred Therapy, Duration of Therapy, Chronic Maintenance	Alternate Therapy	Other Options/Issues
Preferred therapy for severe, nonmeningeal infection (diffuse pulmonary or severely ill patients with extrathoracic disseminated disease): Amphotericin B deoxycholate 0.7–1.0 mg/kg IV daily	Alternative therapy for severe nonmeningeal infection (diffuse pulmonary or disseminated disease): acute phase Certain specialists add triazole to amphotericin B therapy and continue triazole once amphotericin B is stopped.	Therapy should be continued indefinitely for patients with diffuse pulmonary or disseminated diseases as relapse can occur in 25%–33% in HIV-negative patients. It can also occur in HIV-infected patients with CD4 counts > 250 cells/µL.

Coccidioidomycosis (cont'd)

Preferred Therapy, Duration of Therapy, Chronic Maintenance	Alternate Therapy	Other Options/Issues
Lipid formulation amphotericin B 4–6 mg/kg IV daily Duration of therapy: until clinical improvement, then switch to azole		Therapy should be lifelong in patients with meningeal infections as relapse occurred in 80% of HIV-infected patients after discontinuation of triazole therapy.
<u>Preferred therapy for meningeal infections</u> Fluconazole 400–800 mg PO or IV daily	<u>Alternative therapy for meningeal infections</u> Itraconazole 200 mg PO tid for 3 days, then 200 mg PO bid **or** Posaconazole 200 mg PO bid **or** Voriconazole 200–400 mg PO bid **or** Intrathecal amphotericin B deoxycholate, when triazole antifungals are ineffective	
<u>Maintenance therapy (for all cases)</u> Fluconazole 400 mg PO daily **or** Itraconazole 200 mg PO bid	Posaconazole 200 mg PO bid **or** Voriconazole 200 mg PO bid	Itraconazole, posaconazole, and voriconazole may have significant interactions with certain ARV agents. These interactions are complex and can be bidirectional. Refer to Table 5, Guidelines for Prevention and Treatment of Opportunistic Infections in HIV-Infected Adults and Adolescents; http://aidsinfo.nih.gov/contentfiles/lvguidelines/AdultOITablesOnly.pdf, for dosage recommendations.

Coccidioidomycosis (cont'd)

Preferred Therapy, Duration of Therapy, Chronic Maintenance	Alternate Therapy	Other Options/Issues
		Therapeutic drug monitoring and dosage adjustment may be necessary to ensure triazole antifungal and antiretroviral efficacy and reduce concentration-related toxicities.
		Intrathecal amphotericin B should only be given in consultation with a specialist and administered by an individual with experience with the technique.
<u>Preferred therapy for mild infections (focal pneumonia or positive coccidioidal serologic test alone)</u> Fluconazole 400 mg PO daily **or** Itraconazole 200 mg PO bid	<u>Mild infections (focal pneumonia) for patients who failed to respond to fluconazole or itraconazole</u> Posaconazole 200 mg PO bid **or** Voriconazole 200 mg PO bid	Certain patients with meningitis may develop hydrocephalus and require CSF shunting.
<u>Preferred therapy for severe, nonmeningeal infection (diffuse pulmonary or severely ill patients with extrathoracic disseminated disease)</u> Amphotericin B deoxycholate 0.7–1.0 mg/kg IV daily Lipid formulation amphotericin B 4–6 mg/kg IV daily Duration of therapy: until clinical improvement, then switch to azole	<u>Alternative therapy for severe nonmeningeal infection (diffuse pulmonary or disseminated disease):</u> acute phase Certain specialists add triazole to amphotericin B therapy and continue triazole once amphotericin B is stopped.	Therapy should be continued indefinitely for patients with diffuse pulmonary or disseminated diseases as relapse can occur in 25%–33% in HIV-negative patients. It can also occur in HIV-infected patients with CD4 counts > 250 cells/µL. Therapy should be lifelong in patients with meningeal infections as relapse occurred in 80% of HIV-infected patients after discontinuation of triazole therapy.

Coccidioidomycosis (cont'd)

Preferred Therapy, Duration of Therapy, Chronic Maintenance	Alternate Therapy	Other Options/Issues
Preferred therapy for meningeal infections Fluconazole 400–800 mg PO or IV daily	Alternative therapy for meningeal infections Itraconazole 200 mg PO tid for 3 days, then 200 mg PO bid **or** Posaconazole 200 mg PO bid **or** Voriconazole 200–400 mg PO bid **or** Intrathecal amphotericin B deoxycholate, when triazole antifungals are ineffective	Itraconazole, posaconazole, and voriconazole may have significant interactions with certain ARV agents. These interactions are complex and can be bidirectional. Refer to Table 5, Guidelines for Prevention and Treatment of Opportunistic Infections in HIV-Infected Adults and Adolescents; http://aidsinfo.nih.gov/contentfiles/lvguidelines/AdultOITablesOnly.pdf, for dosage recommendations. Therapeutic drug monitoring and dosage adjustment may be necessary to ensure triazole antifungal and antiretroviral efficacy and reduce concentration-related toxicities.
Maintenance therapy (for all cases) Fluconazole 400 mg PO daily **or** Itraconazole 200 mg PO bid	Posaconazole 200 mg PO bid **or** Voriconazole 200 mg PO bid	Intrathecal amphotericin B should only be given in consultation with a specialist and administered by an individual with experience with the technique.

Clinical Presentation: Typically a complication of advanced HIV infection (CD4 cell count < 200/mm³) in endemic areas (southwestern USA or northern Mexico). Most patients present with disseminated disease, which can manifest as fever, diffuse pulmonary infiltrates, adenopathy, skin lesions (multiple forms—verrucous, cold abscesses, ulcers, nodules), and/or bone lesions. Approximately 10% will have spread to the CNS in the form of meningitis (fever, headache, altered mental status).

Diagnostic Considerations: Consider the diagnosis in any patient with advanced HIV-related immunosuppression who has been in a *Coccidioides immitis* endemic area (southwestern United States, northern Mexico) and presents with a systemic febrile syndrome. Diagnosis can be made by culture of the organism, visualization of characteristic spherules on histopathology, or a positive complement-fixation antibody (≥ 1:16). In meningeal cases, cerebrospinal fluid (CSF) profile shows low glucose, high protein, and lymphocytic pleocytosis. A *Coccidiodes* urinary antigen test is available (MiraVista Diagnostics) and may provide a more rapid diagnostic strategy.

Pitfalls: Antibody titers are often negative on presentation. CSF profile of meningitis can be similar to TB. CSF fungal cultures may be negative.

Prognosis: Related to extent of infection and degree of immunosuppression. Clinical response tends to be slow, especially with a high disease burden and advanced HIV disease. Meningeal disease is treated with lifelong fluconazole regardless of CD4 recovery.

Cryptococcal Meningitis

Preferred Therapy, Duration of Therapy, Chronic Maintenance	Alternate Therapy	Other Options/Issues
Preferred induction therapy Liposomal amphotericin B 3–4 mg/kg IV daily + flucytosine 25 mg/kg PO qid (Note: Flucytosine dose should be adjusted in patients with renal dysfunction.)	Alternative induction therapy Amphotericin B deoxycholate 0.7 mg/kg IV daily + flucytosine 25 mg/kg PO qid **or** Amphotericin B lipid complex 5 mg/kg IV daily + flucytosine 25 mg/kg PO qid **or** Liposomal amphotericin B 3–4 mg/kg IV daily + fluconazole 800 mg PO or IV daily **or** Amphotericin B deoxycholate 0.7 mg/kg IV daily + fluconazole 800 mg PO or IV daily **or** Fluconazole 400–800 mg PO or IV daily + flucytosine 25 mg/kg PO qid **or** Fluconazole 1200 mg PO or IV daily	Addition of flucytosine to amphotericin B has been associated with more rapid sterilization of CSF and decreased risk for subsequent relapse.
Preferred consolidation therapy (after at least 2 weeks of successful induction—defined as significant clinical improvement & negative CSF culture) Fluconazole 400 mg PO daily for 8 weeks		Patients receiving flucytosine should have either blood levels monitored (peak level 2 hours after dose should not exceed 30–80 μg/mL), or close monitoring of blood counts for development of cytopenia. Dosage should be adjusted in patients with renal insufficiency. Opening pressure should always be measured when a lumbar puncture (LP) is performed. Repeated LPs or CSF shunting are essential to effectively manage increased intracranial pressure.

Cryptococcal Meningitis(cont'd)

Preferred Therapy, Duration of Therapy, Chronic Maintenance	Alternate Therapy	Other Options/Issues
Preferred maintenance therapy (after at least 8 weeks of consolidation therapy) Fluconazole 200 mg PO daily for at least 12 months	Alternative consolidation therapy (after 2 weeks of successful induction therapy) Itraconazole 200 mg PO bid for 8 weeks—less effective than fluconazole Alternative maintenance therapy No alternative therapy recommendation	Corticosteroids and mannitol are ineffective in reducing intracranial pressure and are NOT recommended. Some specialists recommend a brief course of corticosteroid for management of severe IRIS symptoms.

Clinical Presentation: Often indolent onset of fever, headache, subtle cognitive deficits. Occasional meningeal signs and focal neurologic findings, though nonspecific presentation is most common.

Diagnostic Considerations: Diagnosis usually by cryptococcal antigen of serum and/or CSF; India ink stain of CSF is less sensitive. Diagnosis is essentially excluded with a negative serum cryptococcal antigen (sensitivity of test in AIDS patients approaches 100%). If serum cryptococcal antigen is positive, CSF antigen may be negative in disseminated disease without spread to CNS/meninges. Brain imaging is often normal, but CSF analysis is usually abnormal with elevated opening pressure.

Pitfalls: Be sure to obtain a CSF opening pressure, since reduction of increased intracranial pressure is critical for successful treatment. Remove sufficient CSF during the initial lumbar puncture (LP) to reduce closing pressure to < 200 mm H_2O or 50% of opening pressure. Increased intracranial pressure requires repeat daily lumbar punctures until CSF pressure stabilizes; persistently elevated pressure should prompt placement of a lumbar drain or ventriculo-peritoneal shunting. Adjunctive corticosteroids are not recommended except for the management of severe IRIS. Acetazolamide and mannitol are also not effective.

Therapeutic Considerations: Optimal total dose/duration of amphotericin B prior to fluconazole switch depends on clinical response and rapidity of CSF sterilization (2–3 weeks is reasonable if patient is doing well). Addition of flucytosine to amphotericin B associated with more rapid sterilization of CSF and decreased risk for subsequent relapse. If available, flucytosine levels should be monitored—peak level 2 hours after dose should not exceed 75 mcg/mL. Flucytosine dose must be reduced in renal insufficiency. Fluconazole is preferred over itraconazole for life-long maintenance therapy. Consider discontinuation of chronic maintenance therapy in patients who remain asymptomatic with CD4 > 100–200/mm³ for > 6 months due to ART. Two studies have found that early antiretroviral therapy worsened prognosis, possibly due to IRIS (Clin Infect Dis. 2010;50:1532–1538; N Engl J Med. 2014 Jun 26; 370(26):2487–98), one study did not (PLoS One. 2009;4:e5575); our practice is generally to start ART at approximately week two of treatment after the induction phase of amphotericin and flucytosine if patients are stable.

Prognosis: Variable. Mortality up to 40%. Adverse prognostic factors include increased intracranial pressure, abnormal mental status.

Cryptosporidiosis

Preferred Therapy, Duration of Therapy, Chronic Maintenance	Alternate Therapy	Other Options/Issues
Preferred therapy Initiate or optimize ART for immune restoration to CD4+ count > 100 cells/µL Symptomatic treatment of diarrhea with anti-motility agents Aggressive oral or IV rehydration and replacement of electrolyte loss	Alternative therapy for cryptosporidiosis No therapy has been shown to be effective without ART. Trial of these agents may be used in conjunction with, but not instead of, ART: Nitazoxanide 500–1000 mg PO bid for 14 days **or** Paromomycin 500 mg PO qid for 14–21 days **or** With optimized ART, symptomatic treatment and rehydration and electrolyte replacement	Tincture of opium may be more effective than loperamide in management of diarrhea.

Clinical Presentation: High-volume watery diarrhea with weight loss and electrolyte disturbances, especially in advanced HIV disease.

Diagnostic Considerations: Spore-forming protozoa. Diagnosis by acid-fast bacilli (AFB) smear of stool demonstrating characteristic oocyte, or by cryptosporia stool antigen. Malabsorption may occur.

Pitfalls: No fecal leukocytes; organisms are not visualized on standard ova and parasite exams (need to request special stains).

Therapeutic Considerations: Anecdotal reports of antimicrobial success. Nitazoxanide may be effective in some settings, but no increase in cure rate for nitazoxanide if CD4 < 50/mm³. Immune reconstitution in response to antiretroviral therapy is the most effective therapy, and may induce prolonged remissions and cure. Antidiarrheal agents (Lomotil, Pepto-Bismol) are useful to control symptoms. Hyperalimentation may be required for severe cases.

Prognosis: Related to degree of immunosuppression/response to antiretroviral therapy.

Cytomegalovirus (CMV) Disease

Preferred Therapy, Duration of Therapy, Chronic Maintenance	Alternate Therapy	Other Options/Issues
<u>Preferred therapy for CMV retinitis</u> *For immediate sight-threatening lesions adjacent to the optic nerve or fovea* Intravitreal injections of ganciclovir (2 mg) or foscarnet (2.4 mg) for 1–4 doses over a period of 7–10 days to achieve high intraocular concentration faster Plus one of the listed preferred or alternative systemic therapies <u>Preferred systemic induction therapy</u> • Valganciclovir 900 mg PO bid for 14–21 days *For small peripheral lesions* Administer one of the preferred or alternative systemic therapy. <u>Preferred chronic maintenance therapy (secondary prophylaxis) for CMV retinitis</u> Valganciclovir 900 mg PO daily **or** Ganciclovir implant (may be replaced every 6–8 months if CD4+ count remains < 100 cells/μL) + valganciclovir 900 mg PO daily until immune recovery	<u>Alternative therapy for CMV retinitis</u> Ganciclovir 5 mg/kg IV q12h for 14–21 days, then 5 mg/kg IV daily **or** Foscarnet 60 mg/kg IV q8h or 90 mg/kg IV q12h for 14–21 days **or** Cidofovir 5 mg/kg/week IV for 2 weeks; saline hydration before and after therapy and probenecid 2 g PO 3 hours before the dose followed by 1 g PO 2 hours and 8 hours after the dose (total of 4 g) **Note:** This regimen should be avoided in patients with sulfa allergy because of cross hypersensitivity with probenecid. <u>Alternative chronic maintenance (secondary prophylaxis)</u> Ganciclovir 5 mg/kg IV 5–7 times weekly **or** Foscarnet 90–120 mg/kg IV once daily **or**	The choice of initial therapy for CMV retinitis should be individualized, based on location and severity of the lesion(s), level of immunosuppression, and other factors such as concomitant medications and ability to adhere to treatment. The ganciclovir ocular implant, which is effective for treatment of CMV retinitis is no longer available. For sight-threatening retinitis, intravitreal injections of ganciclovir or foscarnet can be given to achieve higher ocular concentration faster. The choice of chronic maintenance therapy (route of administration and drug choices) should be made in consultation with an ophthalmologist. Considerations should include the anatomic location of the retinal lesion, vision in the contralateral eye, the patient's immunologic and virologic status, and response to ART. Patients with CMV retinitis who discontinue maintenance therapy should undergo regular eye examinations—optimally every 3 months—for early detection of relapse immune reconstitution uveitis (IRU, and then annually after immune reconstitution.

Cytomegalovirus (CMV) Disease (cont'd)

Preferred Therapy, Duration of Therapy, Chronic Maintenance	Alternate Therapy	Other Options/Issues
Preferred therapy for CMV esophagitis or colitis Ganciclovir 5 mg/kg IV q12h; may switch to valganciclovir 900 mg. PO q12h once the patient cantolerate oral therapy Duration: 21–42 days or until symptoms have resolved Maintenance therapy is usually not necessary, but should be considered after relapses. Preferred therapy for documented, histologically confirmed CMV pneumonitis Experience for treating CMV pneumonitis in HIV patients is limited. Use of IV ganciclovir or IV foscarnet is reasonable (doses same as for CMV retinitis). The optimal duration of therapy and the role of oral valganciclovir have not been established. Preferred therapy CMV neurological disease *Treatment should be initiated promptly.* Ganciclovir 5 mg/kg IV q12h + foscarnet (90 mg/kg IV q12h or 60 mg/kg IV q8h) to stabilize disease and maximize response; continue until symptomatic improvement. The optimal duration of therapy and the role of oral valganciclovir have not been established.	Cidofovir 5 mg/kg IV every other week with saline hydration and probenecid as above CMV esophagitis or colitis Foscarnet 90 mg/kg IV q12h or 60 mg/kg q8h for patients with treatment-limiting toxicities to ganciclovir or with ganciclovir resistance **or** Valganciclovir 900 mg PO q12h in milder disease and if able to tolerate PO therapy **or** For mild cases, if ART can be initiated without delay, consider withholding CMV therapy. Duration: 21–42 days or until symptoms have resolved	IRU may develop in the setting of immune reconstitution. Treatment of IRU Periocular corticosteroid or short courses of systemic steroid Initial therapy in patients with CMV retinitis, esophagitis, colitis, and pneumonitis should include initiation or optimization of ART.

CMV Retinitis

Clinical Presentation: Blurred vision, scotomata, field cuts common. Often bilateral, even when initial symptoms are unilateral.

Diagnostic Considerations: Diagnosis by characteristic hemorrhagic ("tomato soup and milk") retinitis on funduscopic exam. Consult ophthalmology in suspected cases.

Pitfalls: May develop immune reconstitution vitreitis after starting antiretroviral therapy.

Therapeutic Considerations: Oral valganciclovir is the preferred option for initial and maintenance therapy. Lifelong maintenance therapy for CMV retinitis is required for CD4 counts < 100/mm^3, but may be discontinued if CD4 counts increase to > 100–150/mm^3 for 6 or more months in response to antiretroviral therapy (in consultation with ophthalmologist). Patients with CMV retinitis who discontinue therapy should undergo regular eye exams to monitor for relapse. Ganciclovir intraocular implants might need to be replaced every 6–8 months for patients who remain immunosuppressed with CD4 < 100–150/mm^3. Immune recovery uveitis (IRU) may develop in the setting of immune reconstitution due to ART and be treated by ophthalmologist with periocular corticosteroid, sometimes systemic corticosteroid.

Prognosis: Good initial response to therapy. High relapse rate unless CD4 improves with antiretroviral therapy.

CMV Encephalitis/Polyradiculitis

Clinical Presentation: Encephalitis presents as fever, mental status changes, and headache evolving over 1–2 weeks. True meningismus is rare. CMV encephalitis occurs in advanced HIV disease (CD4 < 50/mm^3), often in patients with prior CMV retinitis. Polyradiculitis presents as rapidly evolving weakness/sensory disturbances in the lower extremities, often with bladder/bowel incontinence. Anesthesia in "saddle distribution" with T sphincter tone possible.

Diagnostic Considerations: CSF may show lymphocytic or neutrophilic pleocytosis; glucose is often decreased. For CMV encephalitis, characteristic findings on brain MRI include confluent periventricular abnormalities with variable degrees of enhancement. Diagnosis is confirmed by CSF CMV PCR (preferred), CMV culture, or brain biopsy.

Pitfalls: For CMV encephalitis, a wide spectrum of radiographic findings are possible, including mass lesions (rare). Obtain ophthalmologic evaluation to exclude active retinitis. For polyradiculitis, obtain sagittal MRI of the spinal cord to exclude mass lesions, and CSF cytology to exclude lymphomatous involvement (can cause similar symptoms).

Therapeutic Considerations: For any established CMV disease, optimization of antiretroviral therapy is important along with initiating anti-CMV therapy. Ganciclovir plus foscarnet may be beneficial as initial therapy for severe cases. Consider discontinuation of valganciclovir maintenance therapy if CD4 increases to > 100–150/mm^3 × 6 months or longer in response to antiretroviral therapy.

Prognosis: Unless CD4 cell count increases in response to antiretroviral therapy, response to anti-CMV treatment is usually transient, followed by progression of symptoms.

CMV Esophagitis/Colitis

Clinical Presentation: Localizing symptoms, including odynophagia, abdominal pain, diarrhea, sometimes bloody stools.

Diagnostic Considerations: Diagnosis by finding CMV inclusions on biopsy. CMV can affect the entire GI tract, resulting in oral/esophageal ulcers, gastritis, and colitis (most common).

CMV colitis varies greatly in severity, but typically causes fever, abdominal cramping, and sometimes bloody stools.

Pitfalls: CMV colitis may cause colonic perforation and should be considered in any AIDS patient presenting with an acute abdomen, especially if radiography demonstrates free intra-peritoneal air.

Therapeutic Considerations: Initial therapy for any CMV disease should include optimization of antiretroviral therapy. Duration of therapy is dependent on clinical response, typically 3–4 weeks. Consider chronic suppressive therapy for recurrent disease. Screen for CMV retinitis.

Prognosis: Relapse rate is greatly reduced with immune reconstitution due to antiretroviral therapy.

Hepatitis B Virus (HBV)

Preferred Therapy, Duration of Therapy, Chronic Maintenance	Alternate Therapy	Other Options/Issues
ART is recommended for all HIV/HBV-co-infected patients regardless of CD4 cell count. Regimens should include TDF/FTC or TAF/FTC, plus an additional active antiretroviral drug. Duration: Continue treatment indefinitely.	Treatment for patients who refuse or are unable to take ART Assess HBV disease stage and whether HBV treatment should be undertaken. If no indication for treatment of HBV infection, continue to monitor and reassess at a later time. (HBV treatment is indicated for patients with active liver disease, elevated ALT, and HBV DNA > 2,000 international units/mL or significant liver fibrosis.) **or** Peginterferon alfa-2a 180 µg SQ weekly for 48 weeks **or** Peginterferon alfa-2b 1.5 µg/kg SQ once weekly for 48 weeks If tenofovir cannot be used as part of HIV/HBV therapy (because of existing or high risk of renal dysfunction) Use a fully suppressive ART regimen with entecavir (dose adjustment according to renal function).	Adefovir, emtricitabine, entecavir, lamivudine, or tenofovir should not be used for the treatment of HBV infection in patients who are not receiving combination ART. Cross-resistance to emtricitabine or telbivudine should be assumed in patients with suspected or proven lamivudine resistance. When changing ART regimens, continue agents with anti-HBV activity because of the risk of IRIS. If anti-HBV therapy is discontinued and a flare occurs, therapy should be reinstituted, as it can be potentially life saving.

Epidemiology: Hepatitis B virus (HBV) infection is relatively common in patients with HIV, with approximately 60% showing some evidence of prior exposure. Chronic hepatitis B infection interacts with HIV infection in several important ways:

- HBV increases the risk of liver-related death and hepatotoxicity from antiretroviral therapy (Lancet 2002;360:1921–6; Hepatology 2002;35:182–9).
- 3TC, FTC, and tenofovir (both TAF and TDF) all have anti-HBV activity. Thus selection of antiretroviral therapy for patients with HBV can have clinical and resistance implications for HBV as well as HIV. This is most notable with 3TC and FTC, as a high proportion of coinfected patients will develop HBV-associated resistance to these drugs after several years of therapy. This resistance reduces response to subsequent non-3TC or FTC anti-HBV therapy.
- Cessation of anti-HBV therapy may lead to exacerbations of underlying liver disease; in some cases, these flares have been fatal (Clin Infect Dis. 1999;28:1032–5; Scand J Infectious Diseases 2004;36:533–5).
- Immune reconstitution may lead to worsening of liver status, presumably because HBV disease is immune mediated. This is sometimes associated with loss of HBEAg.
- Entecavir can no longer be recommended for HIV/HBV coinfected patients not on ART, as it has anti-HIV activity and may select for HIV resistance mutation M184V (N Engl J Med. 2007;356:2614–21). If needed, it should be used only with a fully suppressive HIV regimen.

Diagnostic Consideration: Obtain HBSAb, HBSAg, and HBCAb at baseline in all patients. If negative, hepatitis B vaccination is indicated. If chronic HBV infection (positive HBSAg) is identified, obtain HBEAg, HBEAb, and HBV DNA levels. As with HCV infection, vaccination with hepatitis A vaccine and counseling to avoid alcohol are important components of preventive care. Isolated hepatitis B core antibody: Some patients with HIV have antibody to hepatitis B core (anti-HBc) but are negative for both HBSAg and HBSAb. This phenomenon appears to be more common in those with HCV coinfection (Clin Infec Dis. 2003 36:1602–6). In this scenario, diagnostic considerations include: (1) recently acquired HBV, before development of HBSAb; (2) chronic HBV, with HBSAg below the levels of detection; (3) immunity to HBV, with HBSAb below the levels of detection; (4) false-positive anti-HBV core. As the incidence of HBV is relatively low in most populations and anti-HBc alone is usually a stable phenomenon over years, recent acquisition of HBV is rarely the explanation. We recommend checking HBV DNA in this situation: If positive, this indicates chronic HBV; if negative, then low-level immunity or false-positive anti-HBV core remain as possible explanations; since distinguishing between these possibilities cannot be done, we recommend immunization with the hepatitis B vaccine series. It is useful to measure HBV serologic markers periodically in this population, as improvement in immune status due to ART may lead to increasing titers of HBSAb and subsequently confirm immunity (Clin Infect Dis. 2007;45:1221–9).

Therapeutic Considerations: HIV treatment guidelines generally recommend starting antiretroviral therapy in all HBV infected patients, regardless of CD4 cell count. In practice, this means using TDF or TAF/FTC (or 3TC) as part of all antiretroviral regimens, as this provides two active drugs against hepatitis B and reduces the risk of inducing FTC or 3TC resistance. Patients being treated with regimens for HBV should be monitored for alanine transaminase (ALT) every 3–4 months during the first year of therapy. HBV DNA levels provide a good marker for efficacy of therapy and should be added to regular laboratory monitoring. The goal of therapy is to reduce HBV DNA to as low a level as possible, preferably below the limits of detection. Time to achieving an undetectable HBV DNA level is much longer for hepatitis B than HIV.

Hepatitis C Virus (HCV)

Treatment of HCV has changed substantially since the last revision of this book, and today there are multiple effective options for HIV/HCV coinfected patients. The following guidelines for therapy are from the combined AASLD/IDSA HCV Guidance, which is available at www. hcvguidelines.org, and are updated regularly.

Rating System Used to Rate the Level of the Evidence and Strength of the Recommendation for Each Recommendation

Recommendations are based on scientific evidence and expert opinion. Each recommended statement includes a Roman numeral (**I**, **II**, or **III**) that represents the level of the evidence that supports the recommendation, and a letter (**A**, **B**, or **C**) that represents the strength of the recommendation.

Classification	Description
Class I	Conditions for which there is evidence and/or general agreement that a given diagnostic evaluation, procedure, or treatment is beneficial, useful, and effective
Class II	Conditions for which there is conflicting evidence and/or a divergence of opinion about the usefulness and efficacy of a diagnostic evaluation, procedure, or treatment
Class IIa	Weight of evidence and/or opinion is in favor of usefulness and efficacy
Class IIb	Usefulness and efficacy are less well established by evidence and/or opinion
Class III	Conditions for which there is evidence and/or general agreement that a diagnostic evaluation, procedure, or treatment is not useful and effective or if it in some cases may be harmful
Level of Evidence	**Description**
Level A*	Data derived from multiple randomized clinical trials, meta-analyses, or equivalent
Level B*	Data derived from a single randomized trial, nonrandomized studies, or equivalent
Level C	Consensus opinion of experts, case studies, or standard of care

Adapted from the American College of Cardiology and the American Heart Association Practice Guidelines. (American Heart Association, 2014); (Shiffman, 2003)

*   In some situations, such as for IFN-sparing HCV treatments, randomized clinical trials with an existing standard-of-care arm cannot ethically or practicably be conducted. The US Food and Drug Administration (FDA) has suggested alternative study designs, including historical controls or immediate versus deferred, placebo-controlled trials. For additional examples and definitions see FDA link: http://www. fda.gov/downloads/Drugs/GuidanceComplianceRegulatoryInformation/Guidances/UCM225333.pdf. In those instances for which there was a single pre-determined, FDA-approved equivalency established, panel members considered the evidence as equivalent to a randomized controlled trial for levels A or B.

Summary of Recommendations for Patients Who Are Initiating Therapy for HCV Infection by HCV Genotype

Genotype 1a Treatment-Naïve Patients Without Cirrhosis – Recommended

Recommended regimens are listed in groups by level of evidence, then alphabetically.

- **Daily fixed-dose combination of elbasvir (50 mg)/grazoprevir (100 mg) for 12 weeks is a recommended regimen for treatment-naïve patients with HCV genotype 1a infection who do not have cirrhosis and in whom no baseline NS5A RAVs§ for elbasvir are detected.**
  Rating: Class I, Level A
- **Daily fixed-dose combination of ledipasvir (90 mg)/sofosbuvir (400 mg) for 12 weeks is a recommended regimen for treatment-naïve patients with HCV genotype 1a infection who do not have cirrhosis.**
  Rating: Class I, Level A
- **Daily fixed-dose combination of paritaprevir (150 mg)/ritonavir (100 mg)/ombitasvir (25 mg) plus twice-daily dosed dasabuvir (250 mg) with weight-based ribavirin for 12 weeks is a recommended regimen for treatment-naïve patients with HCV genotype 1a infection who do not have cirrhosis.**
  Rating: Class I, Level A
- **Daily simeprevir (150 mg) plus sofosbuvir (400 mg) for 12 weeks is a recommended regimen for treatment-naïve patients with HCV genotype 1a infection who do not have cirrhosis.**
  Rating: Class I, Level A
- **Daily fixed-dose combination of sofosbuvir (400 mg)/velpatasvir (100 mg) for 12 weeks is a recommended regimen for treatment-naïve patients with HCV genotype 1a infection who do not have cirrhosis.**
  Rating: Class I, Level A
- **Daily daclatasvir (60 mg*) plus sofosbuvir (400 mg) for 12 weeks is a recommended regimen for treatment-naïve patients with HCV genotype 1a infection who do not have cirrhosis.**
  Rating: Class I, Level B

---

§ Includes G1a polymorphisms at amino acid positions 28, 30, 31, or 93. Amino acid substitutions that confer resistance.
* The dose of daclatasvir may need to increase or decrease when used concomitantly with cytochrome P450 3A/4 inducers and inhibitors, respectively. Please refer to the prescribing information and the section on HIV/HCV coinfection for patients on antiretroviral therapy.

Genotype 1a Treatment-Naïve Patients with Compensated Cirrhosis‡ – Recommended

Recommended regimens are listed in groups by level of evidence, then alphabetically.

- **Daily fixed-dose combination of elbasvir (50 mg)/grazoprevir (100 mg) for 12 weeks is a recommended regimen for treatment-naïve patients with HCV genotype 1a infection who have compensated cirrhosis and in whom no baseline NS5A RAVs§ for elbasvir are detected.**
  Rating: Class I, Level A

Genotype 1a Treatment-Naïve Patients with <u>Compensated Cirrhosis</u>‡ – Recommended (cont'd)

- **Daily fixed-dose combination of ledipasvir (90 mg)/sofosbuvir (400 mg) for 12 weeks is a recommended regimen for treatment-naïve patients with HCV genotype 1a infection who have <u>compensated cirrhosis</u>.**
  Rating: Class I, Level A
- **Daily fixed-dose combination of sofosbuvir (400 mg)/velpatasvir (100 mg) for 12 weeks is a recommended regimen for treatment-naïve patients with HCV genotype 1a infection who have <u>compensated cirrhosis</u>.**
  Rating: Class I, Level A

---

‡   For decompensated cirrhosis, please refer to the appropriate section.
§   Includes G1a polymorphisms at amino acid positions 28, 30, 31, or 93. <u>Amino acid substitutions that confer resistance</u>.

Genotype 1a Treatment-Naïve Patients Without Cirrhosis – Alternative

- **Daily fixed-dose combination of elbasvir (50 mg)/grazoprevir (100 mg) with weight-based ribavirin for 16 weeks is an alternative regimen for patients with HCV genotype 1a infection who do not have cirrhosis but have baseline NS5A RAVs§ for elbasvir.**
  Rating: Class IIa, Level B

---

§   Includes G1a polymorphisms at amino acid positions 28, 30, 31, or 93. <u>Amino acid substitutions that confer resistance</u>.

Genotype 1a Treatment-Naïve Patients with <u>Compensated Cirrhosis</u>‡ – Alternative

Alternative regimens are listed in groups by level of evidence, then alphabetically.
- **Daily fixed-dose combination of paritaprevir (150 mg)/ritonavir (100 mg)/ombitasvir (25 mg) plus twice-daily dosed dasabuvir (250 mg) with weight-based ribavirin for 24 weeks is an alternative regimen for treatment-naïve patients with HCV genotype 1a infection who have <u>compensated cirrhosis</u>.**†
  Rating: Class I, Level A
- **Daily simeprevir (150 mg) plus sofosbuvir (400 mg) with or without weight-based ribavirin for 24 weeks is an alternative regimen for treatment-naïve patients with HCV genotype 1a infection who have <u>compensated cirrhosis</u> and in whom no Q80K polymorphism is detected.**
  Rating: Class II, Level B
- **Daily daclatasvir (60 mg*) plus sofosbuvir (400 mg) with or without weight-based ribavirin for 24 weeks is an alternative regimen for treatment-naïve patients with HCV genotype 1a infection who have <u>compensated cirrhosis</u>.**
  Rating: Class IIa, Level B

- **Daily fixed-dose combination of elbasvir (50 mg)/grazoprevir (100 mg) with weight-based ribavirin for 16 weeks is an alternative regimen for treatment-naïve patients with HCV genotype 1a infection who have <u>compensated cirrhosis</u> and have baseline NS5A RAVs§ for elbasvir.**
  Rating: Class IIa, Level B

Genotype 1a Treatment-Naïve Patients with <u>Compensated Cirrhosis</u>[‡] – Alternative (cont'd)

[‡] <u>For decompensated cirrhosis, please refer to the appropriate section.</u>
[†] Please see statement on FDA <u>warning</u> regarding the use of PrOD or PrO in patients with cirrhosis.
     The dose of daclatasvir may need to increase or decrease when used concomitantly with cytochrome P450 3A/4 inducers and inhibitors, respectively. Please refer to the prescribing information and the section on <u>HIV/HCV coinfection</u> for patients on antiretroviral therapy.
[§] Includes G1a polymorphisms at amino acid positions 28, 30, 31, or 93. <u>Amino acid substitutions that confer resistance</u>.

Genotype 1b Treatment-Naïve Patients Without Cirrhosis – Recommended

Recommended regimens are listed in groups by level of evidence, then alphabetically.

- **Daily fixed-dose combination of elbasvir (50 mg)/grazoprevir (100 mg) for 12 weeks is a recommended regimen for treatment-naïve patients with HCV genotype 1b infection who do not have cirrhosis.**
  Rating: Class I, Level A
- **Daily fixed-dose combination of ledipasvir (90 mg)/sofosbuvir (400 mg) for 12 weeks is a recommended regimen for treatment-naïve patients with HCV genotype 1b infection who do not have cirrhosis.**
  Rating: Class I, Level A
- **Daily fixed-dose combination of paritaprevir (150 mg)/ritonavir (100 mg)/ombitasvir (25 mg) plus twice-daily dosed dasabuvir (250 mg) for 12 weeks is a recommended regimen for treatment-naïve patients with HCV genotype 1b infection who do not have cirrhosis.**
  Rating: Class I, Level A
- **Daily simeprevir (150 mg) plus sofosbuvir (400 mg) for 12 weeks is a recommended regimen for treatment-naïve patients with HCV genotype 1b infection who do not have cirrhosis.**
  Rating: Class I, Level A
- **Daily fixed-dose combination of sofosbuvir (400 mg)/velpatasvir (100 mg) for 12 weeks is a recommended regimen for treatment-naïve patients with HCV genotype 1b infection who do not have cirrhosis.**
  Rating: Class I, Level A
- **Daily daclatasvir (60 mg*) plus sofosbuvir (400 mg) for 12 weeks is a recommended regimen for treatment-naïve patients with HCV genotype 1b infection who do not have cirrhosis.**
  Rating: Class I, Level B

* The dose of daclatasvir may need to increase or decrease when used concomitantly with cytochrome P450 3A/4 inducers and inhibitors, respectively. Please refer to the prescribing information and the section on <u>HIV/HCV coinfection</u> for patients on antiretroviral therapy.

Genotype 1b Treatment-Naïve Patients with <u>Compensated Cirrhosis</u>[‡] – Recommended

Recommended regimens are listed in groups by level of evidence, then alphabetically.

- **Daily fixed-dose combination of elbasvir (50 mg)/grazoprevir (100 mg) for 12 weeks is a recommended regimen for treatment-naïve patients with HCV genotype 1b infection who have <u>compensated cirrhosis</u>.**
  Rating: Class I, Level A

Genotype 1b Treatment-Naïve Patients with <u>Compensated Cirrhosis</u>[‡] – Recommended   (cont'd)

- **Daily fixed-dose combination of ledipasvir (90 mg)/sofosbuvir (400 mg) for 12 weeks is a recommended regimen for treatment-naïve patients with HCV genotype 1b infection who have <u>compensated cirrhosis</u>.**
  Rating: Class I, Level A
- **Daily fixed-dose combination of paritaprevir (150 mg)/ritonavir (100 mg)/ombitasvir (25 mg) plus twice-daily dosed dasabuvir (250 mg) for 12 weeks is a recommended regimen for treatment-naïve patients with HCV genotype 1b infection who have <u>compensated cirrhosis</u>.[†]**
  Rating: Class I, Level A
- **Daily fixed-dose combination of sofosbuvir (400 mg)/velpatasvir (100 mg) for 12 weeks is a recommended regimen for treatment-naïve patients with HCV genotype 1b infection who have compensated cirrhosis.**
  Rating: Class I, Level A

[‡]   <u>For decompensated cirrhosis, please refer to the appropriate section.</u>
[†]   Please see statement on FDA <u>warning</u> regarding the use of PrOD or PrO in patients with cirrhosis.

Genotype 1b Treatment-Naïve Patients with Compensated Cirrhosis[‡] – Alternative

Alternative regimens are listed in groups by level of evidence, then alphabetically.
- **Daily daclatasvir (60 mg*) plus sofosbuvir (400 mg) with or without weight-based ribavirin for 24 weeks is an alternative regimen for treatment-naïve patients with HCV genotype 1b infection who have <u>compensated cirrhosis</u>.**
  Rating: Class IIa, Level B
- **Daily simeprevir (150 mg) plus sofosbuvir (400 mg) with or without weight-based ribavirin for 24 weeks is an alternative regimen for treatment-naïve patients with HCV genotype 1b infection who have <u>compensated cirrhosis</u>.**
  Rating: Class IIa, Level B

[‡]   <u>For decompensated cirrhosis, please refer to the appropriate section.</u>
*   The dose of daclatasvir may need to increase or decrease when used concomitantly with cytochrome P450 3A/4 inducers and inhibitors, respectively. Please refer to the prescribing information and the section on <u>HIV/HCV coinfection</u> for patients on antiretroviral therapy.

Genotype 2 Treatment-Naïve Patients Without Cirrhosis – Recommended

- **Daily fixed-dose combination of sofosbuvir (400 mg)/velpatasvir (100 mg) for 12 weeks is a recommended regimen for treatment-naïve patients with HCV genotype 2 infection who do not have cirrhosis.**
  Rating: Class I, Level A

Genotype 2 Treatment-Naïve Patients Without Cirrhosis – Alternative

- **Daily daclatasvir (60 mg*) plus sofosbuvir (400 mg) for 12 weeks is an alternative regimen for treatment-naïve patients with HCV genotype 2 infection who do not have cirrhosis.**
  Rating: Class IIa, Level B

*   The dose of daclatasvir may need to increase or decrease when used concomitantly with cytochrome P450 3A/4 inducers and inhibitors, respectively. Please refer to the prescribing information and the section on <u>HIV/HCV coinfection</u> for patients on antiretroviral therapy.

Genotype 2 Treatment-Naïve Patients with <u>Compensated Cirrhosis</u>[‡] – Recommended

- **Daily fixed-dose combination of sofosbuvir (400 mg)/velpatasvir (100 mg) for 12 weeks is a recommended regimen for treatment-naïve patients with HCV genotype 2 infection who have <u>compensated cirrhosis</u>.**
  Rating: Class I, Level A

[‡] For decompensated cirrhosis, please refer to the appropriate section.

Genotype 2 Treatment-Naïve Patients with <u>Compensated Cirrhosis</u>[‡] – Alternative

- **Daily daclatasvir (60 mg*) plus sofosbuvir (400 mg) for 16 weeks to 24 weeks is an alternative regimen for treatment-naïve patients with HCV genotype 2 infection who have <u>compensated cirrhosis</u>.**
  Rating: Class IIa, Level B

[‡] For decompensated cirrhosis, please refer to the appropriate section.
* The dose of daclatasvir may need to increase or decrease when used concomitantly with cytochrome P450 3A/4 inducers and inhibitors, respectively. Please refer to the prescribing information and the section on <u>HIV/HCV coinfection</u> for patients on antiretroviral therapy.

Genotype 3 Treatment-Naïve Patients Without Cirrhosis – Recommended

Recommended regimens are listed in groups by level of evidence, then alphabetically.
- **Daily daclatasvir (60 mg*) plus sofosbuvir (400 mg) for 12 weeks is a recommended regimen for treatment-naïve patients with HCV genotype 3 infection who do not have cirrhosis.**
  Rating: Class I, Level A
- **Daily fixed-dose combination of sofosbuvir (400 mg)/velpatasvir (100 mg) for 12 weeks is a recommended regimen for treatment-naïve patients with HCV genotype 3 infection who do not have cirrhosis.**
  Rating: Class I, Level A

* The dose of daclatasvir may need to increase or decrease when used concomitantly with cytochrome P450 3A/4 inducers and inhibitors, respectively. Please refer to the prescribing information and the section on <u>HIV/HCV coinfection</u> for patients on antiretroviral therapy.

Genotype 3 Treatment-Naïve Patients with <u>Compensated Cirrhosis</u>[‡] – Recommended

Recommended regimens are listed in groups by level of evidence, then alphabetically.
- **Daily fixed-dose combination of sofosbuvir (400 mg)/velpatasvir (100 mg) for 12 weeks is a recommended regimen for treatment-naïve patients with HCV genotype 3 infection who have <u>compensated cirrhosis</u>.**
  Rating: Class I, Level A
- **Daily daclatasvir (60 mg*) plus sofosbuvir (400 mg) for 24 weeks with or without weight-based ribavirin is a recommended regimen for treatment-naïve patients with HCV genotype 3 infection who have <u>compensated cirrhosis</u>.[¶]**
  Rating: Class IIa, Level B

[‡] For decompensated cirrhosis, please refer to the appropriate section.
[¶] RAV testing for Y93H is recommended for cirrhotic patients and ribavirin should be included in regimen if present.
* The dose of daclatasvir may need to increase or decrease when used concomitantly with cytochrome P450 3A/4 inducers and inhibitors, respectively. Please refer to the prescribing information and the section on <u>HIV/HCV coinfection</u> for patients on antiretroviral therapy.

Genotype 4 Treatment-Naïve Patients Without Cirrhosis – Recommended

Recommended regimens are listed in groups by level of evidence, then alphabetically.

- **Daily fixed-dose combination of paritaprevir (150 mg)/ritonavir (100 mg)/ombitasvir (25 mg) and weight-based ribavirin for 12 weeks is a recommended regimen for treatment-naïve patients with HCV genotype 4 infection who do not have cirrhosis.**
  Rating: Class I, Level A
- **Daily fixed-dose combination of sofosbuvir (400 mg)/velpatasvir (100 mg) for 12 weeks is a recommended regimen for treatment-naïve patients with HCV genotype 4 infection who do not have <u>cirrhosis</u>.**
  Rating: Class I, Level A
- **Daily fixed-dose combination of elbasvir (50 mg)/grazoprevir (100 mg) for 12 weeks is a recommended regimen for treatment-naïve patients with HCV genotype 4 infection who do not have cirrhosis.**
  Rating: Class IIa, Level B
- **Daily fixed-dose combination of ledipasvir (90 mg)/sofosbuvir (400 mg) for 12 weeks is a recommended regimen for treatment-naïve patients with HCV genotype 4 infection who do not have cirrhosis.**
  Rating: Class IIa, Level B

Genotype 4 Treatment-Naïve Patients with <u>Compensated Cirrhosis</u>[‡] – Recommended

Recommended regimens are listed in groups by level of evidence, then alphabetically.

- **Daily fixed-dose combination of paritaprevir (150 mg)/ritonavir (100 mg)/ombitasvir (25 mg) and weight-based ribavirin for 12 weeks is a recommended regimen for treatment-naïve patients with HCV genotype 4 infection who have <u>compensated cirrhosis</u>.[†]**
  Rating: Class I, Level A
- **Daily fixed-dose combination of sofosbuvir (400 mg)/velpatasvir (100 mg) for 12 weeks is a recommended regimen for treatment-naïve patients with HCV genotype 4 infection who have <u>compensated cirrhosis</u>.**
  Rating: Class I, Level A
- **Daily fixed-dose combination of elbasvir (50 mg)/grazoprevir (100 mg) for 12 weeks is a recommended regimen for treatment-naïve patients with HCV genotype 4 infection who have <u>compensated cirrhosis</u>.**
  Rating: Class IIa, Level B
- **Daily fixed-dose combination of ledipasvir (90 mg)/sofosbuvir (400 mg) for 12 weeks is a recommended regimen for treatment-naïve patients with HCV genotype 4 infection who have <u>compensated cirrhosis</u>.**
  Rating: Class IIa, Level B

[‡]   <u>For decompensated cirrhosis, please refer to the appropriate section.</u>
[†]   Please see statement on FDA <u>warning</u> regarding the use of PrOD or PrO in patients with cirrhosis.

Genotype 5/6 Treatment-Naïve Patients with and Without Cirrhosis – Recommended

- **Daily fixed-dose combination of sofosbuvir (400 mg)/velpatasvir (100 mg) for 12 weeks is a recommended regimen for treatment-naïve patients with HCV genotype 5 or 6 infection regardless of cirrhosis status.**
  Rating: Class I, Level A

> ### Genotype 5/6 Treatment-Naïve Patients with and Without Cirrhosis – Recommended (cont'd)

- **Daily fixed-dose combination of ledipasvir (90 mg)/sofosbuvir (400 mg) for 12 weeks is a recommended regimen for treatment-naïve patients with HCV genotype 5 or 6 infection, regardless of cirrhosis status.**
  Rating: Class II, Level B

American Association for the Study of Liver Diseases, Infectious Diseases Society of America Recommendations for Testing, Managing, and Treating Hepatitis C, last updated July 6, 2016; http://www.hcvguidelines.org/full-report/initial-treatment-box-summary-recommendations-patients-who-are-initiating-therapy-hcv.

Summary of Recommendations for Patients in Whom Previous Treatment Has Failed

> ### Genotype 1a PEG-IFN/Ribavirin Treatment-Experienced Patients Without Cirrhosis – Recommended

Recommended regimens are listed in groups by level of evidence, then alphabetically.
- **Daily fixed-dose combination of elbasvir (50 mg)/grazoprevir (100 mg) for 12 weeks is a recommended regimen for patients with HCV genotype 1a infection who do not have cirrhosis, in whom prior PEG-IFN/ribavirin treatment has failed, and in whom no baseline NS5A RAVs§ for elbasvir are detected.**
  Rating: Class I, Level A
- **Daily fixed-dose combination of ledipasvir (90 mg)/sofosbuvir (400 mg) for 12 weeks is a recommended regimen for patients with HCV genotype 1a infection who do not have cirrhosis, in whom prior PEG-IFN/ribavirin treatment has failed.**
  Rating: Class I, Level A
- **Daily fixed-dose combination of paritaprevir (150 mg)/ritonavir (100 mg)/ombitasvir (25 mg) plus twice-daily dasabuvir (250 mg) and weight-based ribavirin for 12 weeks is a recommended regimen for patients with HCV genotype 1a infection who do not have cirrhosis, in whom prior PEG-IFN/ribavirin treatment has failed.**
  Rating: Class I, Level A
- **Daily simeprevir (150 mg) plus sofosbuvir (400 mg) for 12 weeks is a recommended regimen for patients with HCV genotype 1a infection who do not have cirrhosis, in whom prior PEG-IFN/ribavirin treatment has failed.**
  Rating: Class I, Level A
- **Daily fixed-dose combination of sofosbuvir (400 mg)/velpatasvir (100 mg) for 12 weeks is a recommended regimen for patients with HCV genotype 1a infection who do not have cirrhosis, in whom prior PEG-IFN/ribavirin treatment has failed.**
  Rating: Class I, Level A
- **Daily daclatasvir (60 mg*) plus sofosbuvir (400 mg) for 12 weeks is a recommended regimen for patients with HCV genotype 1a infection who do not have cirrhosis, in whom prior PEG-IFN/ribavirin treatment has failed.**
  Rating: Class I, Level B

§   Includes G1a polymorphisms at amino acid positions 28, 30, 31, or 93. <u>Amino acid substitutions that confer resistance</u>.
*   The dose of daclatasvir may need to increase or decrease when used concomitantly with cytochrome P450 3A/4 inducers and inhibitors, respectively. Please refer to the prescribing information and the section on <u>HIV/HCV coinfection</u> for patients on antiretroviral therapy.

Genotype 1a PEG-IFN/Ribavirin Treatment-Experienced Patients with <u>Compensated Cirrhosis</u>‡ – Recommended (cont'd)

Recommended regimens are listed in groups by level of evidence, then alphabetically.

- **Daily fixed-dose combination of elbasvir (50 mg)/grazoprevir (100 mg) for 12 weeks is a recommended regimen for patients with HCV genotype 1a infection who have <u>compensated cirrhosis</u>, in whom prior PEG-IFN/ribavirin treatment has failed, and in whom no baseline NS5A RAVs§ for elbasvir are detected.**
  Rating: Class I, Level A
- **Daily fixed-dose combination of ledipasvir (90 mg)/sofosbuvir (400 mg) plus weight-based ribavirin for 12 weeks is a recommended regimen for patients with HCV genotype 1a infection who have <u>compensated cirrhosis</u>, in whom prior PEG-IFN/ribavirin treatment has failed.**
  Rating: Class I, Level A
- **Daily fixed-dose combination of sofosbuvir (400 mg)/velpatasvir (100 mg) for 12 weeks is a recommended regimen for patients with HCV genotype 1a infection who have <u>compensated cirrhosis</u>, in whom prior PEG-IFN/ribavirin treatment has failed.**
  Rating: Class I, Level A

‡   <u>For decompensated cirrhosis, please refer to the appropriate section.</u>
§   Includes G1a polymorphisms at amino acid positions 28, 30, 31, or 93. <u>Amino acid substitutions that confer resistance.</u>

Genotype 1a PEG-IFN/Ribavirin Treatment-Experienced Patients Without Cirrhosis – Alternative

- **Daily fixed-dose combination of elbasvir (50 mg)/grazoprevir (100 mg) with weight-based ribavirin for 16 weeks is an alternative regimen for patients with HCV genotype 1a infection who do not have cirrhosis, in whom prior PEG-IFN/ribavirin treatment has failed, and who have baseline NS5A RAVs§ for elbasvir.**
  Rating: Class IIa, Level B

§   Includes G1a polymorphisms at amino acid positions 28, 30, 31, or 93. <u>Amino acid substitutions that confer resistance.</u>

Genotype 1a PEG-IFN/Ribavirin Treatment-Experienced Patients with <u>Compensated Cirrhosis</u>‡ – Alternative

Alternative regimens are listed in groups by level of evidence, then alphabetically.

- **Daily fixed-dose combination of paritaprevir (150 mg)/ritonavir (100 mg)/ombitasvir (25 mg) plus twice-daily dosed dasabuvir (250 mg) and weight-based ribavirin for 24 weeks is an alternative regimen for patients with HCV genotype 1a infection who have <u>compensated cirrhosis</u>, in whom prior PEG-IFN/ribavirin treatment has failed.†**
  Rating: Class I, Level A
- **Daily fixed-dose combination of ledipasvir (90 mg)/sofosbuvir (400 mg) for 24 weeks is an alternative regimen for patients with HCV genotype 1a infection who have <u>compensated cirrhosis</u>, in whom prior PEG-IFN/ribavirin treatment has failed.**
  Rating: Class I, Level A
- **Daily fixed-dose combination of elbasvir (50 mg)/grazoprevir (100 mg) with weight-based ribavirin for 16 weeks is an alternative regimen for patients with HCV**

Genotype 1a PEG-IFN/Ribavirin Treatment-Experienced Patients with <u>Compensated Cirrhosis</u>[‡] – Alternative (cont'd)

genotype 1a infection who have <u>compensated cirrhosis</u>, in whom prior PEG-IFN/ribavirin treatment has failed, and who have baseline NS5A RAVs[§] for elbasvir.
Rating: Class I, Level B

- Daily daclatasvir (60 mg*) plus sofosbuvir (400 mg) with or without weight-based ribavirin for 24 weeks is an alternative regimen for patients with HCV genotype 1a infection who have <u>compensated cirrhosis</u>, in whom prior PEG-IFN/ribavirin treatment has failed.
Rating: Class IIa, Level B

- Daily simeprevir (150 mg) plus sofosbuvir (400 mg) with or without weight-based ribavirin for 24 weeks is an alternative regimen for patients with HCV genotype 1a infection with compensated cirrhosis who are negative for the Q80K variant by commercially available resistance assay, in whom prior PEG-IFN/ribavirin treatment has failed. Other recommended or alternative regimens should be used for patients with <u>compensated cirrhosis</u> and HCV genotype 1a infection in whom the Q80K variant is present.
Rating: Class IIa, Level B

[‡] <u>For decompensated cirrhosis, please refer to the appropriate section.</u>
[†] Please see statement on FDA <u>warning</u> regarding the use of PrOD or PrO in patients with cirrhosis.
[§] Includes G1a polymorphisms at amino acid positions 28, 30, 31, or 93. <u>Amino acid substitutions that confer resistance.</u>
[*] The dose of daclatasvir may need to increase or decrease when used concomitantly with cytochrome P450 3A/4 inducers and inhibitors, respectively. Please refer to the prescribing information and the section on HIV/HCV coinfection for patients on antiretroviral therapy.

Genotype 1b PEG-IFN/Ribavirin Treatment-Experienced Patients Without Cirrhosis – Recommended

Recommended regimens are listed in groups by level of evidence, then alphabetically.

- Daily fixed-dose combination of elbasvir (50 mg)/grazoprevir (100 mg) for 12 weeks is a recommended regimen for patients with HCV genotype 1b infection who do not have cirrhosis, in whom prior PEG-IFN/ribavirin treatment has failed.
Rating: Class I, Level A

- Daily fixed-dose combination of ledipasvir (90 mg)/sofosbuvir (400 mg) for 12 weeks is a recommended regimen for patients with HCV genotype 1b infection who do not have cirrhosis, in whom prior PEG-IFN/ribavirin treatment has failed.
Rating: Class I, Level A

- Daily fixed-dose combination of paritaprevir (150 mg)/ritonavir (100 mg)/ombitasvir (25 mg) plus twice-daily dosed dasabuvir (250 mg) for 12 weeks is a recommended regimen for patients with HCV genotype 1b infection who do not have cirrhosis, in whom prior PEG-IFN/ ribavirin treatment has failed.
Rating: Class I, Level A

- Daily simeprevir (150 mg) plus sofosbuvir (400 mg) for 12 weeks is a recommended regimen for patients with HCV genotype 1b infection who do not have cirrhosis, in whom prior PEG-IFN/ribavirin treatment has failed.
Rating: Class I, Level A

- Daily fixed-dose combination of sofosbuvir (400 mg)/velpatasvir (100 mg) for 12 weeks is a recommended regimen for patients with HCV genotype 1b infection who do not have cirrhosis, in whom prior PEG-IFN/ribavirin treatment has failed.
Rating: Class I, Level A

- **Daily daclatasvir (60 mg*) plus sofosbuvir (400 mg) for 12 weeks is a recommended regimen for patients with HCV genotype 1b infection who do not have cirrhosis, in whom prior PEG-IFN/ribavirin treatment has failed.**
  Rating: Class IIa, Level B

---

* The dose of daclatasvir may need to increase or decrease when used concomitantly with cytochrome P450 3A/4 inducers and inhibitors, respectively. Please refer to the prescribing information and the section on <u>HIV/HCV coinfection</u> for patients on antiretoviral therapy.

Recommended regimens are listed in groups by level of evidence, then alphabetically.
- **Daily fixed-dose combination of elbasvir (50 mg)/grazoprevir (100 mg) for 12 weeks is a recommended regimen for patients with HCV genotype 1b infection who have <u>compensated cirrhosis</u>, in whom prior PEG-IFN/ribavirin treatment has failed.**
  Rating: Class I, Level A
- **Daily fixed-dose combination of ledipasvir (90 mg)/sofosbuvir (400 mg) plus weight-based ribavirin for 12 weeks is a recommended regimen for patients with HCV genotype 1b infection who have <u>compensated cirrhosis</u>, in whom prior PEG-IFN/ribavirin treatment has failed.**
  Rating: Class I, Level A
- **Daily fixed-dose combination of paritaprevir (150 mg)/ritonavir (100 mg)/ombitasvir (25 mg) plus twice-daily dosed dasabuvir (250 mg) for 12 weeks is a recommended regimen for patients with HCV genotype 1b infection who have <u>compensated cirrhosis</u>, in whom prior PEG-IFN/ribavirin treatment has failed.†**
  Rating: Class I, Level A
- **Daily fixed-dose combination of sofosbuvir (400 mg)/velpatasvir (100 mg) for 12 weeks is a recommended regimen for patients with HCV genotype 1b infection who have <u>compensated cirrhosis</u>, in whom prior PEG-IFN/ribavirin treatment has failed.**
  Rating: Class I, Level A

---

‡ <u>For decompensated cirrhosis, please refer to the appropriate section.</u>
† Please see statement on FDA <u>warning</u> regarding the use of PrOD or PrO in patients with cirrhosis.

Alternative regimens are listed in groups by level of evidence, then alphabetically.
- **Daily fixed-dose combination of ledipasvir (90 mg)/sofosbuvir (400 mg) for 24 weeks is an alternative regimen for patients with HCV genotype 1b infection who have <u>compensated cirrhosis</u>, in whom prior PEG-IFN/ribavirin treatment has failed.**
  Rating: Class I, Level A
- **Daily daclatasvir (60 mg*) plus sofosbuvir (400 mg) with or without weight-based ribavirin for 24 weeks is an alternative regimen for patients with HCV genotype 1b infection who have <u>compensated cirrhosis</u>, in whom prior PEG-IFN/ribavirin treatment has failed.**
  Rating: Class IIa, Level B

Genotype 1b PEG-IFN/Ribavirin Treatment-Experienced Patients with <u>Compensated Cirrhosis</u>[‡] – Alternative (cont'd)

- **Daily simeprevir (150 mg) plus sofosbuvir (400 mg) with or without weight-based ribavirin for 24 weeks is an alternative regimen for patients with HCV genotype 1b infection, who have <u>compensated cirrhosis</u>, in whom prior PEG-IFN/ribavirin treatment has failed.**
  Rating: Class IIa, Level B

[‡] For decompensated cirrhosis, please refer to the appropriate section.
The dose of daclatasvir may need to increase or decrease when used concomitantly with cytochrome P450 3A/4 inducers and inhibitors, respectively. Please refer to the prescribing information and the section on <u>HIV/HCV coinfection</u> for patients on antiretroviral therapy.

Genotype 1 Sofosbuvir plus Ribavirin with or Without PEG-IFN Treatment-Experienced Patients – Recommended

- **No cirrhosis:**
  Daily fixed-dose combination of ledipavir (90 mg)/sofosbuvir (400 mg) with weight-based ribavirin for 12 weeks is a recommended regimen for patients with HCV genotype 1 infection, regardless of subtype, who do not have cirrhosis, in whom a previous sofosbuvir plus ribavirin-containing regimen with or without PEG-IFN has failed.
  Rating: Class IIa, Level B
- **<u>Compensated cirrhosis</u>:[‡]**
  Daily fixed-dose combination of ledipasvir (90 mg)/sofosbuvir (400 mg) with weight-based ribavirin for 24 weeks is a recommended regimen for patients with HCV genotype 1 infection, regardless of subtype, who have compensated cirrhosis, in whom a previous sofosbuvir plus ribavirin-containing regimen with or without PEG-IFN has failed.
  Rating: Class IIa, Level B

[‡] <u>For decompensated cirrhosis, please refer to the appropriate section.</u>

Genotype 1 HCV Nonstructural Protein 3 (NS3) Protease Inhibitor (telaprevir, boceprevir, or simeprevir) plus PEG-IFN/Ribavirin Treatment-Experienced Patients Without Cirrhosis – Recommended

Recommended regimens are listed in groups by level of evidence, then alphabetically.
- **Daily fixed-dose combination of ledipasvir (90 mg)/sofosbuvir (400 mg) for 12 weeks is a recommended regimen for patients with HCV genotype 1 infection, regardless of subtype, in whom prior treatment with an HCV protease inhibitor plus PEG-IFN/ribavirin has failed.**
  Rating: Class I, Level A
- **Daily fixed-dose combination of sofosbuvir (400 mg)/velpatasvir (100 mg) for 12 weeks is a recommended regimen for patients with HCV genotype 1 infection, regardless of subtype, who do not have cirrhosis, in whom prior treatment with an HCV protease inhibitor plus PEG-IFN/ribavirin has failed.**
  Rating: Class I, Level A

Genotype 1 HCV Nonstructural Protein 3 (NS3) Protease Inhibitor (telaprevir, boceprevir, or simeprevir) plus PEG-IFN/Ribavirin Treatment-Experienced Patients Without Cirrhosis – Recommended (cont'd)

- **Daily daclatasvir (60 mg*) plus sofosbuvir (400 mg) for 12 weeks is a recommended regimen for patients with HCV genotype 1 infection, regardless of subtype, who do not have cirrhosis, in whom prior treatment with an HCV protease inhibitor plus PEGIFN/ ribavirin has failed.**
  Rating: Class IIa, Level B
- **Daily fixed-dose combination of elbasvir (50 mg)/grazoprevir (100 mg) with weight-based ribavirin for 12 weeks is a recommended regimen for patients with HCV genotype 1 infection, regardless of subtype, who do not have cirrhosis, in whom prior treatment with an HCV protease inhibitor plus PEG-IFN/ribavirin has failed. Genotype 1a patients who have baseline NS5A RAVs[§] for elbasvir should have this treatment extended to 16 weeks.**
  Rating: Class IIa, Level B

  [*] The dose of daclatasvir may need to increase or decrease when used concomitantly with cytochrome P450 3A/4 inducers and inhibitors, respectively. Please refer to the prescribing information and the section on <u>HIV/HCV coinfection</u> for patients on antiretroviral therapy.
  [§] Includes G1a polymorphisms at amino acid positions 28, 30, 31, or 93. <u>Amino acid substitutions that confer resistance.</u>

Genotype 1 HCV Nonstructural Protein 3 (NS3) Protease Inhibitor (telaprevir, boceprevir, or simeprevir) plus PEG-IFN/Ribavirin Treatment-Experienced Patients with <u>Compensated Cirrhosis</u>[‡] – Recommended

Recommended regimens are listed in groups by level of evidence, then alphabetically.
- **Daily fixed-dose combination of ledipasvir (90 mg)/sofosbuvir (400 mg) plus weight-based ribavirin for 12 weeks is a recommended regimen for patients with HCV genotype 1 infection, regardless of subtype, who have <u>compensated cirrhosis</u>, in whom prior treatment with an HCV protease inhibitor plus PEG-IFN/ribavirin has failed.**
  Rating: Class I, Level A
- **Daily fixed-dose combination of ledipasvir (90 mg)/sofosbuvir (400 mg) for 24 weeks is a recommended regimen for patients with HCV genotype 1 infection, regardless of subtype, who have <u>compensated cirrhosis</u>, in whom prior treatment with an HCV protease inhibitor plus PEG-IFN/ribavirin has failed.**
  Rating: Class I, Level A
- **Daily fixed-dose combination of sofosbuvir (400 mg)/velpatasvir (100 mg) for 12 weeks is a recommended regimen for patients with HCV genotype 1 infection, regardless of subtype, who have <u>compensated cirrhosis</u>, in whom prior treatment with an HCV protease inhibitor plus PEG-IFN/ribavirin has failed.**
  Rating: Class I, Level A
- **Daily daclatasvir (60 mg*) plus sofosbuvir (400 mg) with or without weight-based ribavirin for 24 weeks is a recommended regimen for patients with HCV genotype 1 infection, regardless of subtype, who have <u>compensated cirrhosis</u>, in whom prior treatment with an HCV protease inhibitor plus PEG-IFN/ribavirin has failed.**
  Rating: Class IIa, Level B

Genotype 1 HCV Nonstructural Protein 3 (NS3) Protease Inhibitor (telaprevir, boceprevir, or simeprevir) plus PEG-IFN/Ribavirin Treatment-Experienced Patients with <u>Compensated Cirrhosis</u>‡ – Recommended (cont'd)

- **Daily fixed-dose combination of elbasvir (50 mg)/grazoprevir (100 mg) plus weight-based ribavirin for 12 weeks is a recommended regimen for patients with HCV genotype 1 infection, regardless of subtype, who have <u>compensated cirrhosis</u>, in whom a prior treatment with an HCV protease inhibitor plus PEG-IFN/ribavirin has failed. Genotype 1a patients who have baseline NS5A RAVs§ for elbasvir should have this treatment extended to 16 weeks.**
  Rating: Class IIa, Level B

---

‡   <u>For decompensated cirrhosis, please refer to the appropriate section.</u>
*   The dose of daclatasvir may need to increase or decrease when used concomitantly with cytochrome P450 3A/4 inducers and inhibitors, respectively. Please refer to the prescribing information and the section on <u>HIV/HCV coinfection</u> for patients on antiretroviral therapy.
§   Includes G1a polymorphisms at amino acid positions 28, 30, 31, or 93. <u>Amino acid substitutions that confer resistance.</u>

Genotype 1 Simeprevir plus Sofosbuvir Treatment-Experienced Patients – Recommended

---

Recommended regimens are listed in groups by level of evidence, then alphabetically.
- **Deferral of treatment is recommended, pending availability of data, for patients with HCV genotype 1 infection, regardless of subtype, in whom prior treatment with the HCV protease inhibitor simeprevir plus sofosbuvir has failed (no prior NS5A treatment), who do not have cirrhosis, and do not have reasons for urgent retreatment.**
  Rating: Class IIb, Level C
- **Testing for resistance-associated variants that confer decreased susceptibility to NS3 protease inhibitors and to NS5A inhibitors is recommended for patients with HCV genotype 1 infection, regardless of subtype, in whom prior treatment with the HCV protease inhibitor simeprevir plus sofosbuvir has failed (no prior NS5A treatment), who have <u>compensated cirrhosis</u>,‡ or have reasons for urgent retreatment. The specific drugs used in the retreatment regimen should be tailored to the results of this testing as described below.**
  Rating: Class II, Level C
- **When using nucleotide-based (e.g., sofosbuvir) dual direct-acting antiviral (DAA) therapy, a treatment duration of 24 weeks is recommended, and weight-based ribavirin, unless contraindicated, should be added.**
  Rating: Class II, Level C
- **If available, nucleotide-based (e.g., sofosbuvir) triple or quadruple DAA regimens may be considered. In these settings treatment duration ranges from 12 weeks to 24 weeks, and weight-based ribavirin, unless contraindicated, are recommended.**
  Rating: Class II, Level C

---

‡   <u>For decompensated cirrhosis, please refer to the appropriate section.</u>

Genotype 1 HCV NS5A Inhibitor Treatment-Experienced Patients – Recommended

Recommended regimens are listed in groups by level of evidence, then alphabetically.

- **Deferral of treatment is recommended, pending availability of data for patients with HCV genotype 1, regardless of subtype, in whom previous treatment with any HCV nonstructural protein 5A (NS5A) inhibitors has failed, who do not have cirrhosis, and do not have reasons for urgent retreatment.**
  Rating: Class IIb, Level C
- **Testing for resistance-associated variants that confer decreased susceptibility to NS3 protease inhibitors and to NS5A inhibitors is recommended for patients with HCV genotype 1, regardless of subtype, in whom previous treatment with any HCV nonstructural protein 5A (NS5A) inhibitors has failed, and who have <u>compensated cirrhosis</u>‡ or have reasons for urgent retreatment. The specific drugs used in the retreatment regimen should be tailored to the results of this testing as described below.**
  Rating: Class IIb, Level C
- **When using nucleotide-based (e.g., sofosbuvir) dual DAA therapy, a treatment duration of 24 weeks is recommended, and weight-based ribavirin, unless contraindicated, should be added.**
  Rating: Class IIb, Level C
- **If available, nucleotide-based (e.g., sofosbuvir) triple or quadruple DAA regimens may be considered. In these settings treatment duration ranges from 12 weeks to 24 weeks, and weight-based ribavirin, unless contraindicated, are recommended.**
  Rating: Class IIb, Level C

---

‡   <u>For decompensated cirrhosis, please refer to the appropriate section</u>.

Genotype 2 PEG-IFN/Ribavirin Treatment-Experienced Patients Without Cirrhosis – Recommended

- **Daily fixed-dose combination of sofosbuvir (400 mg)/velpatasvir (100 mg) for 12 weeks is a recommended regimen for patients with HCV genotype 2 infection who do not have cirrhosis, in whom prior treatment with PEG-IFN/ribavirin has failed.**
  Rating: Class I, Level A

Genotype 2 PEG-IFN/Ribavirin Treatment-Experienced Patients Without Cirrhosis – Alternative

- **Daily daclatasvir (60 mg*) plus sofosbuvir (400 mg) for 12 weeks is an alternative regimen for patients with HCV genotype 2 infection who do not have cirrhosis, in whom prior treatment with PEG-IFN/ribavirin has failed.**
  Rating: Class IIa, Level B

---

*   The dose of daclatasvir may need to increase or decrease when used concomitantly with cytochrome P450 3A/4 inducers and inhibitors, respectively. Please refer to the prescribing information and the section on <u>HIV/HCV coinfection</u> for patients on antiretroviral therapy.

Genotype 2 PEG-IFN/Ribavirin Treatment-Experienced Patients with <u>Compensated Cirrhosis</u>[‡] – Recommended

- **Daily fixed-dose combination of sofosbuvir (400 mg)/velpatasvir (100 mg) for 12 weeks is a recommended regimen for patients with HCV genotype 2 infection who have <u>compensated cirrhosis</u>, in whom prior treatment with PEG-IFN/ribavirin has failed.**
  Rating: Class I, Level A

[‡] For decompensated cirrhosis, please refer to the appropriate section.

Genotype 2 PEG-IFN/Ribavirin Treatment-Experienced Patients with <u>Compensated Cirrhosis</u>[‡] – Alternative

- **Daily daclatasvir (60 mg*) plus sofosbuvir (400 mg) for 16 weeks to 24 weeks is an alternative regimen for patients with HCV genotype 2 infection who have <u>compensated cirrhosis</u>, in whom prior treatment with PEG-IFN/ribavirin has failed.**
  Rating: Class IIa, Level B

[‡] For decompensated cirrhosis, please refer to the appropriate section.
* The dose of daclatasvir may need to increase or decrease when used concomitantly with cytochrome P450 3A/4 inducers and inhibitors, respectively. Please refer to the prescribing information and the section on <u>HIV/HCV coinfection</u> for patients on antiretroviral therapy.

Genotype 2 Sofosbuvir plus Ribavirin Treatment-Experienced Patients – Recommended

Recommended regimens are listed in groups by level of evidence, then alphabetically.
- **Daily daclatasvir (60 mg*) plus sofosbuvir (400 mg) with or without weight-based ribavirin for 24 weeks is a recommended regimen for patients with HCV genotype 2 infection, regardless of cirrhosis status,[‡] in whom prior treatment with sofosbuvir and ribavirin has failed.**
  Rating: Class IIa, Level C
- **Daily fixed-dose combination of sofosbuvir (400 mg)/velpatasvir (100 mg) with weight-based ribavirin for 12 weeks is a recommended regimen for patients with HCV genotype 2 infection, regardless of cirrhosis status, in whom prior treatment with sofosbuvir and ribavirin has failed.**
  Rating: Class IIa, Level C

[‡] For decompensated cirrhosis, please refer to the appropriate section.
* The dose of daclatasvir may need to increase or decrease when used concomitantly with cytochrome P450 3A/4 inducers and inhibitors, respectively. Please refer to the prescribing information and the section on <u>HIV/HCV coinfection</u> for patients on antiretroviral therapy.

Genotype 3 PEG-IFN/Ribavirin Treatment-Experienced Patients Without Cirrhosis – Recommended

Recommended regimens are listed in groups by level of evidence, then alphabetically.
- **Daily daclatasvir (60 mg*) plus sofosbuvir (400 mg) for 12 weeks is a recommended regimen for patients with HCV genotype 3 infection who do not have cirrhosis, in whom prior treatment with PEG-IFN/ribavirin has failed.[¶]**
  Rating: Class I, Level A

Genotype 3 PEG-IFN/Ribavirin Treatment-Experienced Patients Without Cirrhosis – Recommended (cont'd)

- **Daily fixed-dose combination of sofosbuvir (400 mg)/velpatasvir (100 mg) for 12 weeks is a recommended regimen for patients with HCV genotype 3 infection who do not have cirrhosis, in whom prior treatment with PEG-IFN/ribavirin has failed.¶**
  Rating: Class I, Level A

---

* The dose of daclatasvir may need to increase or decrease when used concomitantly with cytochrome P450 3A/4 inducers and inhibitors, respectively. Please refer to the prescribing information and the section on <u>HIV/HCV coinfection</u> for patients on antiretroviral therapy.

¶ RAV testing for Y93H is recommended and ribavirin should be included in regimen if present.

Genotype 3 PEG-IFN/Ribavirin Treatment-Experienced Patients with <u>Compensated Cirrhosis‡</u> – Recommended

Recommended regimens are listed in groups by level of evidence, then alphabetically.
- **Daily fixed-dose combination of sofosbuvir (400 mg)/velpatasvir (100 mg) with weight-based ribavirin for 12 weeks is a recommended regimen for patients with HCV genotype 3 infection who have <u>compensated cirrhosis</u>, in whom prior treatment with PEG-IFN/ribavirin has failed.**
  Rating: Class I, Level B
- **Daily daclatasvir (60 mg*) plus sofosbuvir (400 mg) with weight-based ribavirin for 24 weeks is a recommended regimen for patients with HCV genotype 3 infection who have <u>compensated cirrhosis</u>, in whom prior treatment with PEG-IFN/ribavirin has failed.**
  Rating: Class IIa, Level B

---

‡ <u>For decompensated cirrhosis, please refer to the appropriate section.</u>
* The dose of daclatasvir may need to increase or decrease when used concomitantly with cytochrome P450 3A/4 inducers and inhibitors, respectively. Please refer to the prescribing information and the section on <u>HIV/HCV coinfection</u> for patients on antiretroviral therapy.

Genotype 3 Sofosbuvir and Ribavirin Treatment-Experienced Patients – Recommended

Recommended regimens are listed in groups by level of evidence, then alphabetically.
- **Daily daclatasvir (60 mg*) plus sofosbuvir (400 mg) with weight-based ribavirin for 24 weeks is a recommended regimen for patients with HCV genotype 3 infection, regardless of cirrhosis status,‡ in whom prior treatment with sofosbuvir and ribavirin has failed.**
  Rating: Class IIa, Level C
- **Daily fixed-dose combination of sofosbuvir (400 mg)/velpatasvir (100 mg) plus weight-based ribavirin for 12 weeks is a recommended regimen for patients with HCV genotype 3 infection, regardless of cirrhosis status,‡ in whom prior therapy with sofosbuvir and ribavirin has failed.**
  Rating: Class IIa, Level C

---

‡ <u>For decompensated cirrhosis, please refer to the appropriate section.</u>
* The dose of daclatasvir may need to increase or decrease when used concomitantly with cytochrome P450 3A/4 inducers and inhibitors, respectively. Please refer to the prescribing information and the section on <u>HIV/HCV coinfection</u> for patients on antiretroviral therapy.

Genotype 4 PEG-IFN/Ribavirin Treatment-Experienced Patients Without Cirrhosis –
Recommended

Recommended regimens are listed in groups by level of evidence, then alphabetically.

- **Daily fixed-dose combination of paritaprevir (150 mg)/ritonavir (100 mg)/ombitasvir (25 mg) (PrO) and weight-based ribavirin for 12 weeks is a recommended regimen for patients with HCV genotype 4 infection who do not have cirrhosis, in whom prior treatment with PEG-IFN/ribavirin has failed.**
  Rating: Class I, Level A
- **Daily fixed-dose combination of sofosbuvir (400 mg)/velpatasvir (100 mg) for 12 weeks is a recommended regimen for patients with HCV genotype 4 infection who do not have cirrhosis, in whom prior treatment with PEG-IFN/ribavirin has failed.**
  Rating: Class I, Level A
- **Daily fixed-dose combination of elbasvir (50 mg)/grazoprevir (100 mg) for 12 weeks is a recommended regimen for patients who have HCV genotype 4 infection who do not have cirrhosis, who experienced virologic relapse after prior PEG-IFN/ribavirin therapy. Genotype 4 patients with prior on-treatment virologic failure (failure to suppress or breakthrough) while on PEG-IFN/ribavirin should be treated for 16 weeks and have weight-based ribavirin added to the treatment regimen.**
  Rating: Class IIa, Level B
- **Daily fixed-dose combination of ledipasvir (90 mg)/sofosbuvir (400 mg) for 12 weeks is a recommended regimen for patients with HCV genotype 4 infection who do not have cirrhosis, in whom prior treatment with PEG-IFN/ribavirin treatment has failed.**
  Rating: Class IIa, Level B

Genotype 4 PEG-IFN/Ribavirin Treatment-Experienced Patients with _Compensated_
Cirrhosis[†] – Recommended

Recommended regimens are listed in groups by level of evidence, then alphabetically.

- **Daily fixed-dose combination of paritaprevir (150 mg)/ritonavir (100 mg)/ombitasvir (25 mg) (PrO) and weight-based ribavirin for 12 weeks is a recommended regimen for patients with HCV genotype 4 infection who have _compensated cirrhosis_, in whom prior treatment with PEG-IFN/ribavirin has failed.[†]**
  Rating: Class I, Level A
- **Daily fixed-dose combination of sofosbuvir (400 mg)/velpatasvir (100 mg) for 12 weeks is a recommended regimen for patients with HCV genotype 4 infection who have _compensated cirrhosis_, in whom prior treatment with PEG-IFN/ribavirin has failed.**
  Rating: Class I, Level A
- **Daily fixed-dose combination of elbasvir (50 mg)/grazoprevir (100 mg) for 12 weeks is a recommended regimen for patients who have HCV genotype 4 infection who have _compensated cirrhosis_, and who experienced virologic relapse after prior PEG-IFN/ribavirin therapy. Genotype 4 patients with prior on-treatment virologic failure (failure to suppress or breakthrough) while on PEG-IFN/ribavirin should be treated for 16 weeks and have weight-based ribavirin added to the treatment regimen.**
  Rating: Class IIa, Level B
- **Daily ledipasvir (90 mg)/sofosbuvir (400 mg) and weight-based ribavirin for 12 weeks is a recommended regimen for patients with HCV genotype 4 infection who have _compensated cirrhosis_, in whom prior treatment with PEG-IFN/ribavirin has failed, and who are eligible for ribavirin.**
  Rating: Class IIa, Level B

Genotype 4 PEG-IFN/Ribavirin Treatment-Experienced Patients with _Compensated Cirrhosis_[‡] – Recommended (cont'd)

[‡]   For decompensated cirrhosis, please refer to the appropriate section.
[†]   Please see statement on FDA <u>warning</u> regarding the use of PrOD or PrO in patients with cirrhosis.

Genotype 4 PEG-IFN/Ribavirin Treatment-Experienced Patients with _Compensated Cirrhosis_[‡] – Alternative

---

- **Daily fixed-dose combination of ledipasvir (90 mg)/sofosbuvir (400 mg) for 24 weeks is an alternative regimen for patients with HCV genotype 4 infection who have <u>compensated cirrhosis</u>, in whom prior treatment with PEG-IFN/ribavirin has failed.**
  Rating: Class IIa, Level B

[‡]   For decompensated cirrhosis, please refer to the appropriate section.

Genotype 5 or 6 PEG-IFN/Ribavirin Treatment-Experienced Patients with or Without Cirrhosis – Recommended

---

Recommended regimens are listed in groups by level of evidence, then alphabetically.
- **Daily fixed-dose combination of sofosbuvir (400 mg)/velpatasvir (100 mg) for 12 weeks is a recommended regimen for patients with HCV genotype 5 or 6 infection regardless of cirrhosis status, in whom prior treatment with PEG-IFN/ribavirin has failed.**
  Rating: Class IIa, Level B

- **Daily fixed-dose combination ledipasvir (90 mg)/sofosbuvir (400 mg) for 12 weeks is a recommended regimen for patients with HCV genotype 5 or 6 infection regardless of cirrhosis status, in whom prior treatment with PEG-IFN/ribavirin has failed.**
  Rating: Class IIa, Level C

Source: American Association for the Study of Liver Diseases, Infectious Diseases Society of America Recommendations for Testing, Managing, and Treating Hepatitis C, last updated July 6, 2016; http://www.hcvguidelines.org/full-report/retreatment-box-summary-recommendations-patients-whom-previous-treatment-has-failed.

Epidemiology: Hepatitis C virus (HCV) infection is transmitted primarily through blood exposure; sexual and perinatal transmission are also possible but less efficient. A notable exception is sexually transmitted HCV among HIV-infected men who have sex with men. Since modes of transmission of HIV and HCV overlap to some extent, there are high rates of HCV coinfection in HIV—an estimated 16% of HIV patients overall, including 80% or more of injected drug users (IDUs) and 5–10% of gay men (Clin Infect Dis. 2002;34:831–7). Genotype 1 accounts for 75% of HCV in the United States. HIV accelerates the progression of chronic HCV infection to cirrhosis, liver failure, and hepatocellular carcinoma (J Infect Dis. 2001;183:1112–5; Clin Infect Dis. 2001;33:562–569). Data are conflicting regarding the independent effect of HCV on HIV disease progression, but several studies have shown a higher rate of antiretroviral therapy-induced hepatotoxicity in those with chronic HCV. In some series, liver failure from HCV is one of the leading causes of death in HIV/HCV coinfected individuals (Clin Infect Dis. 2001;32:492–7).

Clinical Presentation: Persistently elevated liver transaminases; usually asymptomatic. Rarely extrahepatic symptoms or signs (e.g., fatigue, arthralgias, rash consistent with cryoglobulin-induced vasculitis).

Diagnostic Considerations: All HIV-positive patients should be tested for HCV antibody. If the antibody test is negative but the likelihood of HCV infection is high (IDU, unexplained increase in LFTs), obtain an HCV RNA since false-negative antibody tests may occur, especially in advanced HIV disease (J Clin Microbiol. 2000;38:575–7) and since patients with recently-acquired HCV may have a negative HCV antibody due to the window period. Since LFT elevation does not correlate well with underlying HCV activity, other diagnostic strategies are necessary to assess degree of HCV-related liver damage. While liver biopsy is considered the gold standard, most clinicians elect less invasive indirect methods such as fibroelastography (a form of ultrasound that assesses liver stiffness) or algorithms applied to various blood tests (e.g., FibroSure, or AST-to-platelet ratio index). Sexually active men who have sex with men (MSM) are at risk for acquiring HCV; we recommend at least annual screening with HCV antibody for those at risk.

Therapeutic Considerations: Unlike interferon-based therapies, the current interferon-free HCV regimens are just as effective in patients with HIV as they are in those who are HIV negative. The primary challenge is to assess for possible drug interactions with the antiretroviral regimen. If patients are newly diagnosed with HIV/HCV coinfection, an HIV regimen with the fewest possible drug interactions should be selected: TAF/FTC plus DTG, or TAF/FTC plus RAL, or ABC/3TC/DTG. If patients are on other ART regimens and require HCV therapy, close scrutiny for potential drug interactions is essential. A particularly good resource for reviewing interactions is the University of Liverpool Interactions Checker (http://www.hep-druginteractions.org/).

Treatment of hepatitis C and coinfected patients should be reserved for individuals who have stable HIV disease, with virologic suppression, no active HIV related complications, and demonstrated good adherence to therapy and treatment follow-up. HCV therapy should specifically be avoided in those with advanced HIV disease, individuals noncompliant with ART, and patients with other active medical conditions. As HCV therapy is not urgent, HIV treatment should in general be started first.

Once Diagnosis is Established. Recommended evaluations include:

- CBC, INR, renal function, LFTs, albumin
- HCV RNA and genotype
- Hepatitis A and B status, with immunizations done if non-immune. Patients who have chronic HBV (HBSAg positive) should be on HBV therapy prior to HCV treatment, as cases of severe HBV reactivation have occurred during treatment for HCV.
- An accurate list of current medications, with close attention to drug interactions between the HIV regimen and HCV treatments
- Liver fibrosis assessment (usually done with fibroelastography and/or noninvasive blood marker such as APRI, FibroTest, or Fibrosure). If there is evidence of cirrhosis by a non-invasive method, the Child-Turcotte-Pugh (CTP) score should be calculated. HCV regimens that include the protease inhibitors grazoprevir, simeprevir, and paritaprevir should be avoided if the CTP score is 7 or higher.
- Certain regimens may require testing for resistance-associated variants (RAVs). For example, specific RAVS for genotype 1a warrant extending treatment with elbasvir/grazoprevir from 12 to 16 weeks and adding ribavirin.

Choice of Drug Therapy. The full range of recommended options is summarized in the preceding summaries, and updated regularly at www.hcvguidelines.org. Frequently, a specific regimen will be mandated by a patient's insurance plan. However, if there are no restrictions, our preference is to utilize regimen consisting of a single pill daily and, if possible, avoiding the need for ribavirin. The current single pill options include (in order of FDA approval), ledipasvir/sofosbuvir, elbasvir/grazoprevir, and velpatasvir/sofosbuvir. All have demonstrated outstanding efficacy in coinfected patients, with 95% or more cured with 12 weeks of therapy. Velpatasvir/sofosbuvir is preferred for genotypes 2 and 3.

Monitoring. The monitoring plan for HIV/HCV coinfected patients consists of both safety and efficacy evaluations (Table 5.3).

Table 5.3. Monitoring Plan During. Treatment for HCV Infection with Interferon and Ribavirin based treatment duration varies depending on patient characteristics and choice of additional active drug (see Table at start of Hepatitis C section and text for details).

Recommended Monitoring During Antiviral Therapy

- Clinic visits or telephone contact are recommended as clinically indicated during treatment to ensure medication adherence and to monitor for adverse events and potential drug-drug interactions with newly prescribed medications.
- Complete blood count (CBC), creatinine level, calculated glomerular filtration rate (GFR), and hepatic function panel are recommended after 4 weeks of treatment and as clinically indicated. Thyroid-stimulating hormone (TSH) is recommended every 12 weeks for patients receiving IFN. More frequent assessment for drug-related toxic effects (eg, CBC for patients receiving ribavirin) is recommended as clinically indicated. Patients receiving elbasvir/grazoprevir should be monitored with hepatic function panel at 8 weeks (and again at 12 weeks if receiving 16 weeks of treatment).
- A 10-fold increase in alanine aminotransferase (ALT) activity at week 4 should prompt discontinuation of therapy. Any increase in ALT of less than 10-fold at week 4 and accompanied by any weakness, nausea, vomiting, jaundice, or significantly increased bilirubin, alkaline phosphatase, or international normalized ratio, should also prompt discontinuation of therapy. Asymptomatic increases in ALT of less than 10-fold elevated at week 4 should be closely monitored and repeated at week 6 and week 8. If levels remain persistently elevated, consideration should be given to discontinuation of therapy.
  Rating: Class I, Level B
- Quantitative HCV viral load testing is recommended after 4 weeks of therapy and at 12 weeks following completion of therapy. Antiviral drug therapy should NOT be interrupted or discontinued if HCV RNA levels are not performed or available during treatment.
- Quantitative HCV viral load testing can be considered at the end of treatment and 24 weeks or longer following the completion of therapy.
  Rating: Class I, Level B
- Patients with compensated cirrhosis[‡] who are receiving paritaprevir/ritonavir-based regimens should be assessed for clinical signs of decompensated liver disease (eg, ascites, encephalopathy) and for biochemical evidence of liver injury with a hepatic function panel at week 2 and week 4 of treatment, and as needed during the remainder of treatment. Paritaprevir/ritonavir-based regimens should be discontinued if patients develop ascites or encephalopathy or a significant increase in direct bilirubin or ALT or AST.
  Rating: Class I, Level A

Modified from Brown et al. Clinician's Guide to HIV/HCV Coinfection. 2004.

Recommended Monitoring During Antiviral Therapy (cont'd)

- For HBsAg+ patients who are not already on HBV suppressive therapy, monitoring of HBV DNA levels during and immediately after DAA therapy for HCV is recommended and antiviral treatment for HBV should be given if treatment criteria for HBV are met.
  Rating: Class IIa, Level B

An undetectable HCV RNA at week 12 posttreatment is the current standard for assessing a "sustained virologic response" (SVR), which can be equated with cure. Importantly, patients cured of HCV are susceptible to reacquisition and should be cautioned about resuming high-risk behavior.

Herpes Simplex Virus (HSV) Disease

Preferred Therapy, Duration of Therapy, Chronic Maintenance	Alternate Therapy	Other Options/Issues
Preferred therapy for orolabial lesions and initial or recurrent genital HSV Valacyclovir 1 g PO bid, famciclovir 500 mg PO bid, or acyclovir 400 mg PO tid Duration of therapy: Orolabial HSV: 5–10 days Genital HSV: 5–14 days Preferred therapy for severe mucocutaneous HSV infections Initial therapy acyclovir 5 mg/kg IV q8h After lesions began to regress, change to PO therapy as above. Continue therapy until lesions have completely healed.		
Preferred therapy for acyclovir-resistant mucocutaneous HSV infections Foscarnet 80–120 mg/kg/day IV in 2–3 divided doses until clinical response	Alternative therapy for acyclovir-resistant mucocutaneous HSV infections IV cidofovir (dosage as in CMV retinitis) or Topical trifluridine or Topical cidofovir or Topical imiquimod	Patients with HSV infections can be treated with episodic therapy when symptomatic lesions occur, or with daily suppressive therapy to prevent recurrences. Topical formulations of neither trifluridine nor cidofovir are commercially available in the US.

Herpes Simplex Virus (HSV) Disease (*cont'd*)

Preferred Therapy, Duration of Therapy, Chronic Maintenance	Alternate Therapy	Other Options/Issues
Suppressive therapy (For patients with frequent or severe recurrences of genital herpes) Valacyclovir 500 mg PO bid Famciclovir 500 mg PO bid Acyclovir 400 mg PO bid Continue indefinitely regardless of CD4+ cell count.	Duration of therapy: 21–28 days or longer	Extemporaneous compounding of topical products can be prepared using trifluridine ophthalmic solution and the intravenous formulation of cidofovir

Herpes Simplex (genital/oral)
Clinical Presentation: Painful, grouped vesicles on an erythematous base that rupture, crust, and heal within 2 weeks. Lesions may be chronic, severe, ulcerative with advanced immunosuppression.
Diagnostic Considerations: Diagnosis by viral culture of swab from lesion base/roof of blister; alternative diagnostic techniques include Tzanck prep or immunofluorescence staining.
Pitfalls: Acyclovir prophylaxis is not required in patients receiving ganciclovir or foscarnet.
Therapeutic Considerations: In refractory cases, consider acyclovir resistance and treat with foscarnet. Topical trifluridine ophthalmic solution (Viroptic 1%) may be considered for direct application to small, localized areas of refractory disease; clean with hydrogen peroxide, then debride lightly with gauze, apply trifluridine, and cover with bacitracin/polymyxin ointment and nonadsorbent gauze; topical cidofovir (requires compounding) also may be tried. Chronic suppressive therapy with oral acyclovir, famciclovir, or valacyclovir may be indicated for patients with frequent recurrences, dosing similar to HIV-negative patients.
Prognosis: Responds well to treatment except in severely immunocompromised patients, in whom acyclovir resistance may develop.

Herpes Encephalitis (HSV-1)
Clinical Presentation: Acute onset of fever and change in mental status.
Diagnostic Considerations: EEG is abnormal early (< 72 hours), showing unilateral temporal lobe abnormalities. Brain MRI is abnormal before CT scan, which may require several days before a temporal lobe focus is seen. Definitive diagnosis is by CSF PCR for HSV-1 DNA. Profound decrease in sensorium is characteristic of HSV meningoencephalitis. CSF may have PMN predominance and low glucose levels, unlike other viral causes of meningitis. A different clinical entity is HSV meningitis, which is usually associated with HSV-2 and can recur with lymphocytic meningitis. HSV encephalitis is surprisingly rare in HIV patients, but when it occurs, residual neurologic deficits are common; by contrast, HSV meningitis (usually in association with genital HSV outbreaks) has an excellent prognosis.
Pitfalls: Rule out non infectious causes of encephalopathy. Surprisingly, HSV encephalitis is a relatively rare cause of encephalitis in patients with HIV.
Therapeutic Considerations: Treat as soon as possible since neurological deficits may be mild and reversible early on, but severe and irreversible later.
Prognosis: Related to extent of brain injury and early antiviral therapy.

HHV-8 Infection*

Preferred Therapy, Duration of Therapy, Chronic Maintenance	Alternate Therapy	Other Options/Issues
Initiation or optimization of ART should be done for all patients with KS, PEL, or MCD. Preferred therapy for visceral KS, disseminated cutaneous KS, and PEL Chemotherapy + ART Oral valganciclovir or IV ganciclovir might be useful as adjunctive therapy in PEL. Preferred therapy for MCD Valganciclovir 900 mg PO bid for 3 weeks <div align="center">**or**</div>Ganciclovir 5 mg/kg IV q12h for 3 weeks <div align="center">**or**</div>Valganciclovir 900 mg PO bid + zidovudine 600 mg PO q6h for 7–21 days	Alternative therapy for MCD Rituximab, 375 mg/m² given weekly × 4–8 weeks, may be an alternative to or used adjunctively with antiviral therapy.	Patients who receive rituximab for MCD may experience subsequent exacerbation or emergence of KS.

* KS = Kaposi's sarcoma; PEL = primary effusion lymphoma; MDC = multicentric Castleman's disease.

Histoplasma capsulatum

Preferred Therapy, Duration of Therapy, Chronic Maintenance	Alternate Therapy	Other Options/Issues
Preferred therapy for moderately severe to severe disseminated disease *Induction therapy* (for 2 weeks or until clinically improved) Liposomal amphotericin B at 3 mg/kg IV daily Maintenance therapy Itraconazole 200 mg PO TID for 3 days, then BID Preferred therapy for less severe disseminated disease *Induction and maintenance therapy*	Alternative therapy moderately severe to severe disseminated disease *Induction therapy* (for 2 weeks or until clinically improved) Amphotericin B lipid complex 3 mg/kg IV daily <div align="center">**or**</div>Amphotericin B cholesteryl sulfate complete 3 mg/kg IV daily Alternatives to itraconazole for maintenance therapy or treatment of less severe disease	Itraconazole, posaconazole, and voriconazole may have significant interactions with certain ARV agents. These interactions are complex and can be bi-directional. Refer to Table 5, Guidelines for Prevention and Treatment of Opportunistic Infections in HIV-Infected Adults and Adolescents; http://aidsinfo.nih.gov/contentfiles/lvguidelines/AdultOITablesOnly.pdf for dosing recommendations.

Histoplasma capsulatum (cont'd)

Preferred Therapy, Duration of Therapy, Chronic Maintenance	Alternate Therapy	Other Options/Issues
Itraconazole 200 mg PO tid for 3 days, then 200 mg PO bid Duration of therapy: at least 12 months	Voriconazole 400 mg PO bid for 1 day, then 200 mg bid **or**	Therapeutic drug monitoring and dosage adjustment may be necessary to ensure triazole antifungal and ARV efficacy and reduce concentration-related toxicities.
<u>Preferred therapy for meningitis</u> *Induction therapy (4–6 weeks)* Liposomal amphotericin B 5 mg/kg/day *Maintenance therapy* Itraconazole 200 mg PO bid to tid for ≥ 1 year and until resolution of abnormal CSF findings <u>Preferred therapy for long-term suppression therapy</u> In patients with severe disseminated or CNS infection and in patients who relapse despite appropriate therapy Itraconazole 200 mg PO daily	Posaconazole 400 mg PO bid Fluconazole 800 mg PO daily <u>Meningitis</u> No alternative therapy recommendation <u>Long-term suppression therapy</u> Fluconazole 400 mg PO daily	Random serum concentrations of itraconazole + hydroxyitraconazole should be > 1 µg/mL Clinical experience with voriconazole or posaconazole in is limited. Acute pulmonary histoplasmosis in HIV-infected patients with CD4+ count > 300 cells/µL should be managed as non-immunocompromised host.

Clinical Presentation: Two general forms: Mild disease with fever/lymph node enlargement (e.g., cervical adenitis), or severe disease with fever, wasting—also may have diarrhea/meningitis/GI ulcerations.

Diagnostic Considerations: Diagnosis by urine/serum histoplasmosis antigen, sometimes by culture of bone marrow/liver or isolator blood cultures. May occur in patients months to years after having lived/moved from an endemic area.

Pitfalls: Relapse is common after discontinuation of therapy in patients with advanced immunosuppression. Cultures may take 7–21 days to turn positive. Itraconazole has many drug-drug interactions with antiretrovirals, especially PIs.

Therapeutic Considerations: Initial therapy depends on severity of illness on presentation. Extremely sick patients should be started on amphotericin B deoxycholate, with duration of IV therapy dependent on response to treatment. Mildly ill patients can be started on itraconazole. Regardless of disease severity, itraconazole levels should be obtained to ensure adequate absorption. Serum concentrations of itraconazole + hydroxyitraconazole should be > 1 µg/mL. All patients require chronic suppressive therapy, with discontinuation for immune reconstitution with CD4 counts > 100/mm^3 for at least 6 months. HIV patients with CD4 > 500/mm^3 and acute pulmonary histoplasmosis might not require therapy, but a short course of itraconazole (4–8 weeks) is reasonable to prevent systemic spread.

Prognosis: Usually responds to treatment, except in fulminant cases.

Human Papillomavirus (HPV) Disease (see also sections on Cervical and Anal Cancer)

Preferred Therapy, Duration of Therapy, Chronic Maintenance	Alternate Therapy	Other Options/Issues
Treatment of condyloma acuminata (genital warts)		
Patient-applied therapy Podofilox 0.5% solution or 0.5% gel—apply to all lesions bid × 3 consecutive days, followed by 4 days of no therapy, repeat weekly for up to 4 cycles **or** Imiquimod 5% cream—apply to lesion at bedtime and remove in the morning on 3 nonconsecutive nights weekly for up to 16 weeks. Each treatment should be washed with soap and water 6–10 hours after application. **or** Sinecatechins 15% ointment—apply to affected areas tid for up to 16 weeks, until warts are completely cleared and not visible.	Provider-applied therapy Cryotherapy (liquid nitrogen or cryoprobe)—apply until each lesion is thoroughly frozen; repeat every 1–2 weeks. Some providers allow the lesion to thaw, then freeze a second time in each session. **or** Trichloroacetic acid or bichloroacetic acid cauterization—80%–90% aqueous solution, apply to each lesion, repeat weekly for up to 6 weeks until lesions are no longer visible. **or** Surgical excision or laser surgery to external or anal warts. **or** Podophyllin resin 10%–25% suspension in tincture of benzoin—apply to all lesions (up to 10 cm^2), then wash off a few hours later, repeat weekly for up to 6 weeks until lesions are no longer visible.	HIV-infected patients may have larger or more numerous warts and may not respond as well to therapy for genital warts when compared to HIV-uninfected individuals. Topical cidofovir has activity against genital warts, but the product is not commercially available. Intralesional interferon-alpha is usually not recommended because of high cost, difficult administration, and potential for systemic side effects. The rate of recurrence of genital warts is high, despite treatment. There is no consensus on the treatment of oral warts. Many treatments for anogenital warts cannot be used in the oral mucosa. Surgery is the most common treatment for oral warts that interfere with function or for aesthetic reasons.

Genital/Perianal Warts (Condyloma Acuminata)
Clinical Presentation: Single/multiple verrucous genital lesions ± pigmentation usually without inguinal adenopathy.
Diagnostic Considerations: Diagnosis by clinical appearance. Genital warts are usually caused by HPV types 11 and 16. Anogenital warts caused by HPV types 16, 18, 31, 33, and 35 are associated with cervical neoplasia.

Pitfalls: Post HPV infections are asymptomatic.
Therapeutic Considerations: First-line therapy is ablative (cryotherapy or cauterization); if no response to standard treatment, attempt to treat with surgery or cidofovir. Intralesional interferon-alfa generally is not recommended.
Prognosis: The rate of recurrence of anogenital warts is high despite treatment.

Isospora belli Infection

Preferred Therapy, Duration of Therapy, Chronic Maintenance	Alternate Therapy	Other Options/Issues
Preferred therapy for acute infection: TMP-SMX (160 mg/800 mg) PO (or IV) qid for 10 days **or** TMP-SMX (160 mg/800 mg) PO (or IV) bid for 7–10 days Can start with bid dosing first and increase daily dose and/or duration (up to 3–4 weeks) if symptoms worsen or persist. IV therapy may be used for patients with potential or documented malabsorption. Preferred chronic maintenance therapy (secondary prophylaxis) In patients with CD4+ count < 200/μL, TMP-SMX (160 mg/800 mg) PO tiw	Alternative therapy for acute infection Pyrimethamine 50–75 mg PO daily plus leucovorin 10–25 mg PO daily **or** Ciprofloxacin 500 mg PO bid × 7 days as a second-line alternative Alternative chronic maintenance therapy (secondary prophylaxis) TMP-SMX (160 mg/800 mg) PO daily or (320 mg/1600 mg) tiw **or** Pyrimethamine 25 mg PO daily + leucovorin 5–10 mg PO daily **or** Ciprofloxacin 500 mg tiw as a second-line alternative	Fluid and electrolyte management in patients with dehydration. Nutritional supplementation for malnourished patients. Immune reconstitution with ART may result in fewer relapses.

Clinical Presentation: Severe chronic diarrhea without fever/fecal leukocytes.
Diagnostic Considerations: Spore-forming protozoa *(Isospora belli)*. Oocyst on AFB smear of stool larger that cryptosporidium (20–30 microns vs. 4–6 microns). More common in HIV patients from tropical areas. Less common than cryptosporidium or microsporidia. Malabsorption may occur with severe cases. Can be associated with eosinophilia.
Pitfalls: Multiple relapses are possible.
Therapeutic Considerations: Chronic suppressive therapy may be required if CD4 cell count does not increase.
Prognosis: Related to degree of immunosuppression/response to antiretroviral therapy.
Comments: Immune reconstitution with ART results in fewer relapses.

Leishmaniasis, Cutaneous

Preferred Therapy, Duration of Therapy, Chronic Maintenance	Alternate Therapy	Other Options/ Issues
Preferred therapy for acute infection Liposomal amphotericin B 2–4 mg/kg IV daily for × 10 days or interrupted schedule (e.g., 4 mg/kg on days 1–5, 10, 17, 24, 31, 38) to achieve total dose of 20–60 mg/kg **or** Sodium stibogluconate 20 mg/kg IV or IM daily for 3–4 weeks Chronic maintenance therapy May be indicated in immunocompromised patients with multiple relapses.	Alternative therapy for acute infection Oral miltefosine (can be obtained via a treatment IND) **or** Topical paromomycin **or** Intralesional sodium stibogluconate **or** Local heat therapy No data exist for any of these agents in HIV-infected patients; choice and efficacy dependent on species of *Leishmania*.	
Preferred therapy for initial infection Liposomal amphotericin B 2–4 mg/kg IV daily × 10 days or interrupted schedule (e.g., 4 mg/kg on days 1–5, 10, 17, 24, 31, 38) to achieve total dose of 20–60 mg/kg Preferred chronic maintenance therapy (secondary prophylaxis)—especially in patients with CD4+ count < 200 cells/µL Liposomal amphotericin B 4 mg/kg every 2–4 weeks **or** Amphotericin B lipid complex 3 mg/kg every 21 days	Alternative therapy for initial infection Other lipid formulation of amphotericin B, dose and schedule as in preferred therapy **or** Amphotericin B deoxycholate 0.5–1.0 mg/kg IV daily for total dose of 1.5–2.0 g **or** Sodium stibogluconate (pentavalent antimony) 20 mg/kg body weight IV or IM daily for 28 days **or** Miltefosine 100 mg PO daily for 4 weeks (available in the United States under a treatment IND) Alternative chronic maintenance therapy (secondary prophylaxis) Sodium stibogluconate 20 mg/kg IV or IM every 4 weeks	ART should be initiated or optimized. For sodium stibogluconate, contact the CDC Drug Service at (404) 639-3670 or drugservice@ cdc.gov.

Malaria

Preferred Therapy, Duration of Therapy, Chronic Maintenance	Alternate Therapy	Other Options/Issues
Because *Plasmodium falciparum* malaria can progress within hours from mild symptoms or low-grade fever to severe disease or death, all HIV-infected patients with confirmed or suspected *P. falciparum* infection should be hospitalized for evaluation, initiation of treatment, and observation. Treatment recommendations for HIV-infected patients are the same as HIV-uninfected patients. Choice of therapy is guided by the degree of parasitemia, the species of *Plasmodium*, the patient's clinical status, region of infection, and the likely drug susceptibility of the infected species, and can be found at http://www.cdc.gov/malaria.	When suspicion for malaria is low, antimalarial treatment should not be initiated until the diagnosis is confirmed.	For treatment recommendations for specific regions, clinicians should refer to the following web link: http://www.cdc.gov/malaria/ or call the CDC Malaria Hotline: (770) 488-7788: M–F 8 AM–4:30 PM ET, or (770) 488-7100 after hours.

Microsporidiosis

Preferred Therapy, Duration of Therapy, Chronic Maintenance	Alternate Therapy	Other Options/Issues
Initiate or optimize ART; immune restoration to CD4+ count > 100 cells/µL is associated with resolution of symptoms of enteric microsporidiosis. Preferred therapy for gastrointestinal infections caused by *Enterocytozoon bienuesi* Initiate or optimize ART; immune restoration to CD4+ count > 100 cells/µL is associated with resolution of symptoms of enteric microsporidiosis. Manage severe dehydration, malnutrition, and wasting by fluid support and nutritional supplement. Preferred therapy for disseminated (not ocular) and intestinal infection attributed to microsporidia other than *E. bienuesi* and *Vittaforma corneae*	Alternative therapy for gastrointestinal infections caused by *E. bienuesi* Fumagillin 60 mg/day and TNP-470 (a synthetic analog of fumagillin) may be effective, but neither is available in the United States. Nitazoxanide 1000 mg bid with food for 60 days—effects might be minimal for patients with low CD4+ count.	Severe dehydration, malnutrition, and wasting should be managed by fluid support and nutritional supplement. Antimotility agents can be used for diarrhea control if required.

Microsporidiosis (*cont'd*)

Preferred Therapy, Duration of Therapy, Chronic Maintenance	Alternate Therapy	Other Options/Issues
Albendazole 400 mg PO bid, continue until CD4+ count > 200 cells/µL for > 6 months after initiation of ART.		
For ocular infection Topical fumagillin bicylohexylammonium (Fumidil B) 3 mg/mL in saline (fumagillin 70 µg/mL) eye drops—2 drops q2h for 4 days, then 2 drops qid (investigational use only in US) plus albendazole 400 mg PO bid for management of systemic infection Therapy should be continued until resolution of ocular symptoms and CD4 count increase to >200 cells/µL for >6 months in response to ART.	Alternative therapy for disseminated disease Itraconazole 400 mg PO daily plus albendazole 400 mg PO bid for disseminated disease attributed to *Trachipleistophora* or *Anncaliia*.	

Clinical Presentation: Most commonly, intermittent chronic diarrhea without fever/fecal leukocytes; also can disseminate and cause disease in other organs (eyes, lungs).

Diagnostic Considerations: Spore-forming protozoa *(Septata intestinalis, E. bieneusi)*. Diagnosis by modified trichrome or fluorescent antibody stain of stool. Microsporidia can rarely disseminate to sinuses/cornea. Severe malabsorption may occur.

Pitfalls: Microsporidia cannot be detected by routine microscopic examination of stool due to small size.

Therapeutic Considerations: Key to successful resolution is optimizing ART to improve immune function. Albendazole is less effective for *E. bieneusi* than *S. intestinalis*, but speciation is usually not possible. Consider treatment discontinuation for CD4 > 200/mm^3 if patient remains asymptomatic (no signs or symptoms of microsporidiosis). If ocular infection is present, continue treatment indefinitely.

Prognosis: Related to degree of immunosuppression/response to antiretroviral therapy.

Mycobacterium avium Complex (MAC) Disease

Preferred Therapy, Duration of Therapy, Chronic Maintenance	Alternate Therapy	Other Options /Issues
Preferred therapy for disseminated MAC At least two drugs as initial therapy with Clarithromycin 500 mg PO bid + ethambutol 15 mg/kg PO daily (Azithromycin 500–600 mg + ethambutol 15 mg/kg) PO daily if drug interaction or intolerance precludes the use of clarithromycin Duration: at least 12 months of therapy, can discontinue if no signs and symptoms of MAC disease and sustained (>6 months) CD4+ count > 100 cells/μL in response to ART Chronic maintenance therapy (secondary prophylaxis) Same as treatment drugs and regimens Duration: Lifelong therapy, unless in patients with sustained immune recovery on ART	Alternative therapy for disseminated MAC (e.g., when drug interactions or intolerance precludes the use of clarithromycin) Addition of a third or fourth drug should be considered for patients with advanced immunosuppression (CD4+ count < 50 cells/μL), high mycobacterial loads (> 2 log CFU/mL of blood), or in the absence of effective ART. Options include: Amikacin 10–15 mg/kg IV daily **or** Streptomycin 1 gm IV or IM daily **or** RFB 300 mg PO daily (dosage adjustment may be necessary based on drug interactions) **or** Levofloxacin 500 mg PO daily **or** Moxifloxacin 400 mg PO daily	Testing of susceptibility to clarithromycin and azithromycin is recommended. NSAIDs may be used for patients who experience moderate to severe symptoms attributed to ART-associated immune reconstitution inflammatory syndrome (IRIS). If IRIS symptoms persist, short term (4–8 weeks) of systemic corticosteroid (equivalent to 20–40 mg of prednisone) can be used

Clinical Presentation: Typically presents as a febrile wasting illness in advanced HIV disease (CD4 < 50/mm³). Focal invasive disease is possible, especially in patients with advanced immunosuppression after starting antiretroviral therapy. Focal disease likely reflects restoration of pathogen-specific immune response to existing infection ("immune reconstitution inflammatory syndrome" [IRIS]), and typically manifests as fever with lymphadenitis (mesenteric, cervical, thoracic) or rarely disease in the spine mimicking Pott's disease. Immune reconstitution syndrome usually occurs within weeks to months after starting antiretroviral therapy for the first time, but may occur a year or more later.

Diagnostic Considerations: Diagnosis by isolation of organism from a normally sterile body site (blood, lymph node, bone marrow, liver biopsy). Lysis centrifugation (DuPont isolator) is the preferred blood culture method. Anemia and elevated alkaline phosphatase are often seen as laboratory manifestations, reflecting possible liver and bone marrow involvement, respectively.

Pitfalls: Isolator blood cultures may be negative, especially in immune reconstitution inflammatory syndrome initially.

Therapeutic Considerations: Some studies suggest benefit for addition of rifabutin 300 mg (PO) QD, others do not. Rifabutin may require dosage adjustment with NNRTIs and PIs (see p. 126). Monitor carefully for rifabutin drug toxicity (arthralgias, uveitis, leukopenia). Treat IRIS initially with NSAIDs; if symptoms persist, systemic corticosteroids (prednisone 20–40 mg daily) for 4–8 weeks can be used. Some patients will require a more prolonged course of corticosteroids with a slow taper over months. Azithromycin is often better tolerated than clarithromycin and has fewer drug interactions. Optimal long-term management is unknown, though most studies suggest that treatment can be discontinued in asymptomatic patients with > 12 months of therapy and CD4 > 100/mm³ for > 6 months.

Prognosis: Depends on immune reconstitution in response to antiretroviral therapy. Adverse prognostic factors include high-grade bacteremia or severe wasting.

Mycobacterium tuberculosis (TB)

Preferred Therapy, Duration of Therapy, Chronic Maintenance	Alternate Therapy	Other Options /Issues
After collecting specimen for culture and molecular diagnostic tests, empiric treatment should be initiated and continued in HIV-infected individuals with clinical and radiographic presentation suggestive of TB. **Treatment of drug-susceptible active TB disease** <u>Initial phase (2 months)</u> Isoniazid (INH)† + [rifampin (RIF) or rifabutin (RFB)] + pyrazinamide (PZA) + ethambutol (EMB) <u>Continuation phase</u> INH + (RIF or RFB) daily (5–7 times/ week) or tiw	**Treatment for drug-resistant active TB** Resistant to INH (RIF or RFB) + EMB + PZA + (moxifloxacin or levofloxacin) for 2 months; followed by (RIF or RFB) + EMB + (moxifloxacin or levofloxacin) for 7 months	Adjunctive corticosteroid improves survival for TB meningitis and pericarditis. See text for drug, dose, and duration recommendations. RIF is not recommended for patients receiving HIV PI because of its induction of PI metabolism. RFB is a less potent CYP3A4 inducer than RIF and is preferred in patients receiving PIs. Once weekly rifapentine can result in development of rifamycin resistance in HIV- infected patients and is not recommended.

Mycobacterium tuberculosis (TB) (*cont'd*)

Preferred Therapy, Duration of Therapy, Chronic Maintenance	Alternate Therapy	Other Options /Issues
Total duration of therapy (for drug-susceptible TB) Pulmonary TB: 6 months Pulmonary TB and culture-positive after 2 months of TB treatment: 9 months Extra pulmonary TB w/CNS infection: 9–12 months Extra pulmonary TB w/bone or joint involvement: 6 to 9 months Extra-pulmonary TB in other sites: 6 months Total duration of therapy should be based on number of doses received, not on calendar time.	Resistant to rifamycins +/– other drugs Regimen and duration of treatment should be individualized based on resistance pattern, clinical and microbiological responses, and in close consultation with experienced specialists.	Therapeutic drug monitoring should be considered in patients receiving rifamycin and interacting ART. Paradoxical IRIS that is not severe can be treated with NSAIDs without a change in TB or HIV therapy. For severe IRIS reaction, consider prednisone and taper over 4 weeks based on clinical symptoms. For example: If receiving RIF: prednisone 1.5 mg/kg/day for 2 weeks, then 0.75 mg/kg/day for 2 weeks. If receiving RFB: prednisone 1.0 mg/kg/day for 2 weeks, then 0.5 mg/kg/day for 2 weeks. A more gradual tapering schedule over a few months may be necessary for some patients.

† All patients receiving INH should receive pyridoxine 25–50 mg PO daily.

Clinical Presentation: May present atypically. HIV patients with high (> 500/mm³) CD4 cell counts are more likely to have a typical pulmonary presentation, but patients with advanced HIV disease may have a diffuse interstitial pattern, hilar adenopathy, or a normal chest x-ray. Tuberculin skin testing (TST) and interferon gamma release assays (IGRAs) are helpful if positive, but unreliable if negative due to impaired immune response.

Diagnostic Considerations: In many areas, TB is one of the most common HIV-related respiratory illnesses. In other areas, HIV-related TB occurs infrequently except in immigrants or patients arriving from highly TB endemic areas. Maintain a high Index of suspicion for TB in HIV patients with unexplained fevers/pulmonary infiltrates.

Pitfalls: Extrapulmonary and pulmonary TB often coexist, especially in advanced HIV disease.

Therapeutic Considerations: Treatment by directly observed therapy (DOT) is strongly recommended for all HIV patients. If patients have cavitary disease or either positive sputum cultures or lack of clinical response at 2 months, total duration of therapy should be increased up to 9 months or longer depending on clinical response. For CNS disease (meningitis or mass lesions), corticosteroid should be initiated as early as possible (along with TB treatment) and continued for 6–8 weeks. If hepatic transaminases are elevated (AST ≥ 3 times normal) before treatment initiation, treatment options include: (1) standard therapy with frequent monitoring; (2) rifamycin (rifampin or rifabutin) + EMB + PZA for 6 months; or (3) INH + rifamycin + EMB for 2 months, then INH + rifamycin for 7 months.

Once-weekly rifapentine is not recommended for HIV patients. Non severe immune reconstitution inflammatory syndrome (IRIS) may be treated with nonsteroidal anti-inflammatory drugs (NSAIDs); severe cases should be treated with corticosteroids. In all cases of IRIS, antiretroviral therapy should be continued if possible. Monitor carefully for signs of rifabutin drug toxicity (arthralgias, uveitis, leukopenia). In general, ART regimens should avoid protease inhibitors due to interactions with rifamycins; raltegravir, dolutegravir, or efavirenz (in combination with two NRTIs) would be safer options. The optimal timing of ART in the setting of HIV-related TB has recently been clarified by several pivotal studies. ART should be started within 2 weeks of TB treatment when the CD4 cell count is below 50/µL and by 8 to 12 weeks for those with higher CD4 cell counts. The optimal timing for patients with TB meningitis, regardless of CD4 cell count, is less certain, but ART should be started within the first 2 to 8 weeks of diagnosis.

Prognosis: Usually responds to treatment. Relapse rates are related to the degree of immunosuppression and local risk of re-exposure to TB.

Penicilliosis

Preferred Therapy, Duration of Therapy, Chronic Maintenance	Alternate Therapy	Other Options/Issues
Acute infection in severely ill patients Liposomal amphotericin B 3–5 mg/kg/day IV for 2 weeks; followed by itraconazole 200 mg PO bid for 10 weeks, followed by chronic maintenance therapy (as below)	Acute infection in severely ill patients Voriconazole 6 mg/kg IV q12h for 1 day, then 4 mg/kg IV q12h for at least 3 days, followed by 200 mg PO bid for a maximum of 12 weeks, followed by maintenance therapy For mild disease Voriconazole 400 mg PO bid for 1 day, then 200 mg bid for a maximum of 12 weeks, followed by chronic maintenance therapy	ART should be initiated simultaneously with treatment for penicilliosis to improve treatment outcome. Itraconazole and voriconazole may have significant interactions with certain ARV agents. These interactions are complex and can be bidirectional. Refer to Table 5 in Guidelines for Prevention and Treatment of Opportunistic Infections in HIV-Infected Adults and Adolescents; http://aidsinfo.nih.gov/contentfiles/lvguidelines/AdultOITablesOnly.pdf for dosage recommendations.
Mild disease Itraconazole 200 mg PO bid for 8 weeks followed by chronic maintenance therapy (as below) Chronic maintenance therapy (secondary prophylaxis) Itraconazole 200 mg PO daily		Therapeutic drug monitoring and dosage adjustment may be necessary to ensure triazole antifungal and ARV efficacy and reduce concentration-related toxicities.

Penicilliosis (*Penicillium marneffei*)

Clinical Presentation: Papules, pustules, nodules, ulcers, or abscesses. Mostly seen in advanced HIV/AIDS in residents/visitors of Southeast Asia or southern China.

Diagnostic Considerations: Diagnosis by demonstrating organism by stain/culture in tissue specimen. An early presumptive diagnosis can be made several days before the results of fungal cultures are available by microscopic examination of the Wright-stained samples of skin scrapings, bone marrow aspirate, or lymph-node biopsy specimens. Many intracellular and extracellular basophilic, spherical, oval, and elliptical yeast-like organisms can be seen, some with clear central septation, which is a characteristic feature of *P. marneffei*.

Pitfalls: Lesions commonly become umbilicated and resemble molluscum contagiosum.

Therapeutic Considerations: ART should be administered according to standard of care in the community. Requires lifelong suppressive therapy with itraconazole unless CD4 increases to > 100 for ≥ 6 months in response to ART.

Prognosis: Dependent on degree of immune recovery secondary to ART. Without HIV treatment, prognosis is poor, as most affected patients have advanced immunosuppression.

Pneumocystis Pneumonia (PCP)

Preferred Therapy, Duration of Therapy, Chronic Maintenance	Alternate Therapy	Other Options/Issues
Preferred treatment for moderate to severe PCP Trimethoprim-sulfamethoxazole (TMP-SMX): 15–20 mg TMP and 75–100 mg SMX/kg/day IV administered q6h or q8h; may switch to PO after clinical improvement. Duration of therapy: 21 days	Alternative therapy for moderate to severe PCP Pentamidine 4 mg/kg IV daily infused over ≥ 60 minutes; certain specialists reduce dose to 3 mg/kg IV daily because of toxicities. **or** Primaquine 30 mg (base) PO daily plus (clindamycin 600 mg q6h IV or 900 mg IV q8h) or (clindamycin 300 mg PO q6h or 450 mg PO q8h)	Indications for corticosteroids PaO_2 < 70 mmHg at room air or alveolar-arterial O_2 gradient > 35 mmHg Prednisone doses (beginning as early as possible and within 72 hours of PCP therapy): Days 1–5: 40 mg PO bid Days 6–10: 40 mg PO daily
Preferred treatment for mild to moderate PCP Same daily dose of TMP-SMX as above, administered PO in 3 divided doses **or** TMP-SMX (160 mg/800 mg or DS) 2 tablets PO tid Duration of therapy: 21 days	Alternative therapy for mild-to-moderate PCP Dapsone 100 mg PO daily and TMP 5 mg/kg/day PO tid **or** Primaquine 30 mg (base) PO daily plus (clindamycin 300 mg PO q6h or 450 mg PO q8h) **or**	Days 11–21: 20 mg PO daily IV methylprednisolone can be administered as 75% of prednisone dose. Benefits of corticosteroid if started after 72 hours of treatment is unknown, but a majority of clinicians will use it in patients with moderate to severe PCP.

Pneumocystis Pneumonia (PCP) (cont'd)

Preferred Therapy, Duration of Therapy, Chronic Maintenance	Alternate Therapy	Other Options/Issues
<u>Preferred secondary prophylaxis</u> TMP-SMX (160 mg/800 mg or DS) 1 tablet PO daily **or** TMP-SMX (80 mg/400 mg or SS) 1 tablet PO daily	Atovaquone 750 mg PO bid with food <u>Secondary prophylaxis, after completion of PCP treatment</u> TMP-SMX (160 mg/800 mg or DS) 1 tablet PO tiw **or** Dapsone 100 mg PO daily **or** Dapsone 50 mg PO daily + pyrimethamine 50 mg PO weekly + leucovorin 25 mg PO weekly **or** Dapsone 200 mg PO + pyrimethamine 75 mg PO + leucovorin 25 mg PO weekly **or** Aerosolized pentamidine 300 mg every month via Respirgard II™ nebulizer **or** Atovaquone 1500 mg PO daily **or** Atovaquone 1500 mg + pyrimethamine 25 mg + leucovorin 10 mg, each PO daily	Whenever possible, patients should be tested for G6PD deficiency before use of dapsone or primaquine. Alternative therapy should be used in patients found to have G6PD deficiency. Patients who are receivingpyrimethamine/ sulfadiazine for treatment or suppression of toxoplasmosis do not require additional PCP prophylaxis. If TMP-SMX is discontinued because of a mild adverse reaction, reinstitution should be considered after the reaction resolves. The dose can be increased gradually (desensitization), reduced, or the frequency modified. TMP-SMX should be permanently discontinued in patients with possible or definite Stevens-Johnson syndrome or toxicepidermal necrosis.

Clinical Presentation: Fever, cough, dyspnea; often indolent presentation. Physical exam is usually normal. Chest x-ray is variable, but commonly shows a diffuse interstitial pattern. Elevated LDH and exercise desaturation are highly suggestive of PCP.

Diagnostic Considerations: Definitive diagnosis is made by observing the organism on stained specimens of respiratory secretions, obtained by induced sputum or bronchoscopy. Check arterial blood gas (ABG) if O_2 saturation is abnormal or respiratory rate is increased. Serum 1, 3 beta-glucan is usually elevated and may provide additional supportive evidence for the diagnosis of PCP (Clin Infect Dis. 2011 Jul 15;53(2):197–202). PCR of bronchoalveolar lavage fluid is highly sensitive, but may be positive in some patients without clinical disease.

Pitfalls: Slight worsening of symptoms is common after starting therapy, especially if not treated with steroids. Benefits of corticosteroid if started after 72 hours of treatment is unknown, but majority of clinicians will still use it if clinically warranted even after 72 hours. Do not overlook superimposed bacterial pneumonia or other secondary infections, especially in patients with severely depleted CD4 cell counts. Patients receiving second-line agents for PCP prophylaxis—in particular aerosolized pentamidine—may present with atypical radiographic findings, including apical infiltrates, multiple small-walled cysts, pleural effusions, pneumothorax, or single/multiple nodules.

Therapeutic Considerations: Outpatient therapy is possible for mild-moderate disease, but only when close follow-up is assured. Adverse reactions to TMP-SMX (rash, fever, GI symptoms, hepatitis, hyperkalemia, leukopenia, hemolytic anemia) occur in 25–50% of patients, many of whom will need a second-line regimen to complete therapy (e.g., trimethoprim-dapsone or atovaquone). Unless an adverse reaction to TMP-SMX is particularly severe (e.g., Stevens-Johnson syndrome or other life-threatening problem), TMP-SMX may later be considered for PCP prophylaxis, since prophylaxis requires a much lower dose (only 10–15% of treatment dose). Patients being treated for severe PCP with TMP-SMX who do not improve after 1 week may be switched to clindamycin plus primaquine (preferred) or pentamidine. In general, patients receiving antiretroviral therapy when PCP develops should have their treatment continued, since intermittent antiretroviral therapy can lead to drug resistance. For newly diagnosed or antiretroviral-naïve HIV patients, antiretroviral therapy should be started as soon as feasible, preferably within 2 weeks. Steroids should be tapered, not discontinued abruptly. Adjunctive steroids increase the risk of thrush/herpes simplex infection, but probably not CMV, TB, or disseminated fungal infection. Patients should be tested for G6PD deficiency prior to use of primaquine and dapsone.

Prognosis: Usually responds to treatment. Adverse prognostic factors include high A-a gradient, hypoxemia, high LDH.

Progressive Multifocal Leukoencephalopathy (PML)

Preferred Therapy, Duration of Therapy, Chronic Maintenance	Alternate Therapy	Other Options/Issues
There is no specific antiviral therapy for JC virus infection. The main treatment approach is to reverse the immunosuppression caused by HIV. Initiate antiretroviral therapy in ART-naïve patients Optimize ART in patients who develop PML in phase of HIV viremia on antiretroviral therapy.		Corticosteroids may be used for PML-IRIS characterized by contrast enhancement, edema or mass effect, and with clinical deterioration

Clinical Presentation: Hemiparesis, ataxia, aphasia, other focal neurologic defects, which may progress over weeks to months. Usually alert without headache or seizures on presentation.

Diagnostic Considerations: Demyelinating disease caused by reactivation of the latent papovavirus JC virus. Diagnosis by clinical presentation and MRI showing patchy demyelination of white matter, usually without enhancement. Any region of the CNS may be involved, most commonly the occipital lobes (with hemianopia), frontal and parietal lobes (hemiparesis and hemisensory deficits), and cerebellar peduncles and deep white matter (dysmetria and ataxia). JC virus PCR of CSF is useful for non invasive diagnosis. In confusing or atypical presentation, biopsy may be needed to distinguish PML from other opportunistic infections, CNS lymphoma, or HIV encephalitis/encephalopathy.

Pitfalls: Primary HIV-related encephalopathy may have a similar appearance on MRI.

Therapeutic Considerations: The only effective therapy is antiretroviral therapy with immune reconstitution. Treatment should be started promptly if the patient is not on therapy. Some patients experience worsening neurologic symptoms once ART is initiated due to immune reconstitution-induced inflammation. ART should be continued, with consideration of adjunctive steroids especially if neuroimaging shows evidence of inflammation (enhancement or edema). Randomized controlled trials have evaluated cidofovir and vidarabine—neither is effective nor recommended. Adjunctive therapies for PML include mirtazapine, mefloquine, and maraviroc. None has been proven to improve outcomes in PML, but will be used along with ART by some clinicians based on preliminary studies.

Prognosis: Without ART, rapid progression of neurologic deficits over weeks to months is common. Best chance for survival is recovery of the immune system in response to antiretroviral therapy, although some patients will have progressive disease despite immune recovery. (J Infect Dis. 2009;199:77)

Salmonellosis

Preferred Therapy, Duration of Therapy, Chronic Maintenance	Alternate Therapy	Other Options /Issues
All HIV-infected patients with salmonellosis should be treated due to the high risk of bacteremia in these patients.		Oral or IV rehydration if indicated.
Preferred therapy for *Salmonella* gastroenteritis with or without symptomatic bacteremia Ciprofloxacin 500–750 mg PO bid (or 400 mg IV q12h, if susceptible)	Alternative therapy for *Salmonella* gastroenteritis with or without symptomatic bacteremia Levofloxacin 750 mg (PO or IV) q24h	Antimotility agents should be avoided. The role of long-term secondary prophylaxis for patients with recurrent *Salmonella* bacteremia is not well established. Must weigh the benefit against the risks of long-term antibiotic exposure.
Duration of therapy: *For gastroenteritis without bacteremia:* • If CD4 count < 200 cells/μL: 7–14 days • If CD4 count < 200 cells/μL: 2–6 weeks	**or** Moxifloxacin 400 mg (PO or IV) q24h **or** TMP 160 mg-SMX 800 mg (PO or IV) q12h **or** Ceftriaxone 1 g IV q24h **or** Cefotaxime 1 g IV q8h	Effective ART may reduce the frequency, severity, and recurrence of *Salmonella* infections.
For gastroenteritis with bacteremia: • If CD4 count < 200/μL: 14 days; longer duration if bacteremia persists or if the infection is complicated (e.g., if metastatic foci of infection are present) • If CD4 count < 200 cells/μL: 2–6 weeks		
Secondary prophylaxis should be considered for: Patients with recurrent *Salmonella* gastroenteritis +/– bacteremia **or** Patients with CD4 < 200 cells/μL with severe diarrhea		

Clinical Presentation: Patients with HIV are at markedly increased risk of developing salmonellosis. Three different presentations may be seen: (1) self-limited gastroenteritis, as typically seen in immunocompetent hosts; (2) a more severe and prolonged diarrheal disease, associated with fever, bloody diarrhea, and weight loss; or (3) *Salmonella* septicemia, which may present with or without gastrointestinal symptoms.

Diagnostic Considerations: The diagnosis is established through cultures of stool and blood. Given the high rate of bacteremia associated with *Salmonella* gastroenteritis—especially in advanced HIV disease—blood cultures should be obtained in any HIV patient presenting with diarrhea and fever.

Pitfalls: A distinctive feature of *Salmonella* bacteremia in patients with AIDS is its propensity for relapse (rate > 20%).

Therapeutic Considerations: The mainstay of treatment is a fluoroquinolone; greatest experience is with ciprofloxacin, but newer quinolones (moxifloxacin, levofloxacin) may also be effective. For uncomplicated salmonellosis in an HIV patient with CD4 > 200/mm^3, 1–2 weeks of treatment is reasonable to reduce the risk of extraintestinal spread. For patients with advanced HIV disease (CD4 < 200/mm^3) or who have *Salmonella* bacteremia, at least 2–6 weeks of treatment is required. Chronic suppressive therapy, given for several months or until antiretroviral therapy-induced immune reconstitution ensues, is indicated for patients who relapse after cessation of therapy.

Prognosis: Usually responds well to treatment. Relapse rate in AIDS patients in the pre-antiretroviral therapy era with bacteremia was > 20%.

Shigellosis

Preferred Therapy, Duration of Therapy, Chronic Maintenance	Alternate Therapy	Other Options/Issues
Preferred therapy for *Shigella* infection Ciprofloxacin 500–750 mg PO (or 400 mg IV) q12h Duration of therapy: Gastroenteritis: 7–10 days Bacteremia: ≥14 days Recurrent infections: up to 6 weeks	Levofloxacin 750 mg (PO or IV) q24h **or** Moxifloxacin 400 mg (PO or IV) q24h **or** TMP 160 mg-SMX 800 mg (PO or IV) q12h (Note: *Shigella* infections acquired outside of the United States have high rates of TMP-SMX resistance.) **or** Azithromycin 500 mg PO daily for 5 days (Note: not recommended for patients with bacteremia.)	Therapy is indicated both to shorten the duration of illness and to prevent spread of infection. Oral or IV rehydration if indicated. Antimotility agents should be avoided. If no clinical response after 5–7 days, consider follow-up stool culture, alternative diagnosis, or antibiotic resistance. Effective ART may reduce the frequency, severity, and recurrence of *Shigella* infections.

Clinical Presentation: Acute onset of bloody diarrhea/mucus.

Diagnostic Considerations: Diagnosis by demonstrating organism in stool specimens. *Shigella* ulcers in colon are linear, serpiginous, and rarely lead to perforation. More common in gay men.

Therapeutic Considerations: Therapy is indicated to shorten the duration of illness and to prevent spread of infection. Antibiotic resistance an increasing national and global problem.
Prognosis: Good if treated early.

Toxoplasma gondii Encephalitis

Preferred Therapy, Duration of Therapy, Chronic Maintenance	Alternate Therapy	Other Options/Issues
Acute infection Pyrimethamine 200 mg PO × 1, followed by weight-based therapy. If weight < 60 kg: Pyrimethamine 50 mg PO once daily + sulfadiazine 1000 mg PO q6h + leucovorin 10–25 mg PO once daily If weight ≥ 60 kg: Pyrimethamine 75 mg PO once daily + sulfadiazine 1500 mg PO q6h + leucovorin 10–25 mg PO once daily Leucovorin dose can be increased to 50 mg (daily or bid) Duration for acute therapy: At least 6 weeks; longer duration if clinical or radiologic disease is extensive or response is incomplete at 6 weeks Chronic maintenance therapy: Pyrimethamine 25–50 mg PO daily + sulfadiazine 2000–4000 mg PO daily (in 2–4 divided doses) + leucovorin 10–25 mg PO daily Preferred chronic maintenance therapy Pyrimethamine 25–50 mg PO daily plus sulfadiazine 2000–4000 mg PO daily (in 2–4 divided doses) plus leucovorin 10–25 mg PO daily	Acute infection Pyrimethamine (leucovorin)* + clindamycin 600 mg IV or PO q6h **or** TMP-SMX (5 mg/kg TMP and 25 mg/kg SMX) IV or PO bid **or** Atovaquone 1500 mg PO bid with food (or nutritional supplement) + sulfadiazine 1000–1500 mg PO q6h; (weight-based dosing, as in preferred therapy) **or** Atovaquone 1500 mg PO bid with food **or** Pyrimethamine (leucovorin)* plus azithromycin 900–1200 mg PO daily Alternative chronic maintenance therapy/secondary prophylaxis Clindamycin 600 mg PO q8h + pyrimethamine 25–50 mg PO daily + leucovorin 10–25 PO daily **or** Atovaquone 750–1500 mg PO bid +/– [(pyrimethamine 25 mg PO daily plus leucovorin 10 mg PO daily) or sulfadiazine 2000–4000 mg PO] daily	Adjunctive corticosteroids (e.g., dexamethasone) should be administered when clinically indicated only for treatment of mass effect attributed to focal lesions or associated edema; discontinue as soon as clinically feasible. Anticonvulsants should be administered to patients with a history of seizures and continued through the acute treatment; but should not be used prophylactically. If clindamycin is used in place of sulfadiazine, additional therapy must be added to prevent PCP.

* Pyrimethamine and leucovorin doses are the same as for preferred therapy.

Clinical Presentation: Wide spectrum of neurologic symptoms, including sensorimotor deficits, seizures, confusion, and ataxia. Fever and headache are common.

Diagnostic Considerations: Diagnosis by characteristic radiographic appearance and response to empiric therapy in *T. gondii* seropositive patient.

Pitfalls: Use leucovorin (folinic acid) 10 mg (PO) daily with pyrimethamine-containing regimens, not folate/folic acid. Radiographic improvement may lag behind clinical response.

Therapeutic Considerations: Alternate agents include TMP-SMX, atovaquone, azithromycin, clarithromycin, and minocycline (all with pyrimethamine if possible). Decadron 4 mg (PO or IV) q6h is useful for edema/mass effect. Intravenous TMP-SMX useful for critically ill or neurologically compromised patients who cannot take oral therapy. Chronic suppressive therapy can be discontinued if patients are free from signs and symptoms of disease and have a CD4 cell count > 200/mm^3 for > 6 months due to ART. In some centers, TMP-SMX has become the preferred initial therapy given its widespread availability, low cost, and ease of dosing compared with pyrimethamine and sulfadiazine.

Prognosis: Usually responds to treatment if able to tolerate drugs. Clinical response is evident by 1 week in 70%, by 2 weeks in 90%. Radiographic improvement is usually apparent by 2 weeks. Neurologic recovery is variable.

Treponema pallidum (Syphilis)

Preferred Therapy, Duration of Therapy, Chronic Maintenance	Alternate Therapy	Other Options/Issues
Preferred therapy early stage (primary, secondary, and early latent syphilis) Benzathine penicillin G 2.4 million units IM for 1 dose	Alternative therapy early stage (primary, secondary, and early latent syphilis) *For penicillin-allergic patients:* Doxycycline 100 mg PO bid for 14 days **or** Ceftriaxone 1 g IM or IV daily for 10–14 days **or** Azithromycin 2 g PO for 1 dose (Note: azithromycin is not recommended for MSM or pregnant women.)	The efficacy of non-penicillin alternatives has not been evaluated in HIV-infected patients and should be undertaken only with close clinical and serologic monitoring. Combination of procaine penicillin and probenecid is not recommended for patients with history of sulfa allergy.
Preferred therapy late-latent disease (> 1 year or of unknown duration, CSF examination ruled out neurosyphilis) Benzathine penicillin G 2.4 million units IM weekly for 3 doses		
Preferred therapy late-stage (tertiary–cardiovascular or gummatous disease) Benzathine penicillin G 2.4 million units IM weekly for 3 doses (Note: rule out neurosyphilis before initiation of benzathine penicillin, and obtain infectious diseases consultation to guide management.)	Alternative therapy late-latent disease (without CNS involvement) *For penicillin-allergic patients:* Doxycycline 100 mg PO bid for 28 days	The Jarisch-Herxheimer reaction is an acute febrile reaction accompanied by headache and myalgias that might occur within the first 24 hours after therapy for syphilis. This reaction occurs most frequently in patients with early syphilis, high non-treponemal titers, and prior penicillin treatment.

Treponema pallidum (Syphilis) (cont'd)

Preferred Therapy, Duration of Therapy, Chronic Maintenance	Alternate Therapy	Other Options/Issues
Preferred therapy neurosyphilis (including otic and ocular disease) Aqueous crystalline penicillin G, 18–24 million units per day, administered as 3–4 million units IV q4h or by continuous IV infusion for 10–14 days +/– benzathine penicillin G 2.4 million units IM weekly for 3 doses after completion of IV therapy	Alternative therapy neurosyphilis Procaine penicillin 2.4 million units IM daily plus probenecid 500 mg PO qid for 10–14 days +/– benzathine penicillin G 2.4 million units IM weekly for 3 doses after completion of above **or** *For penicillin-allergic patients:* Desensitization to penicillin is the preferred approach; if not feasible, ceftriaxone 2 g IV daily for 10–14 days	

Epidemiology: Syphilis is highly prevalent among some groups with high rates of HIV, notably gay men. Studies have shown that syphilis facilitates HIV transmission, and case reports/series suggest that syphilis in HIV-infected patients is associated with multiple and slower resolving primary chancres, higher titer RPR, slower decline of RPR titers, higher rate of serologic failure, increased frequency of CSF abnormalities and CSF-VDRL positivity, higher incidence of ocular disease, and higher rates of relapse after treatment (Sex Transm Dis. 2001;28:158–65; N Engl J Med. 1997 Jul;337:307–14; Ann Intern Med. 1990;113:872).

Clinical Presentation: The causative organism of syphilis is *Treponema pallidum*, which cannot be cultured in routine clinical laboratories. As a result, the diagnosis of syphilis depends on recognizing the clinical stages and use of serologic tests

- Primary syphilis: Following an incubation period of 2–6 weeks, primary syphilis presents as a papule that later ulcerates to form a syphilitic chancre. These are generally painless and may occur on any mucosal surface. Non-tender regional adenopathy may also be present. Serologic tests for syphilis (RPR or VDRL) can be negative early in primary syphilis, so empiric treatment is indicated in suspected cases, with follow-up testing necessary to confirm the disease.

- Secondary syphilis: Approximately 60–90% of patients with untreated primary syphilis will develop secondary syphilis as a manifestation of *T. pallidum* dissemination. The time course is typically within 6 months of infection acquisition, and the clinical manifestations are highly variable. The most common manifestation of secondary syphilis is a non pruritic macular-papular rash over the entire body, including the palms and soles. Other symptoms and laboratory abnormalities can include condyloma lata (white genital lesions similar in appearance to condyloma acuminata), mucous patches (shallow ulcerations on the oral or genital mucosa), fever, malaise, lymphadenopathy, anorexia, hepatitis, and diminished vision secondary to uveitis.

- Latent syphilis: Defined by a reactive serologic test in the absence of active symptoms, latent syphilis is divided into "early-latent" (< 1 year after exposure) and "late-latent" (> 1 year after exposure). Patients who are unable to give an accurate exposure date are classified as "latent syphilis of unknown duration" and treated as late-latent disease.

- Tertiary (late) syphilis: This develops in 25–40% of patients untreated for earlier disease, usually months to years later. Tertiary syphilis can cause CNS disease, cardiovascular disorders, and gummatous lesions involving the skin and bones. Cardiovascular and gummatous syphilis have become extremely rare, but CNS syphilis still occurs with some frequency and can present in various ways. *Acute syphilitic meningitis* and *meningovascular syphilis* occur relatively early after exposure (typically within the first 1–5 years), sometimes during dissemination of the organism with secondary syphilis. By contrast, *parenchymatous syphilis* usually occurs decades later, and includes general paresis, tabes dorsalis, and focal lesions due to CNS gummas.

Diagnostic Considerations: Diagnostic strategies for syphilis are the same as in HIV-negative patients, and rely mostly on serologic studies since the organism cannot be cultured. Darkfield microscopy on fluid obtained from chancres or condyloma lata may demonstrate the characteristic spiral-shaped organism; however, this technique is of limited utility since it cannot be used in the absence of obvious lesions, and most clinicians do not have access to a darkfield microscope. As a result, a positive serologic test for syphilis (RPR or VDRL or *T. pallidum* ELISA) followed by a positive confirmatory test (MHA-TP, FTA-ABS, or TP-PA) is the most common way to diagnose syphilis in patients with (or without) HIV. Although case reports have cited unusually high titers, false negative results, and delayed onset of seropositivity in patients with HIV infection, no alternative testing strategy is routinely recommended. *Neurosyphilis* is diagnosed via clinical presentation and CSF examination. In symptomatic neurosyphilis, presenting complaints may include cognitive dysfunction, motor or sensory deficits, cranial nerve palsies, ophthalmic or auditory symptoms, and symptoms or signs of meningitis. Diagnostic criteria for neurosyphilis by CSF examination vary, but one commonly used definition is a CSF white blood cell count > 20 cells/mcL or a reactive CSF VDRL. (Although considered highly sensitive, the FTA-ABS test of the spinal fluid is not specific and can be used only to rule out disease.) The diagnosis of neurosyphilis is challenging since the CSF VDRL (the most specific test) is positive in only 30–70%, even in HIV-negative-patients. Furthermore, HIV itself may induce cellular responses independent of syphilis, and clinical manifestations are extremely varied. As a result, there is some debate about which patients with HIV and syphilis should undergo lumbar puncture (LP). One study of 326 HIV-infected patients with syphilis who underwent LP found that 65 (20%) met criteria for neurosyphilis by CSF exam; the risk was substantially higher if the CD4 cell count was ≤ 350 or the RPR was ≥ 1:32 (J Infect Dis. 2004;189:369–76).

Therapeutic Considerations: The treatment of syphilis is generally the same as for HIV-negative patients, with penicillin as the mainstay of therapy. The criteria for treatment response are the same in HIV-infected and HIV-negative individuals. Specifically, the RPR or VDRL titer should decline ≥ 4-fold by 1 year after treatment for early syphilis and by 2–3 years after treatment for latent syphilis. (For HIV patients with early syphilis, there is an increased rate of treatment failure when using serologic criteria; therefore, our practice is to include an RPR as part of monitoring labs performed every 3–4 months unless the titer has reverted to negative.) Failure to achieve ≥ 4-fold decline in titer should prompt investigation of reinfection or a CSF examination to exclude neurosyphilis. For patients with neurosyphilis, follow-up

CSF examinations are performed every 6 months until CSF pleocytosis has normalized; if still abnormal 2 years after treatment, consider retreatment with intravenous penicillin. In general, non-penicillin therapies for syphilis have had limited evaluation in HIV patients; hence these cases warrant close clinical and laboratory follow-up. Procaine penicillin/probenecid options may not be used in patients with severe sulfa allergy.

Table 5.4. Need for Lumbar Puncture (LP) in HIV-Infected Patients with Syphilis

Stage of Syphilis	Recommendation
All stages of syphilis with no neurologic, ophthalmic, or auditory symptoms/signs	No LP; if RPR > 1:32 or CD4 < 350, be especially vigilant for lack of response.
Positive RPR and confirmatory test with neurologic, ophthalmic, or auditory symptoms/ signs	Perform LP.

Varicella-Zoster Virus (VZV) Disease

Preferred Therapy, Duration of Therapy, Chronic Maintenance	Alternate Therapy	Other Options /Issues
Varicella (chickenpox) *Uncomplicated cases* Valacyclovir 1000 mg PO tid for 5–7 days, or famciclovir 500 mg PO tid × 5–7 days *Severe or complicated cases* Acyclovir 10–15 mg/kg IV q8h × 7–10 days May switch to oral acyclovir, famciclovir, or valacyclovir after defervescence if no evidence of visceral involvement. Herpes zoster (shingles) *Acute localized dermatomal* Valacyclovir 1g PO tid for 7–10 days or famciclovir 500 mg PO tid for 7–10 days, longer duration should be considered if lesions are slow to resolve *Extensive cutaneous lesion or visceral involvement*	Primary varicella infection (chickenpox) *Uncomplicated cases (for 5-7 days)* Acyclovir 800 mg PO 5 times/day Herpes zoster (shingles) *Acute localized dermatomal* For 7–10 days; consider longer duration if lesions are slow to resolve. Acyclovir 800 mg PO 5 times/day	Involvement of an experienced ophthalmologist with management of VZV retinitis is strongly recommended. Duration of therapy for VZV retinitis is not well defined, and should be determined based on clinical, virologic, and immunologic responses and ophthalmologic responses. Optimization of ART is recommended for serious and difficult-to-treat VZV infections (e.g., retinitis, encephalitis).

Varicella-Zoster Virus (VZV) Disease (cont'd)

Preferred Therapy, Duration of Therapy, Chronic Maintenance	Alternate Therapy	Other Options /Issues
Acyclovir 10–15 mg/kg IV q8h until clinical improvement is evident. Switch to oral therapy (valacyclovir 1000 mg TID or famciclovir 500 mg TID, or acyclovir 800 mg PO 5x daily) after clinical improvement is evident, to complete a 10–14 day course. Progressive outer retinal necrosis (PORN) (Ganciclovir 5 mg/kg +/– foscarnet 90 mg/kg) IV q12h + (ganciclovir 2 mg/0.05 mL +/– foscarnet 1.2 mg/0.05 mL) intravitreal injection biw Initiate or optimize ART. Acute retinal necrosis (ARN) Acyclovir 10 mg/kg IV q8h + ganciclovir 2 mg/0.05 mL intravitreal injection biw x 1–2 doses × 10–14 days, followed by valacyclovir 1000 mg PO tid × 6 weeks		

Clinical Presentation: Primary varicella (chickenpox) presents as widely disseminated clear vesicles on an erythematous base that heal with crusting and sometimes scarring. Zoster usually presents as painful tense vesicles on an erythematous base in a dermatomal distribution. In patients with HIV, primary varicella is more severe/prolonged, and zoster is more likely to involve multiple dermatomes/disseminate. VZV can rarely cause acute retinal necrosis, which requires close consultation with ophthalmology.

Diagnostic Considerations: Diagnosis is usually clinical. In atypical cases, immunofluorescence can be used to distinguish herpes zoster from herpes simplex.

Pitfalls: Extend treatment beyond 7–10 days if new vesicles are still forming after initial treatment period. Corticosteroids for dermatomal zoster are not recommended in HIV-positive patients.

Therapeutic Considerations: IV therapy is generally indicated for severe disease/cranial nerve zoster.

Prognosis: Usually responds slowly to treatment.

Chapter 6

Complications of HIV Infection*

*   Also see Chapter 5 for Opportunistic Infections and Chapters 3 and 9 for Drug-Induced
    Adverse Effects.

HEMATOLOGIC COMPLICATIONS

A. **Thrombocytopenia.** May be the first and only sign of HIV infection. Treatment is only required for platelet count < 20,000/mm³, active bleeding, or planned procedures. Causes include medications, alcohol, idiopathic thrombocytopenic purpura (ITP), thrombotic thrombocytopenic purpura (TTP), and advanced HIV disease ± marrow infiltration with secondary opportunistic infections (usually accompanied by pancytopenia).

   1. **Idiopathic Thrombocytopenic Purpura (ITP).** Can occur at any stage of HIV disease and sometimes emerges as antiretroviral therapy (ART) induces an immune response. Consultation with a hematologist is advised for platelet count < 20,000 or if rapid recovery of platelet count is required.

      a. **Preferred therapy.** Combination antiretroviral therapy.

      b. **If rapid control of platelet count is needed.** IVIG 1–2 g/kg total dose, over 2–5 days. Duration of response is typically 3–4 weeks. <u>Alternative</u>: Anti-RH D globulin (WinRho) 50–75 µg/kg IV (effective only in RH-positive, non-splenectomized patients). Causes mild hemolysis. Duration of response is similar to IVIG, and may work in some patients who do not respond to IVIG.

      c. **Miscellaneous alternative therapies.** Prednisone 1 mg/kg daily, with taper as tolerated; danazol 400–800 mg (PO) QD; dapsone 100 mg (PO) QD (if not G6PD deficient); alpha-interferon 3 million units 3×/week; splenectomy. Some anecdotal evidence for use of vincristine, splenic irradiation, anti-cd20 antibody (Rituximab).

   2. **Thrombotic Thrombocytopenic Purpura (TTP).** Manifests as microangiopathic hemolytic anemia associated with renal insufficiency and neurologic symptoms. TTP is a **medical emergency**—if it is suspected based on clinical grounds and examination of blood smear, consult hematologist immediately. Standard treatment is prednisone 60–100 mg (PO) QD (or IV equivalent) plus plasmapheresis.

B. **Anemia.** Anemia is associated with a lower quality of life; several studies also suggest it is independently associated with reduced survival (Clin Infect Dis. 1999;29:44–9).

   1. **Etiology**

      a. **Decreased RBC production (low reticulocyte count)**

         • **Direct effect of HIV.** Usually CD4 < 100/mm³; responds well to initiation of antiretroviral therapy.

         • **Infiltration of bone marrow.** In particular MAC—suspect in a patient with advanced AIDS who has fever, weight loss, and anemia out of proportion to drop in other cell lines; can also be due to lymphoma.

- **Iron deficiency (women)**
  - **B12 or folate deficiency:** High MCV is usually related to a side effect of NRTIs (especially ZDV), but need to rule out B12 and folate deficiency, which appears to be more common among patients with HIV.
  - **Certain infections:** <u>Parvovirus B19</u>: Infects and inhibits early RBC precursors, with characteristic bone marrow showing giant pronormoblasts; diagnosed by viral DNA by PCR of blood (not by serology); treated with IVIG. *Mycobacterium avium* complex (<u>MAC</u>): Diagnosed by isolator blood cultures or bone marrow biopsy; treated as described on p. 126.
  - **Drugs:** ZDV (most common in advanced HIV disease, but can occur at any stage; other antiretroviral agents rarely cause anemia); ganciclovir and valganciclovir (lower WBC also); TMP-SMX; amphotericin; interferon.
  b. **Increased RBC destruction (high reticulocyte count)**
    - **Drug-induced:** Dapsone and primaquine if patient is G6PD deficient; ribavirin as part of hepatitis C (HCV) therapy (causes dose-related hemolytic anemia), which may further compromise fatigue associated with HCV therapy.
    - **TTP** (described on p. 143)

2. **Evaluation.** As a minimum work-up, evaluate clinical status, stage of HIV disease, stool for occult blood, CBC/differential, RBC indices, reticulocyte count, iron, total iron binding capacity (TIBC), creatinine, LFTs, B12, folate. Bone marrow aspiration is indicated when above work-up and history fail to identify a cause.

3. **Treatment.** If no reversible cause of anemia is identified, or if the cause cannot be removed (for example, ribavirin-associated anemia during HCV treatment), consider erythropoietin (EPO) for patients with Hgb < 10 g/dL or HCT < 30. Start with 40,000 units (SQ) once weekly with iron supplementation; if at 4 weeks, Hgb has increased by > 1 g/dL, continue same dose until Hgb reaches 11–12 g/dL. Dose can then be reduced to 10,000 units (SQ) once weekly to maintain Hgb at this level. Higher levels have been associated with increased risk of thromboembolic events in non-HIV populations. For non-responders, 60,000 units (SQ) once weekly may be effective. Supplemental iron should also be given.

C. **Neutropenia.** As with anemia, neutropenia is much more common in advanced HIV disease. The risk of infection is increased with lower absolute neutrophil counts (ANC), especially when < 500/mm^3.

1. **Etiology**

   a. **Direct effect of HIV.** Responds well to initiation of antiretroviral therapy.

   b. **Drugs.** ZDV, ganciclovir and valganciclovir (ZDV and ganciclovir given together can cause particularly severe neutropenia), pyrimethamine, TMP-SMX at pneumocystis pneumonia (PCP) treatment doses, interferon, flucytosine. Uncommon causes include other NRTIs, ribavirin, amphotericin, pentamidine, rifabutin. TMP-SMX given at doses used for PCP prophylaxis rarely is the sole cause of neutropenia; if neutropenia does not improve after a trial of an alternative prophylactic regimen, TMP-SMX can be restarted.

   c. **Infections.** MAC, CMV, disseminated fungal diseases (e.g., histoplasmosis).

2. **Treatment.** Only indicated if ANC is consistently < 750/mm³ (some cite 500/mm³).

   After underlying causes are corrected, consider G-CSF (Neupogen) 150–300 µg (SQ) every 1–7 days. Start with 3×/week dosing, then titrate dose to maintain ANC > 1000/mm³.

D. **Eosinophilia**
   1. **Etiology**
      a. **Direct effect of HIV.** Sometimes seen with no apparent cause, especially in advanced HIV disease.
      b. **Drug allergy.** Most commonly to TMP-SMX and other sulfonamides.
      c. **Parasitic infection (rare).** Most HIV-related parasitic infections (e.g., toxo-plasmosis, cryptosporidiosis) do not cause eosinophilia. Rare exceptions include *Isospora belli* and strongyloidiasis (if patient from endemic area).
   2. **Treatment.** Consider withdrawal of offending agent if associated with other allergic phenomena. Check stool for ova and parasites, strongyloides serology.

ONCOLOGIC COMPLICATIONS

Malignancies definitely associated with HIV infection include Kaposi's sarcoma, non-Hodgkin's lymphoma, Hodgkin's disease, lung cancer, squamous cell carcinomas (cervical, anal, head, and neck), and soft tissue sarcoma (in children). Possible associated malignancies include seminoma, lung cancer, and multiple myeloma. Prolonged survival due to ART has led to a greater appreciation of the increased incidence of non-AIDS malignancies in HIV patients (Ann Intern Med. 2008 May 20;148:728); risk appears related to CD4 cell count (AIDS 2008 Oct 18;22:2143).

A. **Kaposi's Sarcoma.** Infection with HHV-8 is a critical viral cofactor; interaction between host immunosuppression, genetic factors, and this virus determine a patient's risk. In North America, Australia, and Western Europe, Kaposi's sarcoma occurs most commonly in gay/bisexual men. The incidence has diminished markedly since the introduction of potent antiretroviral therapy. In developing countries (especially in certain parts of Africa), Kaposi's sarcoma is more evenly distributed among men and women.
   1. **Presentation.** Usually presents as violaceous nodules and plaques on the skin; oral cavity and other mucosal surfaces may be involved. With more advanced immunosuppression, visceral involvement (lungs, gastrointestinal tract) can be life threatening. Invasion of local lymphatics can lead to chronic edema of the limbs, face, and genitals, with increased risk of bacterial superinfection.

2. **Treatment.** Initiation of antiretroviral therapy is often sufficient to cause regression of cutaneous and limited mucosal disease. For disease that progresses despite antivirals, options include local measures (intralesional chemotherapy, radiation therapy) and systemic chemotherapy (liposomal anthracyclines are especially effective). Occasionally clinical disease may temporarily worsen soon after starting ART as a manifestation of the immune reconstitution inflammatory syndrome (IRIS); in these cases, ART should be continued and systemic chemotherapy considered or intensified.

B. **Non-Hodgkin's Lymphoma (NHL).** In patients with HIV infection, NHL is most commonly a manifestation of advanced immunosuppression (CD4 < 100/mm^3) though a minority of cases occur with relatively preserved immune function. Duration of uncontrolled viremia also is a risk factor for NHL.

   1. **Presentation.** Clinical presentation reflects extranodal involvement of the disease: typically, gastrointestinal tract (45%), bone marrow (20%), and CNS (20–30%). Often multiple sites are involved simultaneously. Of note, the patient with AIDS who has diffuse adenopathy and fever will more likely have a systemic infection (most commonly *M. avium* complex, histoplasmosis, cryptococcus) rather than lymphoma. Although the incidence of NHL has declined since the introduction of potent antiretroviral therapy, it has done so to a lesser degree than other opportunistic infections. As a result, NHL in some centers is responsible for a higher proportion of AIDS-related complications compared with the pre-antiretroviral era.

   2. **Treatment.** Generally involves full-dose chemotherapy, with use of recombinant growth factors (G-CSF, erythropoietin) as needed to support cell lines. Initiation of antiretroviral therapy concurrently with chemotherapy may improve outcome by reducing infectious complications and improving recovery time of bone marrow function. It is important to avoid the use of antiviral agents that may have overlapping toxicities with the prescribed chemotherapy (e.g., avoid d4T or ddI when patients are receiving systemic vincristine therapy, as this increases the risk of peripheral neuropathy; avoid ZDV since this may further suppress the bone marrow).

C. **Primary CNS Lymphoma.** Usually a manifestation of advanced HIV disease, with the vast majority of patients having a CD4 cell count < 50/mm^3.

   1. **Presentation.** The typical presentation is one of focal neurologic deficits or seizures, reflecting focal lesion(s) in the brain. MRI findings typically show lesions with irregular enhancement, sometimes involving the corpus callosum and crossing the midline; mass effect is generally evident. Appearance of primary CNS lymphoma is similar to that of CNS toxoplasmosis; in the latter, lesions are often greater in number, but radiographic abnormalities overlap significantly.

   2. **Diagnosis.** If a patient with advanced AIDS presents with focal enhancing lesion(s) on MRI or CT scan and is either toxoplasmosis seronegative or taking TMP-SMX for toxoplasmosis prophylaxis, then primary CNS lymphoma is the most likely diagnosis. While noninvasive testing such as thallium SPECT scan, PET scan, and CSF studies for cytology and Epstein-Barr virus DNA (by PCR) can sometimes be helpful, the definitive diagnosis is generally made through stereotactic brain biopsy. Of note, Epstein-Barr

virus PCR of the CSF in HIV patients without characteristic CNS mass lesions has a very low specificity for CNS lymphoma; a positive test does not invariably indicate this diagnosis (Clin Infect Dis. 2004 Jun 1;38[11]:1629–32).

3. **Treatment.** The prognosis of primary CNS lymphoma remains quite poor, especially for patients who fail antiretroviral therapy. Treatment with steroids and radiation therapy is palliative. Rare patients have experienced sustained remissions after initiating antiretroviral therapy and achieving a significant improvement in immune function.

D. **Cervical Cancer.** Compared to HIV-negative women, the incidence of cervical cancer in HIV-infected women is higher and the disease may be more aggressive. Cervical cancer is strongly associated with human papillomavirus (HPV) infection and progressive immunosuppression. A diagnosis of cervical cancer along with a positive HIV serology is considered AIDS defining. Recommendations for screening include a Pap smear twice the first year after HIV diagnosis, and yearly thereafter if normal. This strategy is associated with a low risk of invasive cervical cancer, comparable to HIV-negative women.

E. **Anal Cancer.** The incidence of anal cancer in HIV-infected men who have sex with men (MSM) is approximately 80 times that of the general population. As with cervical cancer, anal cancer is strongly associated with HPV infection. Although screening for anal cancer using anal Pap smears could identify precancerous lesions much as with cervical cancer, it has not yet been proven that this screening strategy will reduce the incidence of anal cancer. As such, routine screening is not formally recommended in the opportunistic infection (OI) prevention guidelines, but is recommended in the Primary Care Guidelines for HIV, with the caveat that the evidence supporting the screening is weak. Pending results of ongoing studies, a reasonable strategy is as follows:

1. At a minimum, perform annual periodic visual inspection and a digital rectal exam.

2. Perform anal Pap smear for any anorectal complaints; some recommend annual testing on all HIV-positive gay men.

3. For atypical cells of uncertain significance, repeat anal Pap smear in 6–12 months.

4. For squamous intraepithelial lesion (SIL), refer to a colorectal surgeon or other specialist for anoscopy and/or anal colposcopy with biopsy.

ENDOCRINE COMPLICATIONS

A. **Disorders of Adrenal Function.** Although adrenal gland involvement has been documented in up to two-thirds of patients with AIDS on postmortem examination, clinically relevant adrenal insufficiency is rare (~ 3% of patients with AIDS) and is generally a manifestation of late-stage AIDS. Currently the most common cause of adrenal function pathology is iatrogenic, when corticosteroids given by any route (including injected, inhaled, topical) interact with ritonavir or cobicistat.

1. **Etiology.** Potential causes of primary adrenal dysfunction include destruction of the adrenal gland from opportunistic infections (especially cytomegalovirus [CMV]), neoplasms (Kaposi's sarcoma, lymphoma), hemorrhage, and infarction. More commonly, adrenal insufficiency results from the adverse effect of medications, including ketoconazole (decreased steroidogenesis), rifampin/rifabutin (enhanced cortisol metabolism), and corticosteroids/megestrol acetate (suppressed pituitary secretion of corticotropin due to intrinsic glucocorticoid activity; latter may actually induce Cushing's syndrome with prolonged use). A relatively common cause of cortisol excess is the use of inhaled (especially fluticasone), intra-articular, or topical steroids with ritonavir or cobicistat. These pharmacokinetic boosters block the metabolism of many corticosteroids, leading to increased exposure and iatrogenic Cushing's syndrome. Conversely, stopping the inhaled steroid can cause adrenal insufficiency (J Clin Endocrinol Metab. 2005;90:4394–8). If possible, inhaled or injectable steroids should be avoided in patients receiving boosted PIs or cobicistat. Among inhaled steroids, beclomethasone appears to be the safest (J AIDS 2013; 63:355–61).

2. **Diagnosis.** Hypercortisolism should be considered in any patient if they have received corticosteroids by any route and are receiving a boosted PI or cobicistat. Typical symptoms may include fatigue, irritability, sleep disturbance, muscle weakness, facial fullness, erectile dysfunction, new-onset hypertension and labs demonstrating hyperglycemia. The diagnosis is confirmed with a low A.M. cortisol and ACTH. Adrenal insufficiency should be suspected in a patient with advanced HIV disease or recent therapy with steroid-interfering medications who presents with hypotension, profound weakness, or electrolyte abnormalities (hyponatremia, hyperkalemia). Evaluation consists of measurement of A.M. cortisol; if normal and the diagnosis is still suspected, perform a corticotropin stimulation test. If the diagnosis is still suspected despite a normal corticotropin stimulation test, referral to an endocrinologist is warranted since some patients with AIDS have peripheral resistance to glucocorticoid action.

3. **Treatment.** Patients with basal low cortisol levels, even if asymptomatic, require replacement therapy (prednisone 5 mg [PO] at bedtime). For corticotropin hyporesponsiveness, steroid supplementation for stressing conditions (e.g., surgery, intercurrent illness) is indicated. For life-threatening situations, immediate treatment with dexamethasone 4 mg (IV) is indicated; this will not impair the diagnostic utility of the corticotropin stimulation test. Patients with cortisol excess syndromes should have the exogenous steroid discontinued, and be closely monitored for adrenal insufficiency.

B. **Hypogonadism.** Men with HIV infection are more likely to be hypogonadal than HIV-negative controls. The frequency of this abnormality increases with progressive immunodeficiency and may reach 50% in patients with AIDS. In general, there is no detectable underlying etiology. HIV-related hypogonadism is associated with weakness, weight loss, decreased libido, and impaired quality of life. Replacement therapy can improve many of these symptoms, especially when combined with a resistance exercise program. While low testosterone levels have also been observed in HIV-infected women, replacement therapy is experimental. Treatment for men consists of testosterone gel 5 mg QD, testosterone transdermal patch, or injectable testosterone cypionate/enanthate 200 mg every other week. Potential side effects include acne, gynecomastia, and testicular atrophy. Monitor prostate-specific antigen annually for patients on replacement therapy.

C. Thyroid Disease. The thyroid gland is rarely involved in disseminated opportunistic infections (e.g., extrapulmonary pneumocystis). Chronically ill patients with HIV may have low T3, but thyroid-stimulating hormone (TSH) is generally normal. Immune response to antiretroviral therapy may unmask subclinical Grave's disease (as a manifestation of immune reconstitution inflammatory syndrome), leading to clinical hyperthyroidism. Treatment of Grave's disease consists of radioactive thyroid ablation or an anti-thyroid medication (e.g., methimazole) as directed by an endocrinologist. Beta-blockers can be used to ameliorate the symptoms of hyperthyroidism.

D. Pancreatitis. Clinical presentation is similar to HIV-negative patients, with nausea, vomiting, abdominal pain.

    1. Etiology

        a. Medications. The HIV-related medications that commonly were implicated as causes of pancreatitis (didanosine stavudine, and pentamidine) are rarely used today. Less common causes include other NRTIs, TMP-SMX, and protease inhibitors when accompanied by very high triglyceride levels.

        b. Opportunistic infections. Most commonly identified opportunistic infection to cause pancreatitis is CMV, exclusively in those with low CD4 cell counts. Can rarely be caused by TB, MAC, intestinal protozoa (cryptosporidia, microsporidia), widely disseminated toxoplasmosis.

        c. Non-HIV–related complications. Alcohol, obesity, gallstones.

    2. Treatment. Discontinue potentially offending drug; treat identified cause.

E. Hyperglycemia. Patients with HIV appear to be at higher risk of developing insulin resistance and diabetes than HIV-negative controls. Potential contributing factors include lipodystrophy syndrome (especially subcutaneous fat loss) and medications (most notably older ART such as indinavir and the NRTI stavudine).

    1. Diagnosis. For patients on antiretroviral therapy, monitor serum glucose every 3–6 months as part of safety labs. If elevated or abnormal, consider a fasting glucose, insulin level, and hemoglobin A1C. A fasting blood glucose > 126 mg/dL or a glucose level > 200 mg/dL 2 hours after administration of 75 g of glucose is diagnostic of diabetes mellitus.

    2. Treatment. If the patient is on a protease inhibitor and has an undetectable HIV RNA and can switch therapy without risking virologic rebound (see Chapter 4), substitute an NNRTI (e.g., efavirenz, rilpivirine) or an unboosted integrase inhibitor (raltegravir or dolutegravir) for the protease inhibitor. If the patient is not on a protease inhibitor and fasting hyperglycemia persists, follow established guidelines for treatment of diabetes mellitus in the general population, including weight loss, dietary modification, and exercise. Note that dolutegravir increases the exposure to metformin by 2–3 fold; daily doses should not exceed 1000 mg/day.

F. Hypoglycemia. Pentamidine induces hypoglycemia by lysing pancreatic islet cells. Monitor fingerstick glucose levels daily while patients receive this therapy. Prolonged, repeated use of pentamidine may result in diabetes mellitus from irreversible damage to islet cells, leading to insulin deficiency.

G. Ovarian Complications. Amenorrhea is common in women with advanced AIDS who have significant weight loss. Menses may resume with weight gain and improvement in clinical status accompanying antiretroviral therapy.

H. Bone Disease

    1. Osteonecrosis. This complication has been reported in association with HIV infection since the late 1980s, but it appears to be more common since the introduction of effective antiretroviral therapy (J AIDS 2006;42:286–92). It is not clear if the increased incidence is due simply to prolonged survival, or to a direct toxic effect of antiretroviral medications. The most commonly involved sites are the femoral heads, followed by the humeral heads, femoral condyles, proximal tibia, and small bones of the hands and wrists. Most patients will have traditional underlying risk factors, such as a history of corticosteroid use, hyperlipidemia, alcohol abuse, or a hypercoagulable state. The relationship to any specific form of antiretroviral therapy has not been conclusively demonstrated (HIV Med. 2004 Nov;5[6]:421–6).

        a. Diagnosis. Consider osteonecrosis in a patient with refractory hip pain, especially if there are underlying risk factors (see above). If plain film imaging is negative, proceed to MRI, which is more sensitive. Bilateral imaging is indicated since the disease is often bilateral.

        b. Treatment. Conservative management with physical therapy is recommended initially. If pain persists, refer to an orthopedic surgeon for consideration of hip stabilization/hip replacement.

    2. Osteoporosis. Osteopenia and osteoporosis have been reported in 22–50% and 3–21% of patients receiving chronic antiretroviral therapy, respectively. Low bone mineral density appears to be substantially more common in patients with HIV than those who are HIV negative (AIDS 2006 Nov 14;20[17]:2165–74). Spontaneous fractures have also been reported, although the risk is low. Initiation of ART is generally associated with a decline in bone mineral density that then stabilizes; this decrease is greater with tenofovir disoproxil fumarate (TDF)-containing regimens (J Infect Dis. 2011 Jun;203(12):1791–801.)

        a. Diagnosis. Some sources recommend screening for all men older than 50, all postmenopausal women, and for patients with a history of fracture (Clin Infect Dis. 2010 Oct 15;51(8):937–46). The appropriate screening test is regional DEXA scanning. Secondary causes of osteopenia and osteoporosis should be evaluated, including thyrotoxicosis, hyperparathyroidism, hypogonadism, weight loss, alcohol intake, and certain medications (especially corticosteroids). Smoking cessation should be strongly encouraged.

b. **Treatment.** All patients on tenofovir DF who have evidence or risk factors for low bone density should be switched to tenofovir alafenamide, which will increase bone density (Lancet HIV. Lancet HIV 2016 Apr;3(4):e158–65). If osteoporosis is demonstrated on DEXA scan (t-score of –2.5 or lower), consider biphosphonate therapy. Both alendronate and zoledronate have been tested in prospective clinical studies (J Acquir Immune Defic Syndr. 2005 Apr 1;38[4]:426–31; J Clin Endocrinol Metab. 2007 Apr;92[4]:1283–8).

MORPHOLOGIC COMPLICATIONS OF THERAPY

Antiretroviral therapy may be associated with changes in body shape and appearance, with these morphologic alterations sometimes referred to as "lipodystrophy." These consist of two distinct processes: *subcutaneous lipoatrophy*, which is most evident in the face, limbs, and buttocks; and *regional fat accumulation*, which may occur in in the midsection, as a manifestation of visceral adiposity, and less commonly, around the neck and anterior chest. Patients may have predominantly lipoatrophy, fat accumulation, or both. Lipoatrophy has become less common since the principal causative agents stavudine and zidovudine are rarely used today; however, many patients who took these drugs are still living with HIV, and have various degrees of this complication.

These morphologic changes may be accompanied by metabolic derangements, including lipid dysregulation (increased triglycerides and total cholesterol, reduced HDL cholesterol) and insulin resistance. Lipid abnormalities can occur in the absence of body habitus changes, and are more common with certain drugs than others (see Table 6.1).

A. Lipoatrophy

Table 6.1. Treatment and Prevention of Body Habitus Changes Associated with Antiretroviral Therapy

Treatment	• Substitute tenofovir or abacavir for zidovudine, stavudine, or didanosine. • Polylactic acid injections for facial lipoatrophy. • Weight loss and exercise for fat accumulation. • Liposuction for dorsocervical fat accumulation. • Tesamorelin for central fat accumulation.
Prevention	• Start therapy before advanced HIV disease. • Select initial NRTI combinations less likely to induce lipoatrophy (e.g., TAF/FTC, TDF/FTC, or ABC/3TC.). • Switch to TAF/FTC or ABC/3TC if patients are receiving zidovudine even if they do not report lipoatrophy.

Reproduced from Panel on Treatment of HIV-Infected Pregnant Women and Prevention of Perinatal Transmission. Recommendations for use of antiretroviral drugs in pregnant HIV-1-infected women for maternal health and interventions to reduce perinatal HIV transmission in the United States. aidsinfo.nih.gov. June 7, 2016.

1. **Overview.** The most important host risk factor is the stage of HIV disease, as patients with more advanced HIV-related immunosuppression are at greatest risk. Among treatment-related factors, the leading hypothesis for the cause of lipoatrophy is that NRTI-induced mitochondrial toxicity induces fat cell apoptosis, and NRTIs with the highest in vitro inhibition of the mitochondrial enzyme polymerase gamma pose the greatest risk. *Highest risk* is with the dideoxynucleosides (stavudine, didanosine, and zalcitabine); *intermediate risk* is with zidovudine; and *lowest risk* is with tenofovir, abacavir, lamivudine, and emtricitabine. While one study showed a greater degree of mild lipoatrophy with efavirenz versus lopinavir/ritonavir treatment, (AIDS 2009;23:1109–18) in general the NNRTI class of medications has not been implicated in this process, nor have integrase inhibitors.

2. **Treatment.** Treatment strategies for lipoatrophy consist of drug substitutions and cosmetic surgery. Substituting tenofovir or abacavir for stavudine or zidovudine leads to a gradual increase in limb fat that is often accompanied by a subjective improvement in facial appearance (AIDS 2006;20:2043–50). Such improvements occur slowly after antiretroviral switches and may not be evident to the patient for several months or at all. The tenofovir substitution strategy may also improve lipid abnormalities. Substituting an NNRTI for the PI-component of the regimen has had no consistent effect on morphologic changes (AIDS 2005;19:917–25). Although there was initial optimism that insulin-sensitizing agents would help reverse lipoatrophy, the bulk of prospective data do not support a role for this approach, and such drugs are not recommended in the absence of established medical indications (e.g., hyperglycemia). Finally, cosmetic surgery for facial lipoatrophy can often dramatically improve appearance. The most common approach is injection of biologically inert substances such as polylactic acid (Sculptra). Patient satisfaction after polylactic acid injections is extremely high, and thus far the procedure appears safe. The major drawbacks to this treatment approach include the lack of long-term efficacy, relatively high cost, and lack of effect on lipoatrophy of the arms and legs. Patients should be informed that most insurance policies and state-funded programs will not cover the cost of cosmetic surgery for lipoatrophy.

B. **Fat Accumulation and Weight Gain**

1. **Overview.** Weight gain typically accompanies initiation of ART, and in cases where there was HIV-related wasting, this is desirable. However, weight gain and fat accumulation can occur even without pre-ART weight loss, and can be highly disfiguring and uncomfortable to the patient. When fat accumulation is in the form of visceral adiposity, it is associated with increased cardiovascular risk. The neck, upper body, and intra-abdominal (visceral) sites are most often involved. (Neck fat accumulation in the posterior compartment is often referred to as a buffalo hump.) Despite the similarity in some cases to Cushing's syndrome, serum cortisol levels are not elevated. While fat accumulation syndrome is anecdotally linked to PI-based regimens, prospective clinical trials of initial therapy and switch strategies in virologically suppressed patients do not clearly implicate one drug class over another. (Clin Infect Dis. 2016 Apr 1;62(7):853–62.). Overall, the etiology of fat gain and accumulation is poorly

understood, and there are clearly both host and treatment factors. As with lipoatrophy, fat gains are likely to be greatest in patients with high HIV RNA or low CD4 cell counts prior to starting therapy.

2. **Treatment.** No ART treatment modification has consistently led to improvement. A vigorous exercise program may reduce central fat accumulation, and weight loss may reduce neck fat; anecdotally, reducing alcohol intake may also improve outcomes. Recombinant growth hormone reduces central fat accumulation, but treatment is expensive and associated with a risk of other side effects, including glucose intolerance and carpal tunnel syndrome. The injectable growth hormone releasing factor tesamorelin is modestly effective for this indication (J Clin Endocrinol Metab. 2010 Jun 16); it is approved for central fat accumulation at a dose of 2 mg once daily. The beneficial effects of tesamorelin in reducing visceral adiposity wane quickly when the medication is stopped; as such, the optimal duration of therapy is unknown, and some patients continue it indefinitely. Liposuction of neck fat accumulation is the most rapidly effective technique, but recurrences are possible. Insurance coverage for neck liposuction can sometimes be deemed medically necessary if the fat accumulation leads to medical problems such as neck pain or sleep apnea.

C. **Prevention of Lipodystrophy.** Since morphologic changes are only slowly reversible and may be permanent in some patients, the best strategy is to choose treatments that are least likely to induce these abnormalities. None of the currently recommended regimens would be likely to cause lipoatrophy—TAF/FTC, TDF/FTC, and ABC/3TC induce less fat atrophy than zidovudine/lamivudine (Table 6.2). Importantly, providers should proactively switch patients receiving long-term zidovudine/lamivudine to a preferred NRTI combination even if patients are not currently experiencing lipoatrophy. Regimens containing stavudine and didanosine should be avoided.

D. **Lipid Abnormalities.** Multiple abnormalities in lipid metabolism were reported in HIV-infected patients before the availability of combination antiretroviral therapy, including increased levels of very low-density lipoprotein (VLDL) cholesterol and triglycerides and decreased levels of high-density lipoprotein (HDL) cholesterol, low-density lipoprotein (LDL) cholesterol, and apolipoprotein B (JAMA 2003;289:2978–82). However, soon after the introduction of PIs, a dramatic increase in triglyceride levels and, to a lesser extent, total cholesterol levels are evident in PI-treated patients.

1. **Antiretroviral Therapy and Dyslipidemia.** The PIs are all associated to varying degrees with clinically significant dyslipidemia. Among recommended boosted PIs, atazanavir and darunavir appear to have the lowest risk of hyperlipidemia. Other components of the antiretroviral regimen may also induce lipid disturbances: d4T, ZDV, and ABC are all more likely to raise lipids than tenofovir, and efavirenz increases lipids, especially triglycerides, more than nevirapine, etravirine, and rilpivirine. Raltegravir, maraviroc, elvitegravir/cobicistat, and dolutegravir increase lipids less than efavirenz. Treatment of HIV may have the favorable effect of raising HDL cholesterol, particularly with nevirapine and efavirenz. Through unclear mechanisms, tenofovir lowers cholesterol levels (total, LDL, and HDL); since TDF yields higher tenofovir concentrations

Table 6.2. Drug-Induced Dyslipidemia and Switch Therapy

Cause	Switch To	Comments
Protease inhibitors (PIs): ritonavir, indinavir, saquinavir, nelfinavir, lopinavir/ritonavir, tipranavir, fosamprenavir	Atazanavir or atazanavir/ritonavir or darunavir/ ritonavir or rilpivirine or raltegravir or dolutegravir	Need to use boosted atazanavir if patient is also on tenofovir. Do not use unboosted atazanavir if there is any history of PI resistance or PI-related treatment failure; do not use rilpivirine if there is any history of NRTI resistance. If patient is on a proton pump inhibitor, atazanavir and rilpivirine should in general be avoided.
d4T or zidovudine or abacavir	TAF or TDF	Use with caution in patients with impaired renal function. While TDF lowers lipids more than TAF, the latter has a better renal and bone safety profile.
Efavirenz	Rilpivirine or etravirine	

Reproduced from Panel on Treatment of HIV-Infected Pregnant Women and Prevention of Perinatal Transmission. Recommendations for use of antiretroviral drugs in pregnant HIV-1-infected women for maternal health and interventions to reduce perinatal HIV transmission in the United States. aidsinfo.nih.gov. June 7, 2016.

than TAF, the lipid-lowering effect is greater with TDF than TAF, with the total:HDL cholesterol ratio not different between the two.

2. **Treatment of Dyslipidemia.** As for HIV-negative patients, an important step consists of therapeutic lifestyle changes, including dietary counseling, reduction in alcohol intake, smoking cessation, and increased aerobic exercise. Unfortunately, lifestyle changes alone are often insufficient to reverse lipid abnormalities in patients with HIV.

The two most widely used pharmacological strategies are substitution of the potentially offending antiretroviral agent with an alternative antiretroviral and use of lipid-modifying drug therapy. Modification of ART should be done according to the principles outlined in Chapter 4, with careful consideration of past resistance history, potential new drug interactions, and the adverse event profile of the new drug or drugs. If there is more than one possible offending agent, the changes should, if possible, be made sequentially to ensure that the initial change is well tolerated.

Many patients with HIV will be candidates for statin therapy, especially as they age or have other cardiac risk factors. The most important consideration prior to selecting a statin is the potential for drug interactions between certain antiretroviral agents and statins. All PI- and elvitegravir based regimens include ritonavir or cobicistat, which are potent inhibitors of CYP3A4. Since many statins are metabolized predominantly via this enzyme, concomitant administration of ritonavir or cobicistat can lead to elevated statin levels, increasing the risk of statin-related toxicity, including rhabdomyolysis (Clin Infect Dis. 2002;35:e111–2). Conversely, coadministration with efavirenz (a CYP3A4 inducer) can lead to decreased statin efficacy.

Pravastatin, fluvastatin, pitavastatin, and rosuvastatin are not metabolized by CYP3A4, and atorvastatin is to a lesser degree than simvastatin or lovastatin. From a practical standpoint, atorvastatin should generally be the initial statin of choice, since it is potent and available generically. If given with ritonavir or cobicistat, the starting dose should be low (10 mg daily) and the patient closely monitored for hepatic/muscle toxicity. If available, pitavastatin is another good choice for these patients. Simvastatin and lovastatin are contraindicated. Not all statin-ART drug interactions are mediated through CYP3A4: rosuvastatin levels may increase significantly when given with lopinavir/ritonavir through unclear mechanisms, and darunavir increases pravastatin levels. Clinicians should consult drug interaction guides carefully before starting statin therapy (http://www.hiv-druginteractions.org/).

The optimal management of HIV-related hypertriglyceridemia is unclear; for levels greater than 500 mg/dL, aggressive dietary modification and use of fibrates should be implemented to reduce the risk of pancreatitis. If possible, patients should be switched off of ritonavir, cobicistat, or efavirenz, drugs known to induce hypertriglyceridemia.

GASTROINTESTINAL TRACT COMPLICATIONS

A. Anorexia

1. Etiology. Commonly associated with advanced HIV disease, possibly due to high cytokine (especially TNF) levels that correlate with high titer HIV RNA. Other causes include depression, medications, opportunistic infections (especially MAC), and lactic acidosis (related to mitochondrial toxicity).

2. Treatment. <u>Megecetrol acetate</u> (Megace) liquid suspension 400–800 mg (PO) QD improves appetite and quality of life (Ann Intern Med. 1994 Sep 15;121[6]:400–8). Its role in the era of effective ART is limited; should be used as a palliative therapy only. Weight gain that results is generally fat, not lean body mass. Side effects include hypogonadism, deep vein thrombosis (DVT), and gynecomastia. Megecetrol has corticosteroid properties, and therefore can lead to Cushing's-like state (prolonged use) or adrenal insufficiency (when drug is withdrawn). Prolonged use should be avoided; if required, dose should be tapered gradually. <u>Dronabinol</u> (Marinol) 2.5 mg q12h stimulates appetite and reduces nausea. Dronabinol is a synthetic delta-9-tetrahydrocannabinol (THC), the active ingredient in marijuana. The main side effect is oversedation. Patients should start with a dose at bedtime and then increase to q12h as tolerated.

B. Nausea/Vomiting

1. Etiology

    a. Medications. Direct effect of antiretroviral medications (especially PIs, ZDV, ABC hypersensitivity), medication-related pancreatitis (see above), or lactic acidosis from NRTIs.

    b. Opportunistic infections. Intestinal protozoa (e.g., cryptosporidiosis, *Isospora*, giardiasis—all usually accompanied by diarrhea), CMV esophagitis/gastritis, gastrointestinal (GI) tract involvement of MAC.

c. **Others.** Gastric lymphoma, CNS process producing mass effect (toxoplasmosis or lymphoma) or raised intracerebral pressure (cryptococcal meningitis).

2. **Treatment.** Address underlying etiology. If felt to be due to the direct effect of anti-retrovirals, choose an alternate regimen if safe from the virologic perspective (e.g., substitute tenofovir alafenamide for ZDV, integrase inhibitor or NNRTI for PI). If under-lying cause cannot be treated or removed, or for temporary relief of symptoms, thera-peutic options include: prochlorperazine (Compazine) 10 mg (PO) or 25 mg (PR) q12h prn; metoclopramide (Reglan) 10 mg (PO) q6h prn; trimethobenzamide (Tigan) 250 mg (PO) q6h prn; lorazepam 0.5–1.0 mg (PO or IV) q6h prn; ondansetron (Zofran) 4–8 mg (PO) q8h prn or 32 mg (IV or IM) as a single dose; dronabinol (Marinol) 2.5–5.0 mg (PO) q12h. Patients with HIV are at increased risk for phenothiazine-related dystonia, which may occur with prochlorperazine, metoclopramide, and trimethobenzamide. Treat dystonia with diphenhydramine (Benadryl) 50 mg (PO or IV) × 1 dose.

C. **Diarrhea**
   1. **Etiology**
      a. **Infection.** <u>Acute diarrhea</u>: *Salmonella, Shigella, Campylobacter, Clostridium dif-ficile*, giardiasis, *Cyclospora*; <u>subacute/chronic diarrhea</u>: giardiasis, cryptosporidia, microsporidia, *Isospora*, CMV.
      b. **Medication-related.** Especially protease inhibitors; can be part of abacavir hypersensitivity syndrome. Medication-related diarrhea is rarely associated with weight loss or fever (abacavir excluded). Risk of ritonavir-related diarrhea appears to be dose related—several comparative studies have shown lower rates of diar-rhea when the total daily dose is 100 mg rather than 200 mg.
   2. **Treatment.** Treat underlying cause if due to an infection (see Chapter 5). If PI related, consider changing to an alternative PI that is less likely to cause diar-rhea (e.g., atazanavir/ritonavir or darunavir/ritonavir), or to an NNRTI (efavirenz or nevirapine) or integrase inhibitor. Virologic suppression must be maintained, hence switching should be undertaken using the principles outlined in Chapter 4. If diarrhea persists or if medication changes are not possible, offer symptomatic therapy with psyllium 1 tsp q12h–24h, loperamide 2 mg q6h prn, calcium 500 mg q12h; pancreatic enzymes 1–2 tabs with each meal, diphenoxylate/atropine (Lomotil) 1–2 tabs q8h prn, or octreotide 100–500 µg (SQ) q12h. Crofelemer 125 mg PO bid may be helpful in certain patients, in particular those with PI-related diarrhea.

D. **Oral or Esophageal Ulcers**
   1. **Presentation.** Intensely painful ulcers of various size; esophageal ulcers cause severe dysphagia. May occur at any stage of HIV disease (including primary infection), but more common with progressive immunosuppression (CD4 < 100, associated neutro-penia). Most common diagnosis is idiopathic aphthous ulcers; other causes include CMV, herpes simplex virus (HSV), histoplasmosis, and lymphoma. For first-time pre-sentation, culture for HSV and refer for biopsy to exclude other causes.

2. **Treatment.** For idiopathic aphthous ulcers, start with symptom relief, followed by application of local steroids, followed by either systemic steroids or thalidomide (see below). Lesions sometimes respond to immune reconstitution from antiretroviral therapy along with resolution of neutropenia (adjunctive therapy with G-CSF may hasten healing). Therapeutic modalities include:

   a. Symptom reduction with viscous lidocaine (2%).

   b. Topical fluocinonide (Lidex) 0.05% ointment mixed 1:1 with Orobase; apply q6h as needed.

   c. Dexamethasone 0.5/5M elixir mouth rinse q8h–12h.

   d. Local corticosteroid injections by oral surgeon.

   e. Prednisone 40–60 mg/day × 1–2 weeks, tapered as tolerated over 1–2 weeks or longer as needed.

   f. Thalidomide 200 mg (PO) at bedtime × 4–6 weeks, followed by 100 mg (PO) at bedtime twice weekly. Side effects include sedation, constipation, peripheral neuropathy. Severe teratogenicity of thalidomide requires that physicians register with company-sponsored monitoring program before prescribing (see www.thalomid.com). Women of childbearing age must use at least two forms of contraception and have regular pregnancy tests while receiving thalidomide. Informed consent in package insert must be signed before therapy is initiated.

E. HIV Cholangiopathy

   1. **Presentation.** Presents with right upper quadrant pain, fever, and sometimes jaundice. Laboratory evaluation invariably demonstrates increased alkaline phosphatase. Generally occurs with severe immunosuppression (CD4 < 100/mm³). Imaging with ultrasound or ERCP shows dilated or prominent intrahepatic and extrahepatic ducts. Papillary stenosis may also be present.

   2. **Etiology.** Differential diagnosis include cholelithiasis, acalculous cholecystitis, infiltrative infectious or neoplastic diseases of the liver. Screen for infectious etiology, including stool for ova/parasites and/or ERCP aspirates for cryptosporidia, microsporidia, *Cyclospora*, CMV.

   3. **Treatment.** Symptomatic improvement is sometimes seen with endoscopic-guided sphincterotomy or stenting. Treat underlying infectious process, if identified.

RENAL COMPLICATIONS

A. HIV-Associated Nephropathy. A form of progressive glomerulosclerosis, leading to massive proteinuria and progressive renal dysfunction. Over 80% of cases occur in African-Americans. Renal biopsy shows extensive collapsing glomerulosclerosis, tubular ectasia, and tubulo-interstitial disease. Occurs most commonly with low CD4 cell counts

(< 100/mm³), but may occur at any level of immunosuppression. Very uncommon with undetectable HIV RNA (Clin Infect Dis. 2006;43:377–80).

1. **Presentation.** Clinical presentation varies from asymptomatic to symptoms of hypoalbuminemia and renal failure (edema, fatigue, anemia). Hypertension generally is absent. Renal ultrasound demonstrates enlarged or normal-sized kidneys. The cardinal laboratory feature is proteinuria > 1 g/day, usually with rapidly progressive renal failure evolving over weeks to months to end-stage renal disease requiring dialysis.

2. **Diagnostic Considerations.** Biopsy should be considered to rule out other causes of progressive renal disease, such as HCV-associated renal disease, medication-associated toxicity (see below), or a non-HIV-related cause.

3. **Treatment.** Effective options include antiretroviral therapy (case reports suggest PI-based therapy may lead to resolution of disease), ACE inhibitors, and high-dose corticosteroids (60 mg prednisone QD × 1 month followed by gradual taper) (Kidney International 2000;58:1253). Since high-dose steroids are associated with further immune suppression and other complications, a reasonable approach is to begin with antiretroviral therapy plus an ACE inhibitor (e.g., captopril 6.25 mg q8h).

B. **Medication-Related Renal Disease.** HIV-related medications most likely to cause nephrotoxicity are listed below. (See antiretroviral drug summaries in Chapter 9 for dosing in renal insufficiency.)

1. **Tenofovir disoproxil fumarate (TDF).** Can cause tubular injury, leading to increased creatinine. Rarely accompanied by Fanconi's syndrome, with phosphate wasting and acidosis. Renal toxicity is more likely to occur in those with underlying renal disease or advanced HIV infection (Clin Infect Dis. 2005;15:1194–8; J Infect Dis. 2008;197:102). Risk of TDF-related renal disease is higher when given with boosted PIs (J Infect Dis. 2008 Jan 1;197(1):102–8), and a similar incidence is likely when TDF is coadministered with cobicistat. The newer form of tenofovir, tenofovir alafenamide (TAF), leads to a 90% lower plasma concentration of tenofovir, and significantly less effect on estimated GFR and renal tubular proteins (Lancet 2015 April 15; 385(9987): 2606–15). Patients with stable renal impairment can safely receive TAF-based therapies (J Acquir Immune Defic Syndr. 2016 Apr 15; 71(5):530–7). It is unclear whether patients who experienced prior renal toxicity to TDF can receive TAF safely. Our approach is to consider this only after the TDF toxicity has completely resolved.

2. **Atazanavir and indinavir.** Both medications can cause nephrolithiasis, and some studies have linked atazanavir to an increased risk of decreased renal function. For severe nephrolithiasis or other renal complication, change the patient to an alternative PI, generally darunavir.

3. **Pentamidine.** Can cause renal failure in up to 50% of patients; other adverse effects include electrolyte/mineral wasting and hypoglycemia. Risk is related to cumulative dose; monitor creatinine, electrolytes, glucose, calcium, and phosphate during therapy.

4. **Foscarnet.** Induces dose-related renal failure as well as wasting of potassium, calcium, and phosphate. Dose adjustment is necessary for reduced creatinine clearance. Supplement potassium, calcium, and phosphorus as needed.

5. **Cidofovir.** Associated with dose-related renal toxicity, which can be reduced by concomitant administration of probenecid and hydration. Check serum creatinine and urine for protein prior to each dose; if creatinine is > 2 g/dL or there is more than 2+ proteinuria, do not administer further cidofovir as renal toxicity may be irreversible.

6. **Amphotericin B.** Dose-dependent renal toxicity is common. Liposomal preparations are less nephrotoxic.

7. **Trimethoprim-sulfamethoxazole (TMP-SMX).** May cause hyperkalemia through amiloride-like effect from trimethoprim, especially when used at high doses for PCP treatment. Sulfonamide component can rarely cause crystal nephropathy (reversible with hydration).

8. **Acyclovir.** High-dose IV administration can crystalize in kidney and cause acute renal failure. Risk can be reduced with adequate hydration, and renal dysfunction usually responds to hydration and cessation of drug.

C. **HCV-Associated Renal Disease.** Often a manifestation of HCV-associated mixed cryoglobulinemia.

1. **Presentation.** Patients may present with palpable purpura or other dermatologic signs, along with hematuria, proteinuria, and sometimes renal failure. Other related laboratory findings include HCV RNA in plasma, cryoglobulins in blood, and low complement; renal biopsy shows HCV-related immune complexes.

2. **Treatment.** Therapy directed at hepatitis C can lead to improvement in renal disease and other manifestations of cryoglobulinemia.

D. **Heroin Nephropathy.** Can coexist with other forms of renal failure listed above. Results from glomerular injury, presumably from toxic effects of heroin or other contaminants. Distinguished from HIV-associated nephropathy by a slower rate of progression, small (as opposed to large) kidneys on ultrasound, and less proteinuria. Treatment consists of cessation of drug use.

E. **Inhibition of Tubular Secretion of Creatinine.** Several HIV-related drugs block tubular secretion of creatinine, leading to a rapid but small increase in serum creatinine. These drugs include cobicistat, dolutegravir, and TMP-SMX in particular; ritonavir and rilpivirine also induce this effect to a lesser extent. The increase is typically small (< 0.3 mg/dL), occurs shortly after starting treatment, and is not progressive or associated with an actual decline in glomerular function.

CARDIAC COMPLICATIONS

A. **HIV-Related Cardiomyopathy** (JAMA 2008;299:324–31). Biventricular reduction in ejection fraction, with pathologic features typical of myocarditis and/or immune-mediated cardiomyopathy. Prevalence varies widely depending on definition; echocardiogram may show reduced ejection fraction (EF) in up to 50% of patients with AIDS, but symptomatic cardiomyopathy occurs in only 1–3%. More common with progressive immunodeficiency, especially when CD4 cell count < 100.

1. **Etiology.** Usually idiopathic. Differential diagnosis includes several causes, not mutually exclusive: HIV itself, secondary infection (CMV, toxoplasmosis, coxsackie, adenovirus, Chagas), disordered immune response leading to autoimmune myocarditis, nutritional deficiencies (selenium, carnitine), and drug toxicity (older NRTI-associated mitochondrial toxicity, alcohol, and doxorubicin).

2. **Presentation.** Presents as left ventricular failure, with dyspnea, congestive heart failure, elevated jugular venous pressure, and a prominent S_3 on exam. Chest x-ray typically demonstrates an enlarged heart, and echocardiogram shows marked biventricular dysfunction with reduced ejection fraction. Diagnosis is made after exclusion of other common causes of low EF (alcohol, poor nutrition, myocardial ischemia). Cardiac biopsy is rarely useful.

3. **Treatment.** Patients should receive antiretroviral therapy plus usual therapies for heart failure (diuretics, beta-blockers, ACE inhibitors are often quite effective in reducing symptoms). For manifestations of disseminated CMV disease or a positive blood CMV viral load, empiric CMV treatment with valganciclovir 900 mg (PO) q12h × 3 weeks. Although case reports have shown improvement in ejection fraction after cessation of NRTIs, this is a much less common cause of cardiomyopathy than HIV itself.

B. **Pericarditis/Pericardial Effusion**

1. **Etiology.** Pericardial fluid may be due to HIV itself or a complicating malignancy/opportunistic infection. The most common malignancy is lymphoma, where an effusion may be the first manifestation of an extranodal high-grade B-cell lymphoma; Kaposi's sarcoma causes effusions generally only when the disease is widespread elsewhere. In addition, numerous common and opportunistic infections have been reported to cause pericarditis in HIV patients, including pyogenic bacteria (especially *Staphylococcus aureus* and *Streptococcus pneumoniae*), TB, atypical mycobacteria, cryptococcal disease, disseminated histoplasmosis, and CMV.

2. **Presentation and Diagnosis.** Often diagnosed incidentally through enlarged cardiac silhouette and subsequent echocardiogram. May be asymptomatic or cause chest pain, dyspnea, cardiac tamponade, and/or pericardial friction rub. Pericardiocentesis is indicated for large or symptomatic effusions, with fluid sent for cultures (routine, fungal, mycobacterial) and cytology.

3. **Treatment.** Directed at underlying condition. If idiopathic pericarditis, consider starting antiretroviral therapy, and manage symptoms with NSAIDs and corticosteroids (as in HIV-negative patients).

C. **Tricuspid Valve Endocarditis**

1. **Etiology.** Injection drug users (IDUs) with HIV, particularly those with lower CD4 cell counts, are at substantially higher risk for endocarditis than HIV-negative IDUs (J Infect

Dis. 2002;185:1761–6). *Staphylococcus aureus* is the most common pathogen. In one series, rates of infection included *S. aureus* (73%), coagulase-negative *Staphylococcus* species (1%), *Staphylococcus* species not otherwise classified (7%), *Streptococcus* species (13%), *Pseudomonas* species (2%), *Bacillus* species (2%), and other organisms (2%). A significant proportion of the *Staph aureus* isolates will be MRSA.

2. **Presentation and Diagnosis.** Patients typically present with fever, weight loss, and sometimes pulmonary symptoms (dyspnea, chest pain) reflective of septic emboli arising from an infected tricuspid valve. Physical examination usually reveals a heart murmur ± evidence of peripheral septic emboli. Chest x-ray may show multiple septic emboli, some with cavitation. An echocardiogram should be performed to assess for valvular vegetations. Diagnosis is confirmed when a patient with the above clinical presentation has positive blood cultures for an organism known to be associated with endocarditis.

3. **Treatment.** While a short course (2 weeks) of therapy has been effective in HIV-negative IDUs with tricuspid endocarditis, this regimen has not been specifically tested in HIV-positive patients. Recommended regimens include:

   - Methicillin-sensitive *S. aureus* (MSSA): Nafcillin or oxacillin 2 g (IV) q4h × 28 days plus gentamicin 1 mg/kg (IV) q8h × 3–5 days or until blood cultures clear. Cefazolin 2 gm IV q8h may substitute for nafcillin or oxacillin; some clinicians prefer this option as it is generally better tolerated.

   - Methicillin-resistant *S. aureus* or beta-lactam allergy: Vancomycin 1 g (IV) q12h × 28 days plus gentamicin 1 mg/kg (IV) q8h × 3–5 days or until blood cultures clear. Alternative to vancomycin is daptomycin (IV) 6 mg/kg QD × 4 weeks.

   - Unable or unwilling to receive IV therapy: Ciprofloxacin 750 mg (PO) q12h plus rifampin 300 mg (PO) q12h × 4 weeks. This regimen cannot be used with PIs due to rifampin-PI interaction. Linezolid 600 mg (PO) q12h × 4 weeks can be used as an alternative (limited data).

PULMONARY COMPLICATIONS

A. **Pulmonary Hypertension** (JAMA 2008;299:324–31). Idiopathic elevation of pulmonary pressures is sometimes seen in HIV infection. The pathological process is similar to primary pulmonary hypertension (i.e., hypertrophy of vascular endothelium). Pulmonary hypertension is more common in women and can occur at any CD4 cell count.

1. **Presentation.** Dyspnea on exertion, palpitations, chest pain. Exam may reveal elevated jugular venous pressure (JVP) and precordial heave. Diagnosis is supported by echocardiogram and Doppler studies showing right ventricular hypertrophy and elevated pulmonary artery (PA) pressures. Most sensitive test is right heart catheterization, where pressures will exceed 30 mmHg. Recurrent pulmonary emboli should be excluded as a possible cause.

2. **Treatment.** Epoprostenol (FloLan) by continuous infusion. Requires placement of a permanent central venous catheter. Diuretics also help relieve symptoms. Treatment

of pulmonary hypertension should be individualized based on the patient's symptoms and response to vasoreactivity testing. Options include diuretics, calcium antagonists, prostacyclin pathway agonists, endothelin receptor antagonists, and PDE5 inhibitors. Treatments should be chosen based on consultation with experts in pulmonary hypertension.

B. Lymphocytic Interstitial Pneumonitis (LIP). An idiopathic form of diffuse lung disease that is more common in children. Tends to occur with moderate immunosuppression (CD4 cell count 200–400/mm^3) and mimics PCP.

1. **Presentation and Diagnosis.** Cough, dyspnea on exertion, exercise oxygen desaturation. Usually afebrile. Chest x-ray and chest CT show diffuse bilateral reticulonodular infiltrates. Differentiated from PCP by generally higher CD4 cell counts and lower LDH. Diagnosed by bronchioalveolar lavage (BAL) with biopsy, which will exclude PCP and yield the characteristic histopathology of LIP (patchy lymphocytic infiltration and no microorganisms on special stains).

2. **Treatment.** Antiretroviral therapy can either improve LIP or worsen it through enhanced immune activity. Prednisone usually achieves rapid reduction in dyspnea, but tapering dose may be accompanied by a relapse of symptoms.

C. Emphysema. Cigarette smoking is associated with a more rapid progression to bullous emphysema in patients with HIV compared to HIV-negative controls. Clinical presentation and treatment are the same as for the general population.

D. Pulmonary Kaposi's Sarcoma. Generally occurs only in patients with advanced HIV disease and extensive Kaposi's sarcoma elsewhere.

1. **Presentation and Diagnosis.** Chest x-ray demonstrates nodules, masses, and/or pleural effusions. Diagnosed by visual inspection of the airway during bronchoscopy, where typical violaceous plaques may be observed.

2. **Treatment.** Antiretroviral therapy may lead to dramatic improvement in even severe Kaposi's sarcoma, although temporary flares due to immune reconstitution have been reported. Concomitant systemic chemotherapy is also generally required.

HEENT COMPLICATIONS

A. Aphthous Ulcers. See p. 156.

B. Oral Hairy Leukoplakia
1. **Presentation.** Presents as ribbed, "corduroy"-like white patches on the side of the tongue. More common with increased immunosuppression (CD4 < 200/mm^3). Usually painless. Distinguished from oral thrush in that oral hairy leukoplakia does not rub off with tongue depressor. Caused by Epstein-Barr virus.

   2. **Treatment.** No treatment is needed unless the patient is symptomatic. Antiretroviral therapy often leads to resolution. Other treatment options include acyclovir 800 mg (PO) 5×/day or famciclovir 500 mg (PO) q12h or valacyclovir 1000 mg (PO) q8h until resolution. Topical application of podophyllin is sometimes effective.

C. **Salivary Gland Enlargement**
   1. **Presentation.** Can occur at any stage of HIV infection and usually worsens with disease progression. Often accompanied by xerostomia. Biopsy shows lymphoid infiltration, possibly due to HIV itself; may be part of diffuse infiltrative lymphocytosis syndrome (DILS), which can be accompanied by involvement of the lungs, kidneys, and peripheral nerves. For progressive parotid enlargement, a CT scan is recommended to differentiate solid from cystic enlargement. Differential diagnosis includes infectious parotitis, which presents more acutely with fever and local pain.

   2. **Treatment.** Antiretroviral therapy is the preferred approach; will lead to improvement in a majority of cases. Other forms of treatment include repeated aspiration of fluid-filled cysts when symptomatic, local measures for dry mouth (sugarless gum, artificial saliva), and prednisone 40 mg (PO) QD × 1 week followed by gradual taper over 1–2 weeks.

D. **Lymphoepithelial Cysts**
   1. **Presentation.** Presents as enlarged cervical cysts that can mimic lymphadenopathy. Can occur at any CD4 cell count. A biopsy is needed to rule out lymphoma, other malignancies (notably squamous cell carcinoma), or opportunistic infections. Cause is unknown.

   2. **Treatment.** Antiretroviral therapy often causes dramatic reduction in size of cysts.

E. **Gingivitis/Periodontitis**
   1. **Presentation.** Presents as painful gums with easy bleeding, along with erythematous and receding gingiva. May be the initial manifestation of underlying HIV disease. Severity correlates with stage of immunosuppression. Caused by oral anaerobic bacteria (usually polymicrobial), and exacerbated by poor local oral hygiene, smoking, and/or alcoholism.

   2. **Treatment.** Improved local hygiene (brush, floss, antibacterial mouth rinse). Curettage by dentist/periodontist may be helpful. For severe cases, treat for 7–10 days with metronidazole 500 mg (PO) q8h or clindamycin 300 mg (PO) q6h or amoxicillin-clavulanate 850 mg (PO) q12h.

MUSCULOSKELETAL COMPLICATIONS

A. **HIV Arthropathy**
   1. **Presentation.** Presents as painful arthropathy, often involving multiple joints. Pain out of proportion to physical findings. Cause is unknown.

   2. **Treatment.** NSAIDs, other pain relievers.

B. Reiter's Syndrome

1. **Presentation.** Asymmetrical polyarthritis involving the large joints of lower extremities. Arthritis is seen in conjunction with urethritis, skin lesions (circinate balanitis, keratoderma blennorrhagica), and ocular disease. May also occur after gastroenteritis. Appears to occur with greater frequency among HIV patients, usually in association with HLA-B27.

2. **Diagnosis.** Differential diagnosis includes septic arthritis; if joint effusions are present, arthrocentesis with cultures/Gram stain is indicated. Urethral swab for chlamydia and gonorrhea is also recommended.

3. **Treatment.** Consider treatment of urethritis with empiric chlamydia therapy with azithromycin 1 g (PO) × 1 dose. Other measures include NSAIDs and referral to rheumatology for possible immunosuppressive therapy (prednisone, methotrexate, and TNF antagonists).

C. Pyomyositis. Focal infection of muscle often occurring at site of injections, trauma.

1. **Presentation.** Presents as localized pain, swelling, fever. Usually caused by *Staphylococcus aureus* including MRSA, less commonly other pyogenic bacteria, e.g., streptococci, gram-negative rods. More common with advanced HIV immunosuppression (CD4 cell count < 100).

2. **Diagnosis.** Imaging of suspected area with CT followed by diagnostic aspiration for Gram stain/culture.

3. **Treatment.** Antibiotics directed at causative pathogen (usually an anti-staphylococcal penicillin or vancomycin). May also require surgical incision/drainage.

D. HIV Myopathy and NRTI-Related Myopathy. These two conditions may present similarly.

1. **Presentation.** Patients present with myalgias, muscle tenderness, weakness, and elevated CPK levels. Proximal leg muscles are most commonly involved. Condition can occur at any stage of HIV disease.

2. **Diagnosis.** Some experts recommend a biopsy to distinguish between HIV and NRTI-related myopathy. In the former, there is a more prominent inflammatory infiltrate; the latter usually shows evidence of mitochondrial myopathy. NRTI-related myopathy is most commonly associated with zidovudine.

3. **Treatment.** For symptomatic HIV-related myopathy, corticosteroids at high doses (prednisone 1 mg/kg/day) are recommended. Once improvement occurs, this should be tapered over several weeks. For NRTI-related myopathy, change to a regimen that either avoids NRTIs entirely or switches to those NRTIs with lower mitochondrial toxicity (abacavir, emtricitabine, lamivudine, tenofovir).

E. Rhabdomyolysis. Extensive muscle necrosis with myoglobinuria and acute renal failure. May occur as part of medication toxicity (to older NRTIs such as ZDV, d4T, ddI, or rarely to integrase inhibitors) or to HIV itself. Management is by withdrawal of possibly offending agents and hydration—hemodialysis if necessary.

NEUROLOGIC COMPLICATIONS

A. Distal Sensory Neuropathy. Caused by HIV itself and/or neurotoxic effects of medications, in particular the di-deoxy NRTIs no longer in wide use (d4T, ddI, ddC).

    1. Presentation. Typically presents as pain, aching, burning, or tingling of the distal extremities (toes/feet more commonly than fingers/hands). Pain is often worse at night. Principal risk factors include the stage of HIV disease and exposure to the above listed drugs, especially when used in combination.

    2. Diagnosis and Evaluation. Usually clinical, based on patient history. Reduced pin-prick and vibration sense in the involved extremities support the diagnosis, but symptoms often precede objective physical findings. Attempt to identify contributing/other causes, including B_{12} deficiency, syphilis, CMV, multiple myeloma, other neurotoxic agents (dapsone, INH, vincristine; avoid using these drugs if possible with d4T or ddI). If presentation is confusing, refer for electromyogram (EMG) and nerve conduction studies, which will show an axonal neuropathy.

    3. Treatment. Withdraw offending agents, in particular d4T and ddI; symptoms may persist or even worsen for several weeks after cessation of these drugs, and severe neuropathy may be irreversible. Many of the patients currently in care with neuropathy received d4T and/or ddI in the past, and have residual nerve damage. Antiretroviral therapy should be continued and one of several therapies used for neuropathic symptoms can be administered:

- NSAIDs or acetaminophen for mild pain.
- Avoid tight-fitting shoes, extremes of temperature.
- Gabapentin 300 mg at bedtime; increase up to 1200 mg divided q6–8h as needed.
- Nortriptyline 10 mg at bedtime; increase up to 75 mg at bedtime as tolerated.
- Lamictal 25 mg q12h; increase up to 150 mg q12h as tolerated.
- Topical therapy: capsaicin (may make symptoms worse), lidocaine patches.
- Acupuncture.
- Severe pain may require chronic long-acting narcotic pain relievers (e.g., methadone, MS-Contin, transdermal fentanyl).

B. Other Forms of Neuropathy

    1. Types

        a. Acute inflammatory demyelinating neuropathy (AIDP, Guillain-Barré syndrome). Ascending motor weakness usually without sensory involvement. Reported in early and late stage HIV. May evolve into a chronic form with waxing and waning symptoms. Treatment consists of steroids, plasmapheresis, IVIG.

Prognosis is variable for all—tends to be best for mononeuritis especially if due to acute HIV infection.

b. Mononeuritis multiplex. Scattered, asymmetrical, motor and sensory deficits (e.g., facial weakness, foot drop). Reported in acute and chronic HIV. Some cases ascribed to CMV in advanced HIV (CD4 < 50/mm³). Treatment consists of steroids, IVIG. If caused by CMV, treat with valganciclovir at standard doses.

c. HIV-associated neuromuscular weakness syndrome. Rare complication of NRTI-therapy (especially d4T), presenting as progressive ascending paralysis in association with lactic acidosis. When severe, mechanical ventilation may be required. Treatment consists of withdrawal of NRTIs, especially d4T. Residual neurologic impairment is common after recovery.

d. Progressive polyradiculopathy. Complication of advanced HIV disease that typically presents with lower extremity weakness, anaesthesia in a "saddle" distribution (perineal area), and/or bowel and bladder dysfunction. Most common causes include CMV polyradiculitis (p. 93) and lymphoma. Diagnostically, obtain an MRI of the lumbosacral spine to exclude a mass lesion, then proceed to CSF exam. If due to CMV, the usual CSF finding is increased WBC (predominantly polys), increased protein, and positive CMV PCR. If due to lymphoma, the CSF shows increased protein and lymphoma cells on cytology. For CMV polyraduliculitis, treat × 3–4 weeks or until improvement with either ganciclovir 5 mg/kg (IV) q12h or valganciclovir 900 mg (PO) q12h or foscarnet 90 mg/kg (IV) q12h; for severe cases, some advocate ganciclovir plus foscarnet. For lymphoma, treat with chemotherapy plus radiation.

2. Prognosis. Prognosis is variable for all forms of neuropathy but tends to be best for mononeuritis, especially if due to acute HIV infection.

C. HIV-Associated Dementia (AIDS dementia, HIV encephalitis/encephalopathy). Typical presentation at onset consists of short-term memory loss, often with apathy or withdrawal from usual activities. As the disease progresses, cognitive impairment worsens, and speech, motor, and gait disturbances develop. Seizures and akinetic mutism are late-stage manifestations. The incidence of this complication has decreased dramatically since the widespread introduction of combination antiretroviral therapy in 1996. Progression of dementia is gradual (usually over months) and can be arrested/reversed with potent antiretroviral therapy. A more rapidly progressive form has also been reported. HIV dementia almost always occurs in the late stages of HIV disease (CD4 < 100/mm³, HIV RNA > 100,000 copies/mL), but on rare occasions occurs with relatively preserved immune function and low plasma HIV RNA. In the latter case, relatively high HIV RNA levels are often present in the CSF.

1. Diagnosis. Diagnosis is based on a combination of clinical, laboratory, and imaging criteria, as well as exclusion of alternative causes (depression, adverse drug effects, neurosyphilis, CMV encephalitis). HIV-associated dementia should be suspected in a patient with advanced HIV disease and subacute to chronic cognitive impairment, especially short-term memory loss. Administration of the four-step HIV-dementia scale (AIDS Reader 2002;12:29) may help quantify the extent of deficits. MRI shows cerebral atrophy and often non-enhancing white matter abnormalities that can be indistinguishable from progressive multifocal leukoencephalopathy (PML). CSF exam is usually abnormal, with elevated protein and low-level lymphocytic pleocytosis. When HIV RNA in the CSF is measured, it is usually detectable at 1000 copies/mL or higher; an undetectable CSF HIV RNA is unusual in HIV dementia and suggests an alternative diagnosis. Rare cases of "CNS escape" may occur when patients are virologically suppressed based on blood HIV RNA, but still have detectable HIV RNA in the CSF. In such patients, obtain resistance testing of CSF isolate in order to optimize ART.

2. **Treatment.** Potent antiretroviral therapy is the mainstay of therapy and can lead to dramatic improvement, especially in treatment-naïve individuals. Selection of drugs with higher penetration into the CNS is theoretically preferable (Arch Neurol. 2008 Jan;65[1]:65–70), although there are no definitive clinical data to support this approach over choosing alternative agents. As a result, the primary goal should be to choose a regimen with a high likelihood of achieving virologic suppression. In a patient who has failed antiretroviral therapy, treatment is based on resistance testing to maximize antiviral potency.

PSYCHIATRIC COMPLICATIONS

Psychiatric illness is more common in patients with HIV than in those with other medical illnesses of comparable severity. Potential explanations include pre-existing psychiatric illness that predisposes to high-risk behavior for HIV acquisition (substance abuse, sexual addiction), extreme grief reactions from having a stigmatized illness, or neurotoxic effects of HIV manifesting as psychiatric illness. For all psychiatric illnesses, consider starting antiretroviral therapy even if there are otherwise no indications, as therapy is associated with improved neuropsychiatric function. Carefully review package inserts and drug interaction tables at http://www.aidsinfo.nih.gov prior to prescribing any psychotropic agent.

A. **Depression**

1. **Presentation and Diagnosis.** Common symptoms include depressed mood, decreased interest in work/leisure activities, blunted affect, sleep disturbances, alterations in appetite, forgetfulness, and diminished concentration. Key differential is HIV dementia, but depressed mood is usually not a prominent feature of dementia. Among antiretroviral agents, efavirenz is the drug most strongly linked to depression, and one study identified a two-fold increase in risk of suicidal ideation in those randomized to efavirenz (Ann Intern Med. 2014 Jul 1; 161(1):1–10). Consider changing to an different option from the list of recommended initial regimens if a patient develops depression while receiving efavirenz. Other drugs that may be associated with mood changes (albeit to a lesser extent than efavirenz) include rilpivirine, raltegravir, and dolutegravir.

2. **Treatment.** Selective serotonin reuptake inhibitors (SSRIs) or tricyclic antidepressants are the mainstays of therapy, as for HIV-negative patients. In general, start with low doses of all agents and titrate up as needed. Always check treatment guidelines for potential drug interactions with antiretroviral agents. If rapid onset of response is needed, stimulants such as methylphenidate or dextroamphetamine may be tried. Monoamine oxidase (MAO) inhibitors are often contraindicated due to drug interactions.

B. **Mania.** HIV may produce an unusual form of mania as a manifestation of HIV encephalopathy.

   1. **Presentation.** These patients usually have CD4 cell counts < 200/mm^3. It is distinguished from non-HIV-related bipolar disease in that there is no family history of bipolar illness and onset may occur at any age. Symptoms include expansive mood, grandiosity, and diminished sleep.

   2. **Treatment.** Treatment should be undertaken with the assistance of a psychiatrist. Options include lithium 300 mg (PO) q8h or valproic acid 250 mg (PO) q12h or carbamazepine 200 mg (PO) q12h.

C. **Insomnia**

   1. **Etiology.** Sleep disturbance may be a symptom of an underlying medical condition (hepatic encephalopathy, HIV dementia), a psychiatric illness (depression, mania, substance abuse, anxiety), or a medication side effect (efavirenz, dolutegravir, corticosteroids).

   2. **Treatment.** Attempt to identify/treat underlying causes, including "poor sleep hygiene" (excessive caffeine, alcohol, other stimulants). For patients with a history of substance abuse, avoid if possible the chronic use of benzodiazepines, which have addictive potential. As an alternative, trazodone 50–100 mg (PO) at bedtime can be very effective. Short-term insomnia due to anxiety or jet lag can be treated with benzodiazepines such as zolpidem (Ambien) 2.5–5.0 mg (PO) at bedtime or lorazepam 1.0 mg (PO) at bedtime.

DERMATOLOGIC COMPLICATIONS

A. **Viral Infections**

   1. **Herpes Simplex Infection.** Oral/anogenital diseases occur more frequently and are more severe in patients with HIV. Infection may also occur on non-mucosal surfaces (e.g., skin), especially when the patient is severely immunocompromised.

      a. **Diagnosis.** Characteristic vesicles on an erythematous base. Ulcerations may occur in primary disease and more advanced HIV-related immunosuppression. A viral culture for HSV is the diagnostic test of choice and is quite sensitive, especially early during the outbreak and prior to starting anti-herpes therapy.

      b. **Treatment.** See p. 116.

2. **Varicella-Zoster Infection.** Herpes zoster is much more common (20- to 50-fold increased risk) in HIV patients than in age-matched HIV-negative controls and may be first sign of underlying HIV infection. AIDS patients are at increased risk for chronic non-healing zoster, which can last for several weeks. Appearance may also be atypical, with nodular rather than vesicular lesions.

   a. **Diagnosis.** Diagnosed by clinical appearance. Direct fluorescent antibody (DFA) test of a lesion can help distinguish zoster from HSV if the diagnosis is unclear.

   b. **Treatment.** See p. 140.

3. **Molluscum Contagiosum**

   a. **Presentation.** Manifests as clusters of white, umbilicated papules outside the groin/perineal area. Rarely seen except with severe immunosuppression (CD4 < 100/mm³); the number/size of lesions increase as immunosuppression progresses.

   b. **Diagnosis.** Diagnosed by clinical appearance. Biopsy is rarely necessary, but when performed shows large inclusions known as "molluscum bodies." Etiologic virus (a pox virus) cannot be cultured in clinical practice.

   c. **Treatment.** Effective antiretroviral therapy can often lead to dramatic, spontaneous improvement. If this is not possible, or for more immediate control, local cryosurgery or other ablative methods can be effective.

4. **Oral Hairy Leukoplakia (OHL).** See p. 162.

5. **Warts.** Cutaneous and genital warts are extremely common in HIV disease, and in severe cases are disfiguring and difficult to treat. Although usually more severe with progressive HIV disease, in some patients they remain a debilitating problem even with good response to antiretroviral therapy.

   a. **Diagnosis.** Generally a clinical diagnosis. In severe or refractory cases, biopsy is sometimes needed to exclude underlying squamous cell carcinoma.

   b. **Treatment**

      i. **Genital warts.** Imiquimod 5% cream 3×/week at bedtime, wash off in A.M. Alternative: podofilox q12h application with cotton swab for 3 days followed by 4 days without treatment, then repeat. Local inflammation is common with both measures. Provider-applied therapies include cryotherapy and podophyllin resin (severe or bulky cases).

      ii. **Cutaneous warts.** As in HIV-negative patients, spontaneous resolution may occur, especially in relatively immunocompetent patients. Therapy is otherwise similar as in HIV-negative patients, with multiple ablative therapies available (cryotherapy, liquid nitrogen, salicylic acid, bichloracetic acid, and curettage). Refractory cases should be referred to a dermatologist for intra-lesional therapy or wide excision.

B. Bacterial Infections

1. **Staphylococcal Infections.** May cause staphylococcal folliculitis, a pruritic condition associated with small papules. Larger collections of soft tissue staph infection can cause furunculosis or subcutaneous abscesses (more common with advanced HIV-related immunosuppression.) In most parts of the United States, MRSA is the most common cause of purulent soft tissue infection.

   a. **Diagnosis.** Clinical appearance. Culture to exclude MRSA.

   b. **Treatment.** For furunculosis, which is often due to MRSA, treat empirically and modify according to sensitivities; doxycycline or TMP-SMX 1 DS (PO) bid or clindamycin 300 mg PO tid are often effective; vancomycin 1 g IV q12h or linezolid 600 mg (PO) bid are recommended for severe cases. If organism is MSSA, dicloxacillin 500 mg qid or cephalexin 500 mg qid are options. Large furuncles or soft tissue collections must be surgically drained (Antimicrob Agents Chemother. 2007 Nov;51[11]:4044–8). For multiple recurrences, consider decontamination strategies.

      i. **Antibacterials:** Mupirocin nasal ointment anterior nares bid, Bactrim 1 DS bid, ± rifampin 300 mg PO bid—all for 7–10 days (do not use rifampin with protease inhibitors).

      ii. **Household contacts** (including pets) cultured/treated.

      iii. **Local measures**
         — Keep cuts/abrasions covered.
         — Bathe for 10 minutes; 1 tsp bleach/gallon of water.
         — Using a bath sponge, lather armpits, groin, anus, and under the breasts with chlorhexidine topical antiseptic (Hibiclens scrub) after draining bath water.
         — Shower Hibiclens off.

      iv. **Frequent laundering of towels, sheets, clothing.**

2. **Bacillary Angiomatosis.** A cutaneous manifestation of *Bartonella quintanna* and *B. henselae* infection (cat scratch bacillus). Presents as a dome-shaped and often pedunculated papule or papules in a patient with severe immunosuppression. Appearance can mimic Kaposi's sarcoma. Organism can also cause hepatic disease (peliosis hepatitis), fever, encephalopathy, and/or endocarditis. Clinical syndromes due to *Bartonella* infection have become extremely rare since the availability of potent antiretroviral therapy.

   a. **Diagnosis.** Characteristic appearance and biopsy, with pathology showing the characteristic bacillus on Warthin-Starry and Dieterle stains. Organism can be cultured, but laboratory needs to be alerted so special media can be used. Serologies also may be helpful.

   b. **Treatment.** Azithromycin 250–500 mg (PO) qd or clarithromycin 500 mg (PO) q12h or doxycycline 100 mg (PO) q12h. Treatment duration is determined by recovery of immune system in response to antiretroviral therapy.

3. **Syphilis.** See p. 137.

C. Fungal Infections

  1. Disseminated and Invasive Fungal Infections. All disseminated fungal infections can cause skin lesions. Most characteristic are molluscum-like lesions with cryptococcal disease, erythema nodosum with coccidioides, and nodular skin lesions with blastomycosis.

  2. Tinea Corporis, Cruris, or Pedis (jock itch, athlete's foot). Extensive erythematous plaques with severe pruritus.

  a. Diagnosis. Characteristic appearance, with KOH slide preparation showing branched, septated hyphae.

  b. Treatment. Topical therapy with over-the-counter preparations, or by prescription with one of several topical antifungals, including clotrimazole, ciclopirox, or butenafine q12h. For severe disease, use fluconazole 100–200 mg (PO) qd × 7–14 days or terbinafine 250 mg (PO) qd × 14 days.

  3. Candidiasis. In addition to mucosal infections, *Candida* can cause disease in the skin and nails. In the skin, it is often seen in intertriginous areas (groin, under breasts), where it causes a pruritic papular eruption that can coalesce to form large plaques. Web spaces of the fingers and toes may also be involved. Heat and moisture in these areas encourage candidal growth.

  a. Diagnosis. Clinically suspected with papular, sometimes pustular eruption in intertriginous areas. A KOH slide shows yeast and pseudohyphae of *Candida*.

  b. Treatment. Topical therapy with antifungals, such as clotrimazole q12h × 14 days. More severe cases may require systemic therapy with fluconazole 100–200 mg (PO) qd × 7–14 days. It is also important to maintain good hygiene, attempt to aerate and dry involved areas, and avoid tight clothing.

D. Miscellaneous Skin Conditions. All can be the first sign of underlying HIV infection.

  1. Seborrheic Dermatitis. Presents as waxy erythematous and sometimes flaky plaques with scale, usually on face and scalp. Usually worsens with progressive immunodeficiency. May be caused by the yeast *Pityrosporum ovale*. Antiretroviral therapy usually leads to improvement. Symptomatic treatment consists of ketoconazole cream q12h × 7–14 days or a low-potency topical steroid (e.g., hydrocortisone cream 2.5% q12h × 7–14 days). For refractory cases where higher-potency steroids may be indicated, referral to a dermatologist is recommended.

  2. Psoriasis. Severity of psoriasis correlates with the degree of immunosuppression. HIV can sometimes unmask a prior history of mild disease. May be accompanied by arthritis. Antiretroviral therapy is often useful. Other treatments as per HIV-negative patients.

  3. Eosinophilic Folliculitis. In erythematous, papular, severely pruritic eruption, usually on the upper trunk and face. Appearance is similar to bacterial folliculitis, but the rash is unresponsive to antibacterials and biopsy demonstrates an eosinophilic infiltrate. The process becomes more difficult to treat as HIV disease progresses; rubbing/

scratching can lead to ulcerations, prurigo nodularis, secondary staph infections. In darker-skinned individuals, this can ultimately lead to disfiguring post-inflammatory hyperpigmentation.

a. Diagnosis. Skin biopsy is required.

b. Treatment. The disease is characterized by its refractory nature and frequent relapses. Individual treatments may work well in some individuals but not in others. Options include ART, oral/topical corticosteroids, isotretinoin, and phototherapy. Antiretroviral therapy will ultimately lead to improvement in most patients. However, some individuals go through a paradoxical worsening due to a heightened inflammatory response, which can be difficult to distinguish from an adverse drug reaction and can sometimes last for weeks to months. Prednisone 70 mg (PO) qd, tapered by 5–10 mg/d, is also helpful. Intermittent therapy of 60 mg (PO) qd × 2–3 days may be useful to control flares after discontinuation. Potent topical corticosteroids q12h–q8h × 10–14 days can be effective but should not be used on the face. Isotretinoin (Accutane) 1 mg/kg/d or 40 mg (PO) q12h is also of value, with duration determined by response to therapy (associated with skin dryness). Ultraviolet B phototherapy may be used 3×/week until improvement, then maintenance as needed.

4. Xerosis/Ichthyosis. Manifests as dry, flaky, and extremely pruritic skin. Worsens as HIV disease progresses, and exacerbated by some antiretrovirals, particularly indinavir. Treatment consists of antiretroviral therapy (avoid indinavir) and emollients (e.g., Aquaphor, Eucerin, Cetaphil). Short-duration (7–14 days) topical steroids may also be considered for dry/inflamed skin.

Chapter 7

HIV and Pregnancy

OVERVIEW

Antiretroviral therapy reduces the risk of perinatal transmission by lowering maternal HIV RNA and by providing pre- and post-exposure prophylaxis for the infant. The risk of perinatal infection has dropped from 25–30% without intervention to <1% with combination antiretroviral therapy (MMWR Morb Mortal Wkly Rep. 2005;55:592–7), especially when ART reduces HIV RNA to below the levels of detection. Off treatment, although the risk of vertical transmission correlates with maternal viral load, there is no maternal viral load below which the risk of transmission is zero (J Infect Dis. 2001;183:539–45). As a result, combination therapy is indicated for all pregnant women, regardless of baseline HIV RNA or CD4 cell count—the same recommendations that apply to nonpregnant people with HIV, only with a secondary indication of prevention of maternal-to-child transmission (PMTCT).

Treatment recommendations for pregnant women are updated based on clinical studies and data collected by the Antiretroviral Pregnancy Registry (www.apregistry.com/index.htm). The most recent version of the US Public Health Service Task Force treatment guidelines was updated August 6, 2015 and is available at http://aidsinfo.nih.gov. The National Perinatal HIV Hotline (1-888-448-8765) provides free clinical consultation on all aspects of perinatal HIV care. This service is particularly useful in settings where clinicians may not see a large volume of HIV-infected pregnant women.

In settings where safe, affordable, and feasible alternatives are available and culturally acceptable, breastfeeding is not recommended for HIV-infected women. By contrast, in many resource-limited settings, breastfeeding is preferred, with data now strongly supporting the benefits of ongoing ART to the mother in preventing HIV transmission to the newborn during the breastfeeding period (N Engl J Med. 2010 Jun 17;362[24]:2282–94).

INITIAL EVALUATION

Initial evaluation of the HIV-infected pregnant woman requires assessment of the considerations shown in Table 7.1.

Table 7.1. Initial Evaluation of HIV-Infected Pregnant Women

- Degree of immunodeficiency (defined by current and past CD4 cell counts)
- Risk for disease progression and perinatal transmission (determined by HIV RNA)
- If HIV RNA is detectable, whether an antiretroviral resistance is present (determined by resistance testing; previous tests should also be reviewed)
- Need for opportunistic infection prophylaxis
- Baseline hematologic, metabolic, renal, and hepatic parameters
- Complete history of past and current antiretroviral therapy regimens
- Presence of co-infections that might require treatment or special care of the newborn (syphilis, gonorrhea, chlamydia, genital herpes simplex, hepatitis B, hepatitis C)
- Assessment of supportive care needs

REPRODUCTIVE OPTIONS FOR HIV SERODISCORDANT COUPLES

Women with HIV infection may wish to become pregnant even though their male sexual partner does not have HIV. Conversely, HIV uninfected women may have an infected partner. In both of these circumstances, consultation with HIV specialists experienced in management of reproductive options is critical to minimize the likelihood of HIV transmission to the uninfected individual. The guidelines in Table 7.2 below are adapted from the latest revision of the Perinatal Guidelines (https://aidsinfo.nih.gov/Guidelines/HTML/3/perinatal-guidelines/0).

Table 7.2. Reproductive Options for HIV-Concordant and Serodiscordant Couples (Last updated June 7, 2016; last reviewed June 7, 2016)

Panel's Recommendations

For Couples Who Want to Conceive

For Concordant (Both Partners Are HIV-Infected) and Discordant Couples:
- Expert consultation is recommended so that approaches can be tailored to couples' specific needs **(AIII)**.
- Partners should be screened and treated for genital tract infections before attempting to conceive **(AII)**.
- The HIV-infected partner(s) should attain maximum viral suppression before attempting conception **(AIII)**.

For Discordant Couples:
- The HIV-infected partner should be receiving combination antiretroviral therapy and demonstrate sustained suppression of plasma viral load below the limits of detection **(AI)**.
- Periconception administration of antiretroviral pre-exposure prophylaxis for HIV-uninfected partners may offer an additional tool to reduce the risk of sexual transmission **(CIII)**. The utility of pre-exposure prophylaxis for the uninfected partner when the infected partner is receiving combination antiretroviral therapy with maximal viral suppression has not been studied.

Discordant Couples with HIV-Infected Women:
- The safest conception option is artificial insemination, including the option of self-insemination with a partner's sperm during the periovulatory period **(AIII)**.

Discordant Couples with HIV-Infected Men:
- The use of donor sperm from an HIV-uninfected man with artificial insemination is the safest option **(AIII)**.
- When the use of donor sperm is unacceptable, the use of sperm preparation techniques coupled with either intrauterine insemination or in vitro fertilization should be considered **(AII)**.
- Semen analysis is recommended for HIV-infected men before conception is attempted to prevent unnecessary exposure to infectious genital fluid when the likelihood of conception is low because of semen abnormalities **(AIII)**.

Rating of Recommendations: *A = Strong; B = Moderate; C = Optional.*

Rating of Evidence: *I = One or more randomized trials with clinical outcomes and/or validated laboratory endpoints; II = One or more well-designed, nonrandomized trials or observational cohort studies with long-term clinical outcomes; III = Expert opinion.*

Reproduced from Panel on Treatment of HIV-Infected Pregnant Women and Prevention of Perinatal Transmission. Recommendations for use of antiretroviral drugs in pregnant HIV-1-infected women for maternal health and interventions to reduce perinatal HIV transmission in the United States. aidsinfo.nih.gov. June 7, 2016.

The risk of transmission is greatly reduced (and all but eliminated) when the infected partner is receiving suppressive antiretroviral therapy (N Engl J Med. 2011;365:493–505). For further protection, the combination of suppressive ART to the infected partner and PrEP for the uninfected person reduces the need for sperm washing and other advanced reproductive technologies, which are not available to all patients. Given the low risk of HIV transmission with combination ART to the infected partner and PrEP to the seronegative individual, some couples may elect to proceed with conception via unprotected sex timed around the woman's peak fertility period. Such a strategy has been safely employed in some centers.

INITIATION OF ANTIRETROVIRAL THERAPY IN PREGNANCY

Decisions regarding when to start treatment and what regimen to use depends on several factors, including; (1) gestational age of the pregnancy; (2) results of the laboratory testing; and (3) known, suspected, or unknown effects of individual drugs on the fetus and newborn.

HIV-infected women in their first trimester of pregnancy who are not on antiretroviral therapy should begin antiretroviral therapy promptly, as early and sustained virologic suppression diminishes the risk of transmission to the newborn. For women already on ART who become pregnant, treatment should be continued. For pregnant women with acute HIV infection, treatment should be started immediately given the high HIV RNA levels associated with this condition. Before starting treatment, it is important to emphasize the need for adherence to medical therapy. Patients should also be instructed to have a low threshold for reporting any potential side effects early, especially those that may reduce medication compliance, so that treatment can be altered and/or symptomatic relief for the side effect can be provided.

GOALS OF THERAPY AND MONITORING

The goal of treatment is the same as for nonpregnant individuals: to ensure an undetectable HIV RNA using the most sensitive available assay. Once antiretroviral therapy is initiated, monitoring of HIV RNA is recommended at 1–2 weeks, then monthly thereafter until the HIV RNA is undetectable, then every 2–3 months after that. The CD4 cell count should be obtained every 3 months, although treatment should not be changed based solely on CD4 changes provided that virologic suppression is maintained. Laboratory monitoring for toxicity can be performed at the same time as HIV RNA testing.

In the case of virologic failure—i.e., inability to achieve an undetectable HIV RNA or viral rebound occurs—repeat resistance testing is indicated. Subsequent management will depend on assessment of medication adherence and the degree of resistance detected on testing, as described in Chapter 4. For women who have not achieved virologic suppression near the time of delivery, especially if the HIV RNA exceeds 1000 copies/mL, a scheduled cesarean delivery is recommended at 38 weeks gestation. In addition, an elective admission to the hospital for directly observed antiretroviral therapy might enable a greater decline in HIV RNA, further reducing risk of transmission.

PREFERRED AND ALTERNATIVE TREATMENTS FOR PREGNANT WOMEN

An overview of preferred and alternative treatments for pregnant women is shown below in Table 7.4. These recommendations apply to women initiating treatment for the first time during pregnancy, and also to women with virologic suppression who have never had treatment failure or drug resistance. Women who are virologically suppressed on regimens chosen based on prior resistance who then become pregnant should in general continue this regimen to avoid the risk of virologic rebound.

Based on our clinical experience, and these guidelines, our currently preferred regimen for pregnant women is TDF/FTC plus raltegravir. It combines excellent virologic efficacy with low rates of gastrointestinal side effects, the latter an important consideration during pregnancy. Note that data on the use of tenofovir alafenamide in pregnancy are currently limited, and hence regimens using this formulation generally should be avoided pending the results of clinical studies.

Table 7.3. What to Start: Initial Combination Regimens for Antiretroviral-Naive Pregnant Women

Preferred Regimens
Regimens with clinical trial data in adults demonstrating optimal efficacy and durability with acceptable toxicity and ease of use, PK data available in pregnancy, and no evidence to date of teratogenic effects or established adverse outcomes for mother/fetus/newborn. To minimize the risk of resistance, a PI regimen is preferred for women who may stop ART during the postpartum period.

Preferred Two-NRTI Backbones

Drug	Comments
ABC/3TC	Available as FDC. Can be administered once daily. ABC **should not be used** in patients who test positive for HLA-B*5701 because of risk of hypersensitivity reaction. ABC/3TC with ATV/r or with EFV is not recommended if pretreatment HIV RNA > 100,000 copies/mL.
TDF/FTC or 3TC	TDF/FTC available as FDC. Either TDF/FTC or TDF and 3TC can be administered once daily. TDF has potential renal toxicity, thus TDF-based dual-NRTI combinations should be used with caution in patients with renal insufficiency.
ZDV/3TC	Available as FDC. NRTI combination with most experience for use in pregnancy but has disadvantages of requirement for twice-daily administration and increased potential for hematologic toxicities.

Table 7.3. What to Start: Initial Combination Regimens for Antiretroviral-Naive Pregnant Women (cont'd)

Preferred PI Regimens

Drug	Comments
ATV/r plus a Preferred Two-NRTI Backbone	Once-daily administration. Extensive experience in pregnancy. Maternal hyperbilirubinemia.
DRV/r plus a Preferred Two-NRTI Backbone	Better tolerated than LPV/r. PK data available. Increasing experience with use in pregnancy. Must be used twice daily in pregnancy.

Preferred NNRTI Regimen

Drug	Comments
EFV plus a Preferred Two-NRTI Backbone **Note**: May be initiated **after the first 8 weeks of pregnancy.**	Concern because of birth defects seen in primate study; risk in humans is unclear. Postpartum contraception must be ensured. Preferred regimen in women who require co-administration of drugs with significant interactions with PIs or the convenience of co-formulated, single-tablet, once-daily regimen.

Preferred Integrase Inhibitor Regimen

Drug	Comments
RAL plus a Preferred Two-NRTI Backbone	PK data available and increasing experience in pregnancy. Rapid viral load reduction. Useful when drug interactions with PI regimens are a concern. Twice-daily dosing required.

Alternative Regimens
Regimens with clinical trial data demonstrating efficacy in adults but one or more of the following apply: Experience in pregnancy is limited, data are lacking or incomplete on teratogenicity, or regimen is associated with dosing, formulation, toxicity, or interaction issues.

PI Regimen

Drug	Comments
LPV/r plus a Preferred Two-NRTI Backbone	Abundant experience and established PK in pregnancy. More nausea than preferred agents. Twice-daily administration. Once-daily LPV/r is not recommended for use in pregnant women.

Table 7.3. What to Start: Initial Combination Regimens for Antiretroviral-Naive Pregnant Women (cont'd)

NNRTI Regimen

Drug	Comments
RPV/TDF/FTC (or RPV plus a Preferred Two-NRTI Backbone)	RPV not recommended with pretreatment HIV RNA > 100,000 copies/mL or CD4 cell count < 200 cells/mm³. Do not use with PPIs. PK data available in pregnancy but relatively little experience with use in pregnancy. Available in co-formulated, single-pill, once-daily regimen.

<u>Insufficient Data in Pregnancy to Recommend Routine Use in ART-Naive Women</u>
Drugs that are approved for use in adults but lack adequate pregnancy-specific PK or safety data.

Drug	Comments
DTG	No data on use of DTG in pregnancy.
EVG/COBI/TDF/FTC Fixed Drug Combination	No data on use of EVG/COBI component in pregnancy.
FPV	Limited data on use in pregnancy.
MVC	MVC requires tropism testing before use. Few case reports of use in pregnancy.
COBI	No data on use of COBI (including co-formulations with ATV or DRV) in pregnancy.

<u>Not Recommended</u>
Drugs whose use is not recommended because of toxicity, lower rate of viral suppression, or because not recommended in ART-naive populations.

Drug	Comments
ABC/3TC/ZDV	Generally not recommended due to inferior virologic efficacy.
d4T	Not recommended due to toxicity.
ddl	Not recommended due to toxicity.
IDV/r	Nephrolithiasis, maternal hyperbilirubinemia.
NFV	Lower rate of viral suppression with NFV compared to LPV/r or EFV in adult trials.
RTV	RTV as a single PI is not recommended because of inferior efficacy and increased toxicity.

Table 7.3. What to Start: Initial Combination Regimens for Antiretroviral-Naive Pregnant Women (cont'd)

SQV/r	Not recommended based on potential toxicity and dosing disadvantages. Baseline ECG is recommended before initiation of SQV/r because of potential PR and QT prolongation; contraindicated with pre-existing cardiac conduction system disease. Limited data in pregnancy. Large pill burden. Twice-daily dosing required.
ETR	Not recommended in ART-naive populations.
NVP	Not recommended because of greater potential for adverse events, complex lead-in dosing, and low barrier to resistance. NVP should be used with caution when initiating ART in women with CD4 cell count > 250 cells/mm³. Use NVP and ABC together with caution; both can cause hypersensitivity reactions within the first few weeks after initiation.
T20	Not recommended in ART-naive populations.
TPV/r	Not recommended in ART-naive populations.

Key to Acronyms: 3TC = lamivudine; ABC = abacavir; ART = antiretroviral therapy; ARV = antiretroviral; ATV/r = atazanavir/ritonavir; CD4 = CD4 T-lymphocyte cell; COBI = cobicistat; d4T = stavudine; ddl = didanosine; DTG = dolutegravir; DRV/r = darunavir/ritonavir; ECG = electrocardiogram; EFV = efavirenz; ETR = etravirine; EVG = elvitegravir; FDC = fixed-dose combination; FPV = fosamprenavir; FTC = emtricitabine; IDV/r = indinavir/ritonavir; LPV/r = lopinavir/ritonavir; MVC = maraviroc; NFV = nelfinavir; NRTI = nucleoside reverse transcriptase inhibitor; NNRTI = non-nucleoside reverse transcriptase inhibitor; NVP = nevirapine; PI = protease inhibitor; PPI = proton pump inhibitor; PK = pharmacokinetic; RAL = raltegravir; RPV = rilpivirine; RTV = ritonavir; SQV/r = saquinavir/ritonavir; T20 = enfuvirtide; TDF = tenofovir disoproxil fumarate; TPV = tipranavir; ZDV = zidovudine.

Reproduced from Panel on Treatment of HIV-Infected Pregnant Women and Prevention of Perinatal Transmission. Recommendations for use of antiretroviral drugs in pregnant HIV-1-infected women for maternal health and interventions to reduce perinatal HIV transmission in the United States. aidsinfo.nih.gov. June 7, 2016.

INTRAPARTUM CARE

1. DHHS Perinatal Guidelines: Intrapartum Antretroviral Therapy/Prophylaxis:

- Women should continue their antepartum combination antiretroviral therapy (cART) drug regimen on schedule as much as possible during labor and before scheduled cesarean delivery **(AIII)**.
- Intravenous (IV) zidovudine should be administered to HIV-infected women with HIV RNA > 1000 copies/mL (or unknown HIV RNA) near delivery **(AI)**, but is not required for HIV-infected women receiving cART regimens who have HIV RNA ≤ 1000 copies/mL during late pregnancy and near delivery and no concerns regarding adherence to the cART regimen **(BII)**. Scheduled cesarean delivery at 38 weeks gestation (compared to 39 weeks for most indications) is recommended for women who have HIV RNA > 1000 copies/mL near delivery (see Transmission and Mode of Delivery) **(AI)**.
- Women who present in labor with unknown HIV status should undergo expedited HIV testing **(AII)**. If the results are positive, a confirmatory HIV test should be done as soon as possible and maternal (IV zidovudine)/infant (combination antiretroviral [ARV] prophylaxis) ARV drugs should be initiated pending results of the confirmatory test **(AII)**. If the maternal confirmatory HIV test is positive, infant ARV drugs should be managed as discussed in the Infant Antiretroviral Prophylaxis section **(AI)**; if the maternal confirmatory HIV test is negative, the maternal and infant ARV drugs should be stopped.

Rating of Recommendations: A = Strong; B = Moderate; C = Optional.
Rating of Evidence: I = One or more randomized trials with clinical outcomes and/or validated laboratory endpoints; II = One or more well-designed, nonrandomized trials or observational cohort studies with long-term clinical outcomes; III = Expert opinion.

2. DHHS Perinatal Guidelines: Transmission and Mode of Delivery

- Scheduled cesarean delivery at 38 weeks gestation to minimize perinatal transmission of HIV is recommended for women with HIV RNA levels > 1000 copies/mL or unknown HIV levels near the time of delivery, irrespective of administration of antepartum antiretroviral drugs **(AII)**. Scheduled cesarean delivery performed solely for prevention of perinatal transmission in women receiving combination antiretroviral therapy with HIV RNA ≤ 1000 copies/mL is not routinely recommended due to the low rate of perinatal transmission in this group and the potential for increased complications following cesarean delivery in HIV-infected women **(AII)**. In women with HIV RNA levels < 1000 copies/mL, cesarean delivery performed for standard obstetrical indications should be scheduled at 39 weeks gestation **(AII)**.

- Because there is insufficient evidence to determine whether cesarean delivery after rupture of membranes or onset of labor reduces the risk of perinatal HIV transmission, management of women originally scheduled for cesarean delivery who present with ruptured membranes or in labor must be individualized at the time of presentation **(BII)**. In these circumstances, consultation with an expert in perinatal HIV (e.g., telephone consultation with the National Perinatal HIV/AIDS Clinical Consultation Center at [888] 448–8765) may be helpful in rapidly developing an individualized plan.
- Women with HIV infection should be counseled that HIV infection may put them at higher risk of surgical complications of cesarean delivery **(AII)**.

Rating of Recommendations: A = Strong; B = Moderate; C = Optional.
Rating of Evidence: I = One or more randomized trials with clinical outcomes and/or validated laboratory endpoints; II = One or more well-designed, nonrandomized trials or observational cohort studies with long-term clinical outcomes; III = Expert opinion.

3. DHHS Perinatal Guidelines: Other Intrapartum Management Considerations

- The following should generally be avoided because of a potential increased risk of transmission, unless there are clear obstetric indications:
  » Artificial rupture of membranes **(BIII)**
  » Routine use of fetal scalp electrodes for fetal monitoring **(BIII)**
  » Operative delivery with forceps or a vacuum extractor and/or episiotomy **(BIII)**
- The antiretroviral drug regimen a woman is receiving should be taken into consideration when treating excessive postpartum bleeding resulting from uterine atony:
  » In women who are receiving a cytochrome P450 (CYP) 3A4 enzyme inhibitor such as a protease inhibitor, methergine should be used only if no alternative treatments for postpartum hemorrhage are available and the need for pharmacologic treatment outweighs the risks. If methergine is used, it should be administered in the lowest effective dose for the shortest possible duration **(BIII)**.
  » In women who are receiving a CYP3A4 enzyme inducer such as nevirapine, efavirenz, or etravirine, additional uterotonic agents may be needed because of the potential for decreased methergine levels and inadequate treatment effect **(BIII)**.

Rating of Recommendations: A = Strong; B = Moderate; C = Optional.
Rating of Evidence: I = One or more randomized trials with clinical outcomes and/or validated laboratory endpoints; II = One or more well-designed, nonrandomized trials or observational cohort studies with long-term clinical outcomes; III = Expert opinion.

POSTPARTUM MANAGEMENT

Children born to HIV-infected women need to be assessed for the possibility of HIV infection and for short- and long-term toxicities due to in utero exposure to antiretroviral agents (Table 7.5). Exposure to antiretroviral agents should become a part of the child's permanent medical record. Breastfeeding is not recommended for HIV-infected women provided there is safe and culturally acceptable formula feeding available.

Further arrangements are needed for long-term care of the woman, including primary and HIV-specialty care appointments, made prior to hospital discharge, and family planning counseling. The postpartum period poses significant challenges to some women for ART adherence, and hence this should be closely monitored. Mental health status and the possibility of postpartum depression also need to be assessed, and appropriate supports need to be put into place. Case management services best assure adequate support and compliance with healthcare needs.

REFERENCES AND SUGGESTED READINGS

Antiretroviral Pregnancy Registry Steering Committee. Antiretroviral pregnancy registry international interim report for 1 Jan 1989–31 January 2012. Wilmington, NC: Registry Coordinating Center; 2012. Available at http://www. APRegistry.com.

Aweeka F, Lizak P, Frenkel L, et al. Steady state nevirapine pharmacokinetics during 2nd and 3rd trimester pregnancy and postpartum: PACTG 1022. Paper presented at: 11th Conference on Retroviruses and Opportunistic Infections (CROI); February 8–11, 2004; San Francisco, CA. Abstract 932.

Baylor MS, Johann-Liang R. Hepatotoxicity associated with nevirapine use. J Acquir Immune Defic Syndr. 2004;35(5):538–539. Available at http://www.ncbi.nlm.nih.gov/entrez/query.fcgi?cmd=Retrieve&db=pubmed&dopt=Abstract&list_uids=15021321.

Best BM, Capparelli EV, Stek A, et al. Raltegravir pharmacokinetics during pregnancy. Paper presented at: 50th Interscience Conference on Antimicrobial Agents and Chemotherapy (ICAAC); September 12–15, 2010; Boston, MA.

Best BM, Mirochnick M, Capparelli EV, et al. Impact of pregnancy on abacavir pharmacokinetics. AIDS. Feb 28 2006;20(4):553–560. Available at http://www.ncbi.nlm.nih.gov/pubmed/16470119.

Best BM, Stek AM, Mirochnick M, et al. Lopinavir tablet pharmacokinetics with an increased dose during pregnancy. J Acquir Immune Defic Syndr. Aug 2010;54(4):381–388. Available at http://www.ncbi.nlm.nih.gov/pubmed/20632458.

Brennan-Benson P, Pakianathan M, Rice P, et al. Enfurvitide prevents vertical transmission of multidrug-resistant HIV-1 in pregnancy but does not cross the placenta. AIDS Jan 9 2006;20(2):297–299. Available at http://www.ncbi.nlm.nih.gov/pubmed/16511429.

Bristol-Myers Squibb Company. Healthcare provider important drug warning letter. January 5, 2001. Available at http://www.bms.com.

Bryson YJ, Mirochnick M, Stek A, et al. Pharmacokinetics and safety of nelfinavir when used in combination with zidovudine and lamivudine in HIV-infected pregnant women: Pediatric AIDS Clinical Trials Group (PACTG) Protocol 353 HIV Clin Trials. Mar-Apr 2008;9(2):115–125. Available at http:// www.ncbi.nlm.nih.gov/pubmed/18474496.

Burchett SK, Best B, Mirochnick M, et al. Tenofovir pharmacokinetics during pregnancy, at delivery and postpartum. Paper presented at: 14th Conference on Retroviruses and Opportunistic Infections (CROI); February 25–28, 2007; Los Angeles, CA. Abstract 738b.

Capparelli EV, Aweeka F, Hitti J, et al. Chronic administration of nevirapine during pregnancy: impact of pregnancy on pharmacokinetics. HIV Med. Apr 2008;9(4):214–220. Available at http://www.ncbi.nlm.nih.gov/pubmed/18366444.

Capparelli EV, Best BM, Stek A, et al. Pharmacokinetics of darunavir once or twice daily during pregnancy and postpartum. Paper presented at: 3rd International Workshop on HIV Pediatrics; July 15–16, 2011; Rome, Italy.

Capparelli EV, Stek A, Best B, et al. Boosted fosamprenavir pharmacokinetics during Pregnancy. Paper presented at: 17th Conference on Retroviruses and Opportunistic Infections (CROI); February 16–19, 2010; San Francisco, CA. Abstract 908.

Conradie F, Zorrilla C, Josipovic D, et al. Safety and exposure of once-daily ritonavir-boosted atazanavir in HIV-infected pregnant women. HIV Med. Oct 2011;12(9):570–579. Available at http://www.ncbi.nlm.nih.gov/pubmed/21569187

Cressey TR, Jourdain G, Rawangban B, et al. Pharmacokinetics and virologic response of zidovudine/lopinavir/ritonavir initiated during the third trimester of pregnancy. AIDS. Sep 10 2010;24(14):2193–2200. Available at http://www.ncbi.nlm.nih.gov/pubmed/20625263.

Cressey TR, Stek A, Capparelli E, et al. Efavirenz pharmacokinetics during the third trimester of pregnancy and postpartum. J Acquir Immune Defic Syndr. Mar 1 2012;59(3):245–252. Available at http://www.ncbi.nlm.nih.gov/pubmed/22083071.

De Santis M, Carducci B, De Santis L, Cavaliere AF, Straface G. Periconceptional exposure to efavirenz and neural tube defects. Arch Intern Med. Feb 11 2002;162(3):355. Available at http://www.ncbi.nlm.nih.gov/pubmed/11822930.

Dieterich DT, Robinson PA, Love J, Stern JO. Drug-induced liver injury associated with the use of non-nucleoside reverse-transcriptase inhibitors. Clin Infect Dis. 2004;38 (Suppl 2):S80–89. Available at http://www.ncbi.nlm.nih.gov/entrez/query.fcgi?cmd=Retrieve&db=pubmed&dopt=Abstract&list_uids=14986279.

Flynn PM, Mirochnick M, Shapiro DE, et al. Pharmacokinetics and safety of single-dose tenofovir disoproxil fumarate and emtricitabine in HIV-1-infected pregnant women and their infants. Antimicrob Agents Chemother. Dec 2011;55(12):5914–5922. Available at http://www.ncbi.nlm.nih.gov/pubmed/21896911.

Fundaro C, Genovese O, Rendeli C, Tamburrini E, Salvaggio E. Myelomeningocele in a child with intrauterine exposure to efavirenz. AIDS. Jan 25 2002;16(2): 299–300. Available at http://www.ncbi.nlm.nih.gov/pubmed/11807320.

Gafni RI, Hazra R, Reynolds JC, et al. Tenofovir disoproxil fumarate and an optimized background regimen of antiretroviral agents as salvage therapy: impact on bone mineral density in HIV-infected children. Pediatrics. Sep 2006;118(3):e711–718. Available at http://www.ncbi.nlm.nih.gov/pubmed/16923923.

Ghosn J, De Montgolfier I, Cornelie C, et al. Antiretroviral therapy with a twice-daily regimen containing 400 milligrams of indinavir and 100 milligrams of ritonavir in human immunodeficiency virus type 1-infected women during pregnancy. Antimicrob Agents Chemother. Apr 2008;52(4):1542–1544. Available at http://www.ncbi.nlm.nih.gov/pubmed/18250187.

Hayashi S, Beckerman K, Homma M, Kosel BW, Aweeka FT. Pharmacokinetics of indinavir in HIV-positive pregnant women. AIDS. May 26 2000;14(8):1061–1062. Available at http://www.ncbi.nlm.nih.gov/pubmed/10853990.

Hirt D, Urien S, Ekouevi DK, et al. Population pharmacokinetics of tenofovir in HIV-1-infected pregnant women and their neonates (ANRS 12109). Clin Pharmacol Ther. Feb 2009;85(2):182–189. Available at http://www.ncbi.nlm.nih.gov/pubmed/18987623.

Izurieta P, Kakuda TN, Feys C, Witek J. Safety and pharmacokinetics of etravirine in pregnant HIV-1-infected women. HIV Med. Apr 2011;12(4):257–258. Available at http://www.ncbi.nlm.nih.gov/pubmed/21371239.

Lambert JS, Else LJ, Jackson V, et al. Therapeutic drug monitoring of lopinavir/ritonavir in pregnancy. HIV Med. Mar 2011;12(3):166–173. Available at http://www.ncbi.nlm.nih.gov/pubmed/20726906.

Mallal S, Phillips E, Carosi G, et al. HLA-B*5701 screening for hypersensitivity to abacavir. N Engl J Med. Feb 7 2008;358(6):568–579. Available at http://www.ncbi.nlm.nih.gov/pubmed/18256392.

McKeown DA, Rosenvinge M, Donaghy S, et al. High neonatal concentrations of raltegravir following transplacental transfer in HIV-1 positive pregnant women. AIDS. Sep 24 2010;24(15):2416–2418. Available at http://www.ncbi.nlm.nih.gov/pubmed/20827058.

Meyohas MC, Lacombe K, Carbonne B, Morand-Joubert L, Girard PM. Enfuvirtide prescription at the end of pregnancy to a multi-treated HIV-infected woman with virological breakthrough. AIDS. Sep 24 2004;18(14):1966–1968. Available at http://www.ncbi.nlm.nih.gov/pubmed/15353987.

Mirochnick M, Best BM, Stek AM, et al. Atazanavir pharmacokinetics with and without tenofovir during pregnancy. J Acquir Immune Defic Syndr. Apr 15 2011;56(5):412–419. Available at http://www.ncbi.nlm.nih.gov/pubmed/21283017.

Mirochnick M, Kafulafula G, et al. The pharmacokinetics (PK) of tenofovir disoproxil fumarate (TDF) after administration to HIV-1 infected pregnant women and their newborns. Paper presented at: 16th Conference on Retroviruses and Opportunistic Infections (CROI); February 8–11, 2009; Montreal, Canada. Abstract 940.

Mirochnick M, Kunwenda N, Joao E, et al. Tenofovir disoproxil fumarate (TDF) pharmacokinetics (PK) with increased doses in HIV-1 infected pregnant women and their newborns (HPTN 057). Paper presented at: 11th International Workshop on Clinical Pharmacology of HIV Therapy; April 7–9, 2010; Sorrento, Italy. Abstract 3.

Mirochnick M, Siminski S, Fenton T, Lugo M, Sullivan JL. Nevirapine pharmacokinetics in pregnant women and their infants after in utero exposure. Pediatr Infect Dis J. Aug 2001;20(8):803–805. Available at http://www.ncbi.nlm.nih.gov/pubmed/11734746.

Mirochnick M, Stek A, Capparelli EV, et al. Pharmacokinetics of increased dose atazanavir with and without tenofovir during pregnancy. Paper presented at: 12th International Workshop on Clinical Pharmacology of HIV Therapy; April 13–16, 2011; Miami, FL.

Moodley J, Moodley D, Pillay K, et al. Pharmacokinetics and antiretroviral activity of lamivudine alone or when coadministered with zidovudine in human immunodeficiency virus type 1-infected pregnant women and their offspring. J Infect Dis. Nov 1998;178(5):1327–1333. Available at http://www.ncbi.nlm.nih.gov/pubmed/9780252.

Natha M, Hay P, Taylor G, et al. Atazanavir use in pregnancy: a report of 33 cases. Paper presented at: 14th Conference on Retoviruses and Opportunistic Infections (CROI); February 25–28, 2007; Los Angeles, CA. Abstract 750.

O'Sullivan MJ, Boyer PJ, Scott GB, et al. The pharmacokinetics and safety of zidovudine in the third trimester of pregnancy for women infected with human immunodeficiency virus and their infants: phase I acquired immunodeficiency syndrome clinical trials group study (Protocol 082). Zidovudine Collaborative Working Group. Am J Obstet Gynecol. 1993;168(5):1510–1516. Available at http://www.ncbi.nlm.nih.gov/entrez/query.fcgi?cmd=Retrieve&db=pubmed&dopt=Abstract&list_uids=8098905.

Read JS, Best BM, Stek AM, et al. Pharmacokinetics of new 625 mg nelfinavir formulation during pregnancy and postpartum. HIV Med. Nov 2008;9(10):875–882. Available at http://www.ncbi.nlm.nih.gov/pubmed/18795962.

Ripamonti D, Cattaneo D, Maggiolo F, et al. Atazanavir plus low-dose ritonavir in pregnancy: pharmacokinetics and placental transfer. AIDS. Nov 30 2007;21(18):2409–2415. Available at http://www.ncbi.nlm.nih.gov/pubmed/18025877.

Saag M, Balu R, Phillips E, et al. High sensitivity of human leukocyte antigen-b*5701 as a marker for immunologically confirmed abacavir hypersensitivity in white and black patients. Clin Infect Dis. Apr 1 2008;46(7):1111–1118. Available at http://www.ncbi.nlm.nih.gov/pubmed/18444831.

Sarner L, Fakoya A. Acute onset lactic acidosis and pancreatitis in the third trimester of pregnancy in HIV-1 positive women taking antiretroviral medication. Sex Transm Infect. Feb 2002;78(1):58–59. Available at http://www.ncbi.nlm.nih.gov/pubmed/11872862.

Schooley RT, Ruane P, Myers RA, et al. Tenofovir DF in antiretroviral-experienced patients: results from a 48-week, randomized, double-blind study. AIDS. Jun 14 2002;16(9):1257–1263. Available at http://www.ncbi.nlm.nih.gov/pubmed/12045491.

Scott GB, Rodman JH, Scott WA, et al. for the PACTG 354 Protocol Team. Pharmacokinetic and virologic response to ritonavir (RTV) in combination with zidovudine (XDV) and lamivudine (3TC) in HIV-1 infected pregnant women and their infants. Paper presented at: 9th Conference on Retroviruses and Opportunistic Infections (CROI); February 24–28, 2002; Seattle, WA. Abstract 794-W. Available at http://www.retroconference.org/2002/.

Stek AM, Mirochnick M, Capparelli E, et al. Reduced lopinavir exposure during pregnancy. AIDS. Oct 3 2006;20(15):1931–1939. Available at http://www.ncbi.nlm.nih.gov/pubmed/16988514.

Tarantal AF, Castillo A, Ekert JE, Bischofberger N, Martin RB. Fetal and maternal outcome after administration of tenofovir to gravid rhesus monkeys (Macaca mulatta). J Acquir Immune Defic Syndr. Mar 1 2002;29(3):207–220. Available at http://www.ncbi.nlm.nih.gov/pubmed/11873070.

Unadkat JD, Wara DW, Hughes MD, et al. Pharmacokinetics and safety of indinavir in human immunodeficiency virus-infected pregnant women. Antimicrob Agents Chemother. Feb 2007;51(2):783–786. Available at http://www.ncbi.nlm.nih.gov/pubmed/17158945.

van der Lugt J, Colbers A, Molto J, et al. The pharmacokinetics, safety and efficacy of boosted saquinavir tablets in HIV type-1-infected pregnant women. Antivir Ther. 2009;14(3):443–450. Available at http://www.ncbi.nlm.nih.gov/pubmed/19474478.

Villani P, Floridia M, Pirillo MF, et al. Pharmacokinetics of nelfinavir in HIV-1-infected pregnant and nonpregnant women. Br J Clin Pharmacol. Sep 2006;62(3):309–315. Available at http://www.ncbi.nlm.nih.gov/pubmed/16934047.

Wade NA, Unadkat JD, Huang S, et al. Pharmacokinetics and safety of stavudine in HIV-infected pregnant women and their infants: Pediatric AIDS Clinical Trials Group Protocol 332. J Infect Dis. Dec 15 2004;190(12):2167–2174. Available at http://www.ncbi.nlm.nih.gov/pubmed/15551216.

Wang Y, Livingston E, Patil S, et al. Pharmacokinetics of didanosine in antepartum and postpartum human immunodeficiency virus–infected pregnant women and their neonates: an AIDS clinical trials group study. J Infect Dis. 1999;180(5):1536–1541. Available at http://www.ncbi.nlm.nih.gov/entrez/query.fcgi?cmd=Retrieve&db=pubmed&dopt=Abstract&list_uids=10515813.

Weizsaecker K, Kurowski M, Hoffmeister B, Schurmann D, Feiterna-Sperling C. Pharmacokinetic profile in late pregnancy and cord blood concentration of tipranavir and enfuvirtide. Int J STD AIDS. May 2011;22(5):294-295. Available at http://www.ncbi.nlm.nih.gov/pubmed/21571982.

Chapter 8

Post-Exposure and Pre-Exposure Prophylaxis

OCCUPATIONAL POST-EXPOSURE PROPHYLAXIS (PEP)

The Centers for Disease Control and Prevention (CDC) estimates approximately 600,000 significant exposures to blood borne pathogens occur yearly. Of 56 confirmed cases of HIV acquisition in healthcare workers, more than 90% involved percutaneous exposure, with the remaining cases due to mucous membrane/non intact skin exposure (Table 8.1). Estimates of HIV seroconversion rates after percutaneous and mucous membrane exposure to HIV-infected blood are 0.3% and 0.09%, respectively; lower rates of transmission occur after non intact skin exposure, and no transmission has thus far been reported to occur through intact skin. By comparison, the risks of seroconversion after percutaneous exposure to Hepatitis B (HBV) and Hepatitis C viruses (HCV) are 30% (without immunization of exposed individual) and 3%, respectively. Without PEP, risk factors for increased risk of HIV transmission after percutaneous exposure include deep injury (odds ratio 16.1), visible blood on device (odds ratio 5.2), source patient is terminally ill (odds ratio 6.4), or needle was in source patient's artery/vein (odds ratio 5.1); ZDV prophylaxis reduces the risk of transmission (odds ratio 0.2). All guidelines suggest PEP should be administered as soon as possible after exposure, but there is no absolute window (e.g., within 1–2 weeks) after which PEP should be withheld following serious exposure.

In the United States, occupationally acquired HIV has become increasingly rare. From 1985–2013, there were 58 confirmed and 150 possible cases of occupationally acquired HIV infection among healthcare personnel (HCP). Since 1999, only one confirmed case (a laboratory technician sustaining a needle puncture while working with a live HIV culture in 2008) has been reported. The decreasing incidence of occupational HIV acquisition likely relates to several factors, including: 1) greater emphasis on workplace protection from blood and body fluids (barrier protection, improved needle safety designs, universal use of gloves); 2) widespread adaptation of PEP with combination antiretroviral regimens; and 3) source patients may be on HIV therapy, reducing HIV RNA levels in blood.

National guidelines for occupational post-exposure prophylaxis were updated in 2013 (Infect Control Hosp Epidemiology 2013;34:875–892). They are available online free of charge (http://www.jstor.org/stable/10.1086/672271). These guidelines replaced a 2005 version with several substantial changes, including: 1) All PEP regimens should consist of three antiviral drugs; 2) the preferred PEP regimen is TDF/FTC plus raltegravir, with several alternative choices listed; 3) if a fourth-generation combination HIV p24 antigen–HIV antibody test is utilized for follow-up HIV testing of exposed HCP, HIV testing may be concluded 4 months after exposure.

The content in this chapter is adapted from both these updated guidelines, the National Clinician Consultation Center (http://nccc.ucsf.edu/clinical-consultation/pep-post-exposure-prophylaxis/), and those issued by New York State (http://www.hivguidelines.org/clinical-guidelines/post-exposure-prophylaxis/hiv-prophylaxis-following-occupational-exposure/). For consultation or assistance with HIV PEP, contact the National Clinicians' Post-Exposure Prophylaxis Hotline at telephone number 888-448-4911 9AM to 2AM EST, 7 days a week, or visit its website at http://nccc.ucsf.edu/clinician-consultation/pep-post-exposure-prophylaxis/. Occupationally acquired HIV infections and PEP failures should be reported to the CDC at 404-639-2050.

Table 8.1. Estimated Per-Act Probability of Acquiring HIV from an Infected Source, by Exposure Act[1]

Type of Exposure	Risk per 10,000 Exposures
Parenteral	
Blood transfusion	9000[2]
Needle sharing during injection drug use	67[3]
Percutaneous (needle-stick)	30[4]
Sexual	
Receptive anal intercourse	50[5, 6]
Receptive penile-vaginal intercourse	10[5, 6, 7]
Insertive anal intercourse	6.5[5, 6]
Insertive penile-vaginal intercourse	5[5, 6]
Receptive oral intercourse	Low[5, 9]
Insertive oral intercourse	Low[5, 9]
Other[8]	
Biting	Negligible[10]
Spitting	Negligible
Throwing body fluids (including semen or saliva)	Negligible
Sharing sex toys	Negligible

[1] Factors that increase the risk of HIV transmission include sexually transmitted infections, early and late-stage HIV infection, and a high level of HIV in the blood. Factors that reduce the risk of HIV transmission include condom use, male circumcision, and use of antiretrovirals.

[2] Donegan E, Stuart M, Niland JC, et al. Infection with human immunodeficiency virus type 1 (HIV-1) among recipients of antibody-positive blood donations. *Ann Intern Med*. 1990;113(10):733–739.

[3] Kaplan EH, Heimer R. A model-based estimate of HIV infectivity via needle sharing. *J Acquir Immune Defic Syndr*. 1992;5(11):1116–1118.

[4] Bell DM. Occupational risk of human immunodeficiency virus infection in healthcare workers: an overview. *Am J Med*. 1997;102(5B):9–15.

[5] Varghese B, Maher JE, Peterman TA, Branson BM, Steketee RW. Reducing the risk of sexual HIV transmission: quantifying the per-act risk for HIV on the basis of choice of partner, sex act, and condom use. *Sex Transm Dis*. 2002;29(1):38–43.

[6] European Study Group on Heterosexual Transmission of HIV. Comparison of female to male and male to female transmission of HIV in 563 stable couples. *BMJ*. 1992;304(6830):809–813.

[7] Leynaert B, Downs AM, de Vincenzi I; European Study Group on Heterosexual Transmission of HIV. Heterosexual transmission of HIV: variability of infectivity throughout the course of infection. *Am J Epidemiol*. 1998;148(1):88–96.

[8] HIV transmission through these exposure routes is technically possible but extremely unlikely and not well documented.

[9] HIV transmission through oral sex has been documented, but rare. Accurate estimates of risk are not available.

[10] Pretty LA, Anderson GS, Sweet DJ. Human bites and the risk of human immunodeficiency virus transmission. *Am J Forensic Med Pathol*. 1999;20(3):232–239.

Data from: MMWR Recomm Rep. 2005 Jan 21; 54 (RR-2):1–20.

Quick Guide for PEP after Occupational Exposures

(adapted from http://nccc.ucsf.edu/clinical-resources/pep-resources/pep-quick-guide/, last revised December 2, 2014)

Initial Evaluation: Assessing Exposures and Testing

What is considered to be a potential exposure to HIV, HBV, or HCV?

For transmission of bloodborne pathogens (HIV, HBV, and HCV) to occur, an exposure must include both of the following:

1. **Infectious body fluid**
   - Blood, semen, vaginal fluids, amniotic fluids, breast milk, cerebrospinal fluid, pericardial fluid, peritoneal fluid, pleural fluid and synovial flood can transmit HIV, HBV, and HCV.
   - Note that saliva, vomitus, urine, feces, sweat, tears, and respiratory secretions do not transmit HIV (unless visibly bloody). The risk of HBV and HCV transmission from non bloody saliva is negligible.

2. **A portal of entry** (percutaneous, mucous membrane, cutaneous with non intact skin). If both of these factors are not present, there is no risk of transmission and further evaluation is not required.

What baseline testing should be performed after an exposure?

(If no exposure occurred or source person tests negative, no testing is clinically indicated. Testing may be considered for other purposes including medicolegal concerns or as per institutional protocols.)

1. **Source person (SP):**
   - HIV Ab (rapid HIV Ab testing preferred if available).* Note that informed consent is required in some states before all HIV testing, even SP of occupational exposures. If patient lacks the capacity to give consent, some states permit testing on blood samples already obtained for other diagnostic purposes.
   - HCV Ab
   - HBV surface Ag

   If source person's rapid HIV Ab test is positive, assume this is a true positive and send confirmatory testing using standard HIV testing protocol (see Chapter 2). See below.

2. **Exposed person (EP):**
   - HIV Ab
   - HCV Ab
   - HBV testing: Depends on immunization status.

Note that most healthcare and public safety personnel have been vaccinated against hepatitis B. If previously vaccinated and they know they responded to the vaccination series (a positive titer is > 10 mIU/mL, but most do not know their titer), they are considered to have lifelong immunity and require no further testing or treatment. Similarly, if employee health records indicate they responded to the vaccination series, they are considered to be immune.

* *Is the rapid HIV test accurate enough to decide on whether to give PEP?*

Yes, the rapid HIV test is extremely sensitive and specific and can be used to determine whether to offer PEP. A positive rapid HIV test should be considered a true positive for the purposes of PEP decision-making. A negative rapid test should be considered a true negative. Investigation of whether a source might be in the "window period" is unnecessary for determining whether HIV PEP is indicated unless acute retroviral syndrome (see Chapter 1) is clinically suspected.

Deciding Whether to Give PEP

What is the time frame for using PEP?

Efficacy is time sensitive: first dose should be given as soon as possible (Figure 8.1). Optimal time to start PEP is within hours of exposure, rather than days. Do not wait for source patient test results (unless results of rapid test will be available within an hour or two) to proceed with a PEP decision and treatment, when indicated. Most consider 72 hours post-exposure as the outer limit of opportunity to initiate PEP; however, a delay of that scale is believed to compromise PEP efficacy. The 72-hour outside limit recommendation is based on animal studies; no human data are available.

HIV PEP: What to Give

How to choose a PEP regimen

Three-drug PEP regimens are now the recommended regimens for all exposures (Tables 8.3 and 8.4). The new guidelines no longer require assessing the degree of risk for the purpose of choosing a "basic" two-drug regimen vs. an "expanded" three-drug regimen, which was confusing for many treating clinicians. Consultation with an expert can help determine if the exposure poses a "negligible risk"; in negligible risk cases, PEP is not recommended.

PREFERRED HIV 3-DRUG PEP REGIMEN:

Truvada [Tenofovir DF, (TDF) 300 mg + emtricitabine (FTC) 200 mg]
1 PO once daily

PLUS

Raltegravir (Isentress; RAL) 400 mg PO twice daily or Dolutegravir (Tivicay) 50 mg PO once Daily. See Table 8.5 for additional information.

How long is PEP given?

PEP is given for 28 days. If source person testing is negative for HIV, PEP can be stopped before 28 days.

How to monitor and manage side effects of PEP

Side effects can be a limiting factor in PEP adherence. Side effects are generally self-limited but sometimes can last the duration of the 28-day PEP course. Gastrointestinal side effects (nausea, vomiting, diarrhea) are most common. Headache, fatigue, insomnia, and gastrointestinal upset are other side effects. Antiemetic and antidiarrheal medications can be prescribed to help with PEP adherence. If side effects are severe, consider changing to a different regimen. Toxicities are rare with the current preferred PEP regimens, are generally not life-threatening, and are reversible.

The most important side effect of the preferred regimen is renal toxicity from tenofovir. This regimen should be used with caution in patients with impaired renal function.

Table 8.2. Situations for which Expert Consultation for Human Immunodeficiency Virus (HIV) Post-Exposure Prophylaxis (PEP) Is Recommended

Delayed (i.e., later than 72 hours) exposure report
• Interval after which benefits from PEP are undefined.

Unknown source (e.g., needle in sharps disposal container or laundry)
• Use of PEP to be decided on a case-by-case basis.
• Consider severity of exposure and epidemiologic likelihood of HIV exposure.
• Do not test needles or other sharp instruments for HIV.

Known or suspected pregnancy in the exposed person
• Provision of PEP should not be delayed while awaiting expert consultation.

Breast feeding in the exposed person
• Provision of PEP should not be delayed while awaiting expert consultation.

Known or suspected resistance of the source virus to antiretroviral agents
• If source person's virus is known or suspected to be resistant to one or more of the drugs considered for PEP, selection of drugs to which the source person's virus is unlikely to be resistant is recommended.
• Do not delay initiation of PEP while awaiting any results of resistance testing of the source person's virus.

Toxicity of the initial PEP regimen
• Symptoms (e.g., gastrointestinal symptoms and others) are often manageable without changing PEP regimen by prescribing antimotility or antiemetic agents.
• Counseling and support for management of side effects is very important, as symptoms are often exacerbated by anxiety.

Serious medical illness in the exposed person
• Significant underlying illness (e.g., renal disease) or an exposed provider already taking multiple medications may increase the risk of drug toxicity and drug-drug interactions.

Expert consultation can be made with local experts or by calling the National Clinicians' Post-Exposure Prophylaxis Hotline (PEPline) at 888-448-4911.

Modified from Centers for Disease Control and Prevention. Updated U.S. public health service guidelines for the management of occupational exposures to HIV and recommendations for postexposure prophylaxis. MMWR Recomm Rep. 2005;54(RR09);1–17.

Lab monitoring for drug toxicity: Test CBC, renal and hepatic function tests at baseline and 2 weeks after starting PEP (see Table 8.3).

How should HIV exposures in pregnant and breastfeeding women be managed?

• Starting PEP in pregnant/breastfeeding exposed persons should be based on considerations similar to those of non pregnant exposed persons.
• When deciding to start PEP, a pregnant exposed person should discuss with the treating clinician the potential risks of exposing her fetus to antiretroviral (ARV) medications.

- All pregnant women starting ARVs should be entered in the Antiretroviral Pregnancy Registry, a database designed to collect information on the outcomes of ARV-exposed pregnancies regardless of HIV status: http://www.apregistry.com..

Special considerations

- The pregnant exposed person and her fetus are at risk for HIV acquisition.
- Acute HIV in pregnancy incurs a high risk of vertical transmission.
- The use of most PEP medications can be justified when the benefits outweigh the risk of infant exposure to ARVs.
- Based on limited data, use of ARVs in pregnancy, including in the first trimester, does not appear to increase the risk of birth defects compared to the general population.
- Toxicities from currently recommended PEP drugs are not thought to be increased in pregnancy.

What drugs should be used for PEP in pregnancy?

Tenofovir/emtricitabine (Truvada, TDF/FTC) 1 tab daily + raltegravir (RAL) 400 mg twice daily. Since this is a preferred regimen in the Pregnancy Guidelines, we recommend it over use of alternatives if possible.

What Follow-Up Testing Should be Performed?

Standard follow-up for an exposed person (EP) should include the following (see Table 8.6):

HIV

- If source patient is HIV positive, check a fourth-generation Ag/Ab test or HIV RNA test at 6 weeks and at 3–4 months. If an antibody-only test is used, standard antibody testing should be performed at 3 and 6 months. Symptoms of acute HIV (see Chapter 1) should prompt immediate evaluation.
- If source patient cannot be tested for HIV or source patient has unknown HIV status, testing should be as above.
- If source patient tests negative for HIV, no follow-up HIV testing is recommended for the EP.

HBV

- Serologic follow-up testing for HBV exposures is only required for persons who do not have baseline positive HBV surface Ab. Testing at 6 months consists of HBsAg and HBcAb (total).

HCV

- If source patient is HCV RNA positive or has risk factors for HCV but unknown HCV status, obtain HCV RNA PCR viral load at 6 weeks and HCVAb at 4–6 months.
- Symptoms of acute hepatitis should prompt immediate evaluation.
- If source patient is HCV negative, no follow-up testing is recommended for EP.

Table 8.3. Monitoring Recommendations After Initiation of PEP Regimens Following Occupational Exposure[a]

	Baseline	Week 1	Week 2	Week 3	Week 4–6	Week 12
Clinic visit	÷	÷ Or by telephone	÷ Or by telephone	÷ Or by telephone	÷	
Pregnancy test	÷					
Serum liver enzymes, BUN, creatinine, CBC[b]	÷		÷		÷	
HIV test[c]	÷				÷	÷

Source: New York State Department of Health AIDS Institute 2014. HIV prophylaxis following occupational exposure. http://www.hivguidelines.org/wp-content/uploads/2016/03/HIV-Prophylaxis-Following-Occupational-Exposure_3-28-16.pdf (Table 6, page 18).

[a] For post-exposure management for hepatitis B and C, see Section XI in Guidelines: Occupational Exposures to Hepatitis B and C.

[b] CBC should be obtained for all exposed workers at baseline. Follow-up CBC is indicated only for those receiving a zidovudine-containing regimen.

[c] Recommended even if PEP is declined.

NONOCCUPATIONAL POST-EXPOSURE PROPHYLAXIS (nPEP)

The CDC issued an update on the management of nonoccupational post-exposure prophylaxis (nPEP) in 2016 (https://stacks.cdc.gov/view/cdc/38856). An additional resource for clinicians is the New York State Department of Health AIDS Institute (http://www.hivguidelines.org/clinical-guidelines/post-exposure-prophylaxis/hiv-prophylaxis-following-non-occupational-exposure/). Both of these resources are used to inform the summary below.

A. Evaluation. Risk assessment and initiation of nPEP should occur in clinical settings that can provide the following:

- Assessment of HIV risk following exposure
- HIV and sexually transmitted infection STI testing and treatment
- Prevention and risk-reduction counseling
- Clinicians with expertise in the use of ART
- Timely access to care and initiation of nPEP

If all of these services are not available, clinicians should assess the exposure and initiate nPEP when indicated according to the criteria and recommendations in these guidelines.

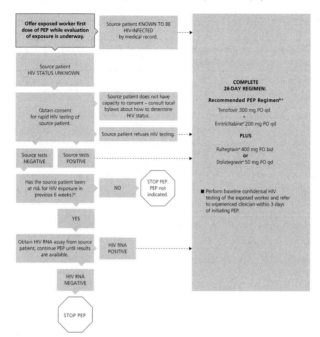

a Depending on the test used, the window period may be shorter than 6 weeks. Clinicians should contact appropriate laboratory authorities to determine the window period for the test that is being used.

b If the source is known to be HIV-infected, information about his/her viral load, ART medication history, and history of antiretroviral drug resistance should be obtained when possible to assist in selection of a PEP regimen.* **Initiation of the first dose of PEP should not be delayed while awaiting this information and/or results of resistance testing.** When this information becomes available, the PEP regimen may be changed if needed in consultation with an experienced provider.

c See Chapter 10 for dosing recommendations in patients with renal impairment.

d Lamivudine 300 mg PO qd may be substituted for emtricitabine. A fixed-dose combination is available when tenofovir is used with emtricitabine (Truvada 1 PO qd).

e See Chapter 10 for drug-drug interactions, dosing adjustments, and contraindications associated with raltegravir and dolutegravir.

Figure 8.1. PEP Following Occupational Exposure

Reproduced from New York State Department of Health AIDS Institute. HIV prophylaxis following occupational exposure. 2014. This material was accessed on 10/6/16 on the HIV Clinical Resource website (www.hivguidelines. org). The HIV Clinical Guidelines Program is a collaborative effort of the New York State Department of Health AIDS Institute and the Johns Hopkins University Division of Infectious Diseases.

*Infect Control Hosp Epidemiol. 2003; 24:724–730.

Table 8.4. Human Immunodeficiency Virus (HIV) Postexposure Prophylaxis (PEP) Regimens

RECOMMENDED AND ALTERNATIVE REGIMEN FOR HIV PEP FOLLOWING OCCUPATIONAL OR NON-OCCUPATIONAL EXPOSURE[a]

Recommended Regimen

Tenofovir disoproxil fumarate[b] 300 mg PO daily + emtricitabine[b,c] 200 mg PO daily

plus

Raltegravir[d] 400 mg PO twice daily or dolutegravir[d] 50 mg PO daily

[a] When the source is known to be HIV-infected, past and current ART experience, viral load data, and genotypic or phenotypic resistance data (if available) may indicate the use of an alternative PEP regimen. Consult with a clinician experienced in managing PEP.

[b] The dosing of tenofovir disoproxil fumarate and emtricitabine/lamivudine should be adjusted in patients with baseline creatinine clearance < 50 mL/min (see Chapter 10 for dosing recommendations). Tenofovir disoproxil fumarate should be used with caution in exposed workers with renal insufficiency or who are taking concomitant nephrotoxic medications. Fixed-dose combinations should not be used in patients who need dose adjustment due to renal failure.

[c] Lamivudine 300 mg PO daily may be substituted for emtricitabine. However, a fixed-dose combination is available when tenofovir disoproxil fumarate is used with emtricitabine (Truvada 1 PO daily).

Alternative HIV PEP Regimen

Tenofovir disoproxil fumarate[a] 300 mg PO daily + emtricitabine[a,b] 200 mg PO daily

plus

Darunavir 800 mg PO daily,[c] or atazanavir 300 mg PO daily,[c] or fosamprenavir 1400 mg PO daily[c]

and

Ritonavir 100 mg PO daily[c]

[a] The dosing of lamivudine/emtricitabine, and tenofovir disoproxil fumarate should be adjusted in patients with baseline creatinine clearance < 50 mL/min (see Chapter 9 for dosing recommendations). Tenofovir disoproxil fumarate should be used with caution in exposed workers with renal insufficiency or who are taking concomitant nephrotoxic medications. Fixed-dose combinations should not be used in patients who need dose adjustment due to renal failure.

[b] Lamivudine 300 mg PO daily may be substituted for emtricitabine. However, a fixed-dose combination is available when tenofovir disoproxil fumarate is used with emtricitabine (Truvada 1 PO daily).

[c] See Chapter 9 for dosing recommendations for protease inhibitors in exposed workers with hepatic impairment.

Note: Use of regimens other than those described above should be done in consultation with an expert in PEP.

Modified from New York State Department of Health AIDS Institute. HIV prophylaxis following occupational exposure. http://www.hivguidelines.org/clinical-guidelines/post-exposure-prophylaxis/hiv-prophylaxis-following-occupational-exposure/. 2014. This material was accessed on 10/6/16 on the HIV Clinical Resource website (www.hivguidelines.org). The HIV Clinical Guidelines Program is a collaborative effort of the New York State Department of Health AIDS Institute and the Johns Hopkins University Division of Infectious Diseases.

Table 8.5. Drugs to Avoid in PEP Regimens

Drug(s) to Avoid	Rationale
Efavirenz (EFV)	• Poor adherence anticipated due to CNS side effects, which are common. • CNS side effects may impair work after the initial and subsequent doses. • EFV should be avoided in first 6 weeks of pregnancy and in women of childbearing potential who are not using effective contraception. • Substantial EFV resistance in community HIV isolates.
Nevirapine	Contraindicated for use in PEP due to potential for severe hepatotoxicity.
Abacavir	Potential for hypersensitivity reactions.
Stavudine, didanosine	Possibility of toxicities.
Nelfinavir, indinavir	Poorly tolerated.
CCR5 co-receptor antagonists	Lack of activity against potential CXCR4 tropic virus.

Data from New York State Department of Health AIDS Institute. HIV prophylaxis following occupational exposure. http://www.hivguidelines.org/clinical-guidelines/post-exposure-prophylaxis/hiv-prophylaxis-following-occupational-exposure/. 2014. This material was accessed on 10/6/16 on the HIV Clinical Resource website (www .hivguidelines.org). The HIV Clinical Guidelines Program is a collaborative effort of the New York State Department of Health AIDS Institute and the Johns Hopkins University Division of Infectious Diseases.

[a] MMWR Morb Mortal Wkly Rep. 2001;49:1153–56.

The patient should then be referred for follow-up care to a clinician who has experience in the use of antiretroviral agents and who can provide ongoing prevention counseling.

Treating clinicians who do not have access to experienced HIV clinicians should call the National Clinicians' Consultation Center PEPline at 1-888-448-4911 to review the case.

Patients who present for nPEP should be evaluated as soon as possible in order to initiate therapy, if indicated, within recommended timeframes (preferably < 72 hours) (Figure 8.2). When an HIV exposure occurs, the events and the subsequent interventions should be clearly documented in order to facilitate determination of the effectiveness of nPEP.

Laboratory and clinical evaluations for patients initiating nPEP are outlined in Table 8.6. Note that the New York State Guidelines do not recommend a 6-month follow-up, since delayed seroconversions have not been reported since 1990; the CDC guidelines recommend a 6-month follow-up only if hepatitis C is acquired at the same time as HIV, as this concurrent infection has delayed HIV seroconversion.

The recommended and alternative regimens for nPEP are outlined in Table 8.4. The treatment duration is 28 weeks. In certain circumstances, healthcare providers may choose different strategies from these if the source patient is known to harbor resistance to the drugs in the recommended or alternative regimens. Such choices should only be undertaken with expert consultation. Note Table 8.5 for drugs to avoid as part of nPEP regimens.

It is important for clinicians to facilitate adherence, as studies show that pill taking is irregular in nPEP, especially for those who are victims of sexual assault.

Some individuals provided nPEP may be repeatedly at high risk for HIV acquisition. When nPEP is completed, they should be evaluated as candidates for pre-exposure prophylaxis, or PrEP, a strategy which is covered in the next section.

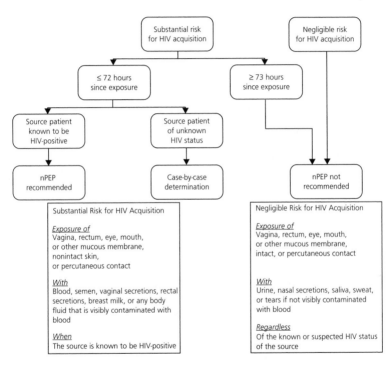

Figure 8.2. Algorithm for Evaluation and Treatment of Possible Nonoccupational HIV Exposures

From: CDC, U.S. Department of Health and Human Services April 18, 2016. Updated Guidelines for Antiretroviral Postexposure Prophylaxis After Sexual, Injection Drug Use, or Other Nonoccupational Exposure to HIV—United States, 2016; https://stacks.cdc.gov/view/cdc/38856

Table 8.6. Recommended Schedule of Laboratory Evaluations of Source and Exposed Persons for Providing nPEP with Preferred Regimens

Test	Source Baseline	Exposed Persons Baseline	4–6 weeks after exposure	3 months after exposure	6 months after exposure
		For all persons considered for or prescribed nPEP for any exposure			
HIV Ag/Ab testing[a] (or antibody testing if Ag/Ab test unavailable)	√	√	√	√	√[b]
Hepatitis B serology, including: Hepatitis B surface antigen Hepatitis B surface antibody Hepatitis B core antibody	√	√	—	—	√[c]
Hepatitis C antibody test	√	√	—	—	√[d]
		For all persons considered for or prescribed nPEP for sexual exposure			
Syphilis serology[e]	√	√	√	—	√
Gonorrhea[f]	√	√	√[g]	—	—
Chlamydia[f]	√	√	√[g]	—	—
Pregnancy[h]	—	√	√	—	—
		For persons prescribed tenofovir DF+ emtricitabine + raltegravir or tenofovir DF+ emtricitabine + dolutegravir			
Serum creatinine (for calculating estimated creatinine clearance[i])		√	√	—	—
Alanine transaminase, aspartate aminotranferase		√	√	—	—
		For all persons with HIV infection confirmed at any visit			
HIV viral load	√	√[j]			
HIV genotypic resistance	√	√[j]			

Abbreviations: Ag/Ab, antigen/antibody combination test; HIV, human immunodeficiency virus; nPEP, nonoccupational postexposure prophylaxis; tenofovir DF, tenofovir disoproxil fumarate.

Table 8.6. Recommended Schedule of Laboratory Evaluations of Source and Exposed Persons for Providing nPEP with Preferred Regimens (Cont'd)

[a] Any positive or indeterminate HIV antibody test should undergo confirmatory testing of HIV infection status.

[b] Only if hepatitis C infection was acquired during the original exposure; delayed HIV seroconversion has been seen in persons who simultaneously acquire HIV and hepatitis C infection.

[c] If exposed person susceptible to hepatitis B at baseline.

[d] If exposed person susceptible to hepatitis C at baseline.

[e] If determined to be infected with syphilis and treated, should undergo serologic syphilis testing 6 months after treatment.

[f] Testing for chlamydia and gonorrhea should be performed using nucleic acid amplification tests. For patients diagnosed with a chlamydia or gonorrhea infection, retesting 3 months after treatment is recommended.

- For men reporting insertive vaginal, anal, or oral sex, a urine specimen should be tested for chlamydia and gonorrhea.
- For women reporting receptive vaginal sex, a vaginal (preferred) or endocervical swab or urine specimen should be tested for chlamydia and gonorrhea.
- For men and women reporting receptive anal sex, a rectal swab specimen should be tested for chlamydia and gonorrhea.
- For men and women reporting receptive oral sex, an oropharyngeal swab should be tested for gonorrhea. (http://www.cdc.gov/std/tg2015/tg-2015-print.pdf)

[g] If not provided presumptive treatment at baseline, or if symptomatic at follow-up visit.

[h] If woman of reproductive age, not using effective contraception, and with vaginal exposure to semen.

[i] eCrCl = estimated creatinine clearance calculated by the Cockcroft-Gault formula; eCrClCG = [(140 – age) × ideal body weight] ÷ (serum creatinine × 72) (× 0.85 for females).

[j] At first visit where determined to have HIV infection.

Reproduced from: CDC, U.S. Department of Health and Human Services April 18, 2016. Updated Guidelines for Antiretroviral Postexposure Prophylaxis After Sexual, Injection Drug Use, or Other Nonoccupational Exposure to HIV—United States, 2016, Table 2.

PRE-EXPOSURE PROPHYLAXIS

Pre-exposure prophylaxis (PrEP) refers to the practice of giving individuals who are HIV negative but at high risk antiretroviral therapy to reduce the risk of acquiring HIV. Several clinical trials have established that preexposure prophylaxis with tenofovir DF/emtricitabine is effective, especially when taken as directed.

The first study demonstrating that PrEP is effective was the iPrEx study, which included nearly 2500 HIV-negative men who have sex with men (MSM) in South America, the U.S., Thailand, and South Africa, and randomized them in a double-blinded fashion to receive once-daily oral TDF/FTC or placebo (N Engl J Med 2010; 363:2587–2599). Those receiving active PrEP had a 44% reduction in the risk of acquiring HIV, with the efficacy much better in those with good medication adherence. No major toxicity was seen in the TDF/FTC group. Subsequently, additional studies conducted in sub-Saharan Africa among heterosexual men and women have also shown PrEP to be effective provided medication adherence is adequate. Studies that have failed to demonstrate the efficacy of PrEP have invariably shown very low rates of pill taking by the participants.

Table 8.7. Summary of Guidance for PrEP Use

	Men Who Have Sex with Men	Heterosexual Women and Men	Injection Drug Users
Detecting substantial risk of acquiring HIV infection	HIV-positive sexual partner Recent bacterial STI High number of sex partners History of inconsistent or no condom use Commercial sex work	HIV-positive sexual partner Recent bacterial STI High number of sex partners History of inconsistent or no condom use Commercial sex work In high-prevalence area or network	HIV-positive injecting partner Sharing injection equipment Recent drug treatment
Clinically eligible	Documented negative HIV test result before prescribing PrEP No signs/symptoms of acute HIV infection Normal renal function; no contraindicated medications Documented hepatitis B virus infection and vaccination status		

Reproduced from CDC and Prevention. Preexposrue prophylaxis for the prevention of HIV infection in the United State: 2014. A clinical practice guideline.

Two follow-up studies done in high risk men who have sex with men demonstrated exceptionally high levels of protection, with no clear failures among those taking the medication as directed (N Engl J Med. 2015; 373:2237–46; Lancet January 2, 2016; 387:53–60). While preexposure prophylaxis is not 100% effective (a single case of multidrug resistant HIV was acquired even with adherence to PrEP), patients who elect to start PrEP can be informed that protection exceeds 90%.

Based on the results of these studies, the CDC has issued a guidance on the use of PrEP in clinical practice (Figure 8.3). Note that in the United States, these recommendations apply only to high- risk individuals; the incidence of HIV among heterosexuals at "community risk" in the United States is too low to warrant PrEP. Similarly, some MSM and injection drug users who are at low risk for HIV would not be candidates for PrEP. Table 8 below highlights those individuals for whom PrEP should be strongly considered as part of a comprehensive HIV prevention strategy.

Before initiating PrEP

Determine eligibility
- Document negative HIV antibody test(s) immediately before starting PrEP medication.
- Test for acute HIV infection if patient has symptoms consistent with acute HIV infection.
- Confirm that patient is at substantial, ongoing, high risk for acquiring HIV infection.
- Confirm that calculated creatinine clearance is ≥ 60 mL per minute (via Cockcroft–Gault formula).

Other recommended actions
- Screen for hepatitis B infection; vaccinate against hepatitis B if susceptible, or treat if active infection exists, regardless of decision about prescribing PrEP.
- Screen and treat as needed for STIs.

Beginning PrEP medication regimen

- Prescribe 1 tablet of Truvada* (TDF [300 mg] plus FTC [200 mg]) daily.
- In general, prescribe no more than a 90-day supply, renewable only after HIV testing confirms that patient remains HIV uninfected.
- If active hepatitis B infection is diagnosed, consider using TDF/FTC for both treatment of active hepatitis B infection and HIV prevention.
- Provide risk-reduction and PrEP medication adherence counseling and condoms.

Follow-up while PrEP medication is being taken

- Every 2–3 months, perform an HIV antibody test; document negative result.
- Evaluate and support PrEP medication adherence at each follow-up visit, more often if inconsistent adherence is identified.
- Every 2–3 months, assess risk behaviors and provide risk-reduction counseling and condoms. Assess STI symptoms and, if present, test and treat for STI as needed.
- Every 6 months, test for STI even if patient is asymptomatic, and treat as needed.
- 3 months after initiation, then yearly while on PrEP medication, check blood urea nitrogen and serum creatinine.

On discontinuing PrEP (at patient request, for safety concerns, or if HIV infection is acquired)

- Perform HIV test(s) to confirm whether HIV infection has occurred.
- If HIV positive, order and document results of resistance testing and establish linkage to HIV care.
- If HIV negative, establish linkage to risk-reduction support services as indicated.
- If active hepatitis B is diagnosed at initiation of PrEP, consider appropriate medication for continued treatment of hepatitis B.

Abbreviations: HIV = human immunodeficiency virus; STI = sexually transmitted infection; TDF = tenofovir disoproxil fumarate; FTC = emtricitabine.

Modified from Centers for Disease Control and Prevention. CDC fact sheet: PrEP: A new tool for HIV prevention. http://www.cdc.gov/hiv/pdf/prevention_prep_factsheet.pdf. 2012.

Pre-prescription visit:

- Discuss PrEP use; clarify misconceptions.
- Perform following laboratory tests:
  - HIV test (see text for guidance on what type of test to use)
  - Metabolic panel
  - Urinalysis
  - Hepatitis A, B, and C serology
  - STI screening
  - Pregnancy test

After confirmation of negative HIV test:
Prescribe 30-day supply of PrEP
Follow up in 2 weeks to assess side effects
(in person or by phone)

Adherence and commitment should be assessed at each visit. Schedule visits every 30 days for patients who report poor adherence or intermittent use.

30-day visit:

Assess:

- Side effects.
- Serum creatinine and calculated creatinine clearance for patients with borderline renal function or at increased risk for kidney disease (> 65 years of age, black race, hypertension, or diabetes).
- Discuss risk reduction and provide condoms.

Prescribe 60-day refill; patient must come in for 3-month visit for HIV test and follow-up assessments, then 90-day schedule can begin.

3-month visit
- HIV test.
- Ask about STI symptoms.
- Discuss risk reduction and provide condoms.
- Serum creatinine and calculated creatinine clearance.
- Pregnancy test.

6-month visit
- HIV test.
- Obtain STI screening tests.
- Pregnancy test.
- Discuss risk reduction and provide condoms.

9-month visit
- HIV test.
- Ask about STI symptoms.
- Discuss risk reduction and provide condoms.
- Serum creatinine and calculated creatinine clearance.
- Pregnancy test.

12-month visit
- HIV test.
- Obtain STI screening tests.
- HCV serology for MSM, IDUs, and those with multiple sexual partners.
- Discuss risk reduction and provide condoms.
- Pregnancy test.
- Urinalysis.

Figure 8.3. Flowsheet for Starting and Monitoring PrEP

Reproduced from New York State Department of Health AIDS Institute. Guidance for the use of pre-exposure prophylaxis (PrEP) to prevent HIV transmission. http://www.hivguidelines.org/clinical-guidelines/pre-exposure-prophylaxis/guidance-for-the-use-of-pre-exposure-prophylaxis-prep-to-prevent-hiv-transmission/. 2015. This material was accessed on 10/6/16 on the HIV Clinical Resource website (www.hivguidelines.org). The HIV Clinical Guidelines Program is a collaborative effort of the New York State Department of Health AIDS Institute and the Johns Hopkins University Division of Infectious Diseases.

Chapter 9

Antiretroviral, Anti-HBV, and Anti-HCV Drug Summaries

David W. Kubiak, PharmD, BCPS
Kari J. Furtek, PharmD, MPH, BCPS

This section contains prescribing information pertinent to the clinical use of antiretroviral agents in adults, as compiled from a variety of sources, including Micromedex®, Micromedex 2.0 online version 21.2®, Department of Health and Human Services Guidelines for the Use of Antiretroviral Agents in HIV-1-Infected Adults and Adolescents (http://www.aidsinfo.nih.gov/guidelines/), accessed September 27, 2016, HCV Guidance: Recommendations for Testing, Managing, and Treating Hepatitis C (http://www.hcvguidelines.org), accessed September 27, 2016, and manufacturers' product information, among others. The information provided is not exhaustive, and the reader is referred to other drug information references and the manufacturer's product literature for further information. Clinical use of the information provided and any consequences that may arise from its use are the responsibilities of the prescribing physician. The authors, editors, and publisher do not warrant or guarantee the information contained in this section, and do not assume and expressly disclaim any liability for errors or omissions or any consequences that may occur from such. **The use of any drug should be preceded by careful review of the package insert, which provides indications and dosing approved by the U.S. Food and Drug Administration. This information can be obtained on the Website provided at the end of the reference list for each drug summary.**

Drugs are listed alphabetically by generic name; trade names follow in parentheses. To search by trade name, consult the index. Each drug summary contains the following information:

Usual Dose. Represents the usual dose to treat HIV infection in adult patients with normal hepatic and renal function. Additional information can be found in the manufacturer's package insert and product literature.

Bioavailability. Refers to the percentage of the dose reaching the systemic circulation from the site of administration (PO or IM). For PO antibiotics, bioavailability refers to the percentage of dose absorbed from the gastrointestinal (GI) tract.

Excreted Unchanged. Refers to the percentage of drug excreted unchanged, and provides an indirect measure of drug concentration in the urine/feces.

Serum Half-Life (normal/ESRD). The serum half-life ($T_{1/2}$) is the time (in hours) in which serum concentration falls by 50%. Serum half-life is useful in determining dosing interval. If the half-life of drugs eliminated by the kidneys is prolonged in end-stage renal disease (ESRD), then the total daily dose is reduced in proportion to the degree of renal dysfunction. If the half-life in ESRD is similar to the normal half-life, then the total daily dose does not change.

Plasma Protein Binding. Expressed as the percentage of drug reversibly bound to serum albumin. It is the unbound (free) portion of a drug that equilibrates with tissues and imparts antiviral activity. Plasma protein binding is not typically a factor in antimicrobial effectiveness unless binding exceeds 95%. Decreases in serum albumin (nephrotic syndrome, liver disease) or competition for protein binding from other drugs or endogenously produced substances (uremia, hyperbilirubinemia) will increase the percentage of free drug available for antimicrobial activity, and may require a decrease in dosage. Increases in serum binding proteins (trauma, surgery, critical illness) will decrease the percentage of free drug available for antimicrobial activity, and may require an increase in dosage.

Volume of Distribution (V_d). Represents the apparent volume into which the drug is distributed, and is calculated as the amount of drug in the body divided by the serum concentration (in liters/kilogram). V_d is related to total body water distribution (V_d H_2O = 0.7 L/kg). Hydrophilic (water soluble) drugs are restricted to extracellular fluid and have a $V_d \leq 0.7$ L/kg. In contrast, hydrophobic (highly lipid soluble) drugs penetrate most fluids/tissues of the body and have a large V_d. Drugs that are concentrated in certain tissues (e.g., liver) can have a V_d greatly exceeding total body water. V_d is affected by organ profusion, membrane diffusion/permeability, lipid solubility, protein binding, and state of equilibrium between body compartments. For hydrophilic drugs, increases in V_d may occur with burns, heart failure, dialysis, sepsis, cirrhosis, or mechanical ventilation; decreases in V_d may occur with trauma, hemorrhage, pancreatitis (early), or GI fluid losses. Increases in V_d may require an increase in total daily drug dose for antimicrobial effectiveness; decreases in V_d may require a decrease in drug dose. In addition to drug distribution, V_d reflects binding avidity to cholesterol membranes and concentration within organ tissues (e.g., liver).

Mode of Elimination. Refers to the primary route of inactivation/excretion of the drug, which impacts dosing adjustments in renal/hepatic failure.

Dosage Adjustments. Each grid provides dosing adjustments based on renal and hepatic function. Antimicrobial dosing for hemodialysis (HD)/peritoneal dialysis (PD) patients is the same as indicated for patients with a creatinine clearance (CrCl) < 10 mL/min. Some antimicrobial agents require a supplemental dose immediately after hemodialysis (post-HD)/peritoneal dialysis (post-PD); following the supplemental dose, antimicrobial dosing should once again resume as indicated for a CrCl < 10 mL/min. "No change" indicates no change from the usual dose. "Avoid" indicates the drug should be avoided in the setting described. "None" indicates no supplemental dose is required. "No information" indicates there are insufficient data from which to make a dosing recommendation. Dosing recommendations are based on data, experience, or pharmacokinetic parameters. Continuous venovenous hemofiltration (CVVH) dosing recommendations represent general guidelines, since antibiotic removal is dependent on area/type of filter, ultrafiltration rates, and sieving coefficients; replacement dosing should be individualized and guided by serum levels, if possible. Creatinine clearance (CrCl) is used to gauge the degree of renal insufficiency, and can be estimated by the following calculation: CrCl (mL/min) = [(140 – age) × weight (kg)] / [72 × serum creatinine (mg/dL)]. The calculated value is multiplied by 0.85 for females. It is important to recognize that due to age-dependent decline in renal function, elderly patients with "normal" serum creatinine may have low CrCl, requiring dosage adjustments. (For example, a 70-year-old, 50-kg female with a serum creatinine of 1.2 mg/dL has an estimated CrCl of 34 mL/min.) "Antiretroviral Dosage Adjustment" grids indicate recommended dosage adjustments when protease inhibitors (PIs) and non-nucleoside reverse transcriptase inhibitors (NNRTIs) are combined or used in conjunction with rifampin or rifabutin. These grids were compiled, in part, from Guidelines for the Use of Antiretroviral Agents in HIV-Infected Adults and Adolescents, Panel on Clinical Practices for Treatment of HIV Infection, Department of Health and Human Services, http://www.aidsinfo.nih.gov/guidelines/, accessed September 27, 2016.

Drug Interactions. Refers to common/important drug interactions, as compiled from various sources. If a specific drug interaction is well-documented, then other drugs from the same drug class (e.g., atorvastatin) may also be listed, based on theoretical considerations. Drug interactions may occur as a consequence of altered absorption (e.g., metal ion chelation of tetracycline), altered distribution (e.g., sulfonamide displacement of barbiturates from serum albumin), altered metabolism (e.g., rifampin-induced hepatic P-450 metabolism of theophylline/warfarin; chloramphenicol inhibition of phenytoin metabolism), or altered excretion (e.g., probenecid competition with penicillin for active transport in the kidney).

Adverse Side Effects. Common/important side effects are indicated.

Allergic Potential. Described as low or high. Refers to the likelihood of a hypersensitivity reaction to a particular agent.

Safety in Pregnancy. Designated by the U.S. Food and Drug Administration's (FDA) use-in-pregnancy letter code (Table 9.1) for agents approved prior to 2015. These categories were eliminated in 2015 in accordance with the Pregnancy and Lactation Labeling Rule and were substituted with narratives describing existing data with aims to assist practitioners and patients with making informed decisions about risk versus benefit of therapy. (Further details can be found on the FDA Website: http://www.fda.gov/Drugs/DevelopmentApprovalProcess/DevelopmentResources/Labeling/ucm093307.htm, accessed September 27, 2016. Drugs approved after 2015 will include a brief narrative. Readers should be directed to prescribing information or to contact pregnancy registries for more information.

Antiretroviral Pregnancy Registry. To monitor maternal-fetal outcomes of pregnant women exposed to antiretroviral drugs, an Antiretroviral Pregnancy Registry has been established. Clinicians who are treating HIV-infected pregnant women are strongly encouraged to report cases of prenatal exposure to antiretroviral drugs (either administered alone or in combinations). The registry collects observational, nonexperimental data regarding antiretroviral exposure during pregnancy for the purpose of assessing potential teratogenicity. Telephone: 910-251-9087 or 1-800-258-4263;Website: http://www.apregistry.com;e-mail: registries@kendle.com.

Comments. Includes useful information for each antiretroviral agent.

Selected References. These references are classic, important, or recent. When available, the Website containing the manufacturer's prescribing information/package insert is provided.

Table 9.1. FDA Use-in-Pregnancy Letter Code

Category	Interpretation
A	Controlled studies show no risk. Adequate, well-controlled studies in pregnant women have not shown a risk to the fetus in any trimester of pregnancy
B	No evidence of risk in humans. Adequate, well-controlled studies in pregnant women have not shown increased risk of fetal abnormalities despite adverse findings in animals, or, in the absence of adequate human studies, animal studies show no fetal risk. The chance of fetal harm is remote, but remains a possibility
C	Risk cannot be ruled out. Adequate, well-controlled human studies are lacking, and animal studies have shown a risk to the fetus or are lacking. There is a chance of fetal harm if the drug is administered during pregnancy, but potential benefit from use of the drug may outweigh potential risk
D	Positive evidence of risk. Studies in humans or investigational or post marketing data have demonstrated fetal risk. Nevertheless, potential benefit from use of the drug may outweigh potential risk. For example, the drug may be acceptable if needed in a life-threatening situation or serious disease for which safer drugs cannot be used or are ineffective
X	Contraindicated in pregnancy. Studies in animals or humans or investigational or post marketing reports have demonstrated positive evidence of fetal abnormalities or risk which clearly outweigh any possible benefit to the patient

Data from: U.S. Food and Drug Administration.

Abacavir (Ziagen) (ABC)

Drug Class: Antiretroviral NRTI (nucleoside reverse transcriptase inhibitor)
Usual Dose: HLA-B*5701 negative patients—300 mg (PO) bid
How Supplied: Oral solution: 20 mg/mL, Oral tablet: 300 mg
Pharmacokinetic Parameters:
Peak serum level: 3 mcg/mL
Bioavailability: 83%
Excreted unchanged (urine): 1.2%
Serum half-life (normal/ESRD): 1.5/8 h
Plasma protein binding: 50%
Volume of distribution (V_d): 0.86 L/kg
Primary Mode of Elimination: Hepatic
Dosage Adjustments*

CrCl 50–80 mL/min	No change
CrCl 10–50 mL/min	No change
CrCl < 10 mL/min	No change
Post-HD dose	None
Post-PD dose	None
CVVH dose	No change
Mild hepatic insufficiency	200 mg (PO) QD
Moderate or severe hepatic insufficiency	Avoid

Drug Interactions: Methadone (↑ methadone clearance with abacavir 600 mg bid); ethanol (↑ abacavir serum levels by 41% and may ↑ toxicity).
Adverse Effects: *Abacavir may cause severe hypersensitivity reactions (see comments), usually during the first 4–6 weeks of therapy,* **which may be fatal.** Drug fever/rash, abdominal pain/ diarrhea, nausea, vomiting, anorexia, insomnia, weakness, headache, ↑SGOT/ SGPT, hyperglycemia, hypertriglyceridemia, lactic acidosis with hepatic steatosis (rare, but potentially life-threatening toxicity with use of NRTIs). Potential for increased cardiovascular events, especially in patients with cardiovascular risk factors.
Allergic Potential: High (~ 5%)
Safety in Pregnancy: C
Comments: May be taken with or without food. **HLA-B*5701 testing should precede the use of abacavir or an abacavir-containing regimen to reduce the risk of hypersensitivity reaction. Immediately and permanently discontinue if a hypersensitivity reaction occurs; never restart abacavir sulfate following a hypersensitivity reaction or if hypersensitivity cannot be ruled out, which may include fever, rash, fatigue, nausea, vomiting, diarrhea, abdominal pain, anorexia, respiratory symptoms, which may include fever, rash, fatigue, nausea, vomiting, diarrhea, abdominal pain, anorexia, respiratory symptoms.**
Cerebrospinal Fluid Penetration: 27–33%

REFERENCES:

Cutrell A, Brothers C, Yeo J, Hernandez J, Lapierre D. Abacavir and the potential risk of myocardial infarction. Lancet 2008 Apr 26;371(9622):1413 (E-pub ahead of print).

Mallal S, Phillips E, Carosi G, et al. HLA-B*5701 screening for hypersensitivity to abacavir. N Engl J Med. 2008; 358:568–79.

Panel on Antiretroviral Guidelines for Adults and Adolescents. Guidelines for the use of antiretroviral agents in HIV-1-infected adults and adolescents, updated July 14, 2016. Department of Health and Human Services; 1–288. Available at https://aidsinfo.nih.gov/contentfiles/lvguidelines/adultandadolescentgl.pdf.

Product Information: Ziagen oral tablets, oral solution, abacavir oral tablets, oral solution. ViiV Healthcare, Research Triangle Park, NC, 2015.

"Usual dose" assumes normal renal/hepatic function. * For renal insufficiency, give usual dose × 1 followed by maintenance dose per CrCl. For dialysis patients, dose the same as for CrCl < 10 mL/min and give supplemental (post-HD/PD dose) immediately after dialysis. CrCl = creatinine clearance; CVVH = continuous venovenous hemofiltration; HD/PD = hemodialysis/peritoneal dialysis. See pp. 204–207 for explanations, pp. xi–xii for abbreviations.

Abacavir + Lamivudine (Epzicom) (ABC/3TC)

Drug Class: Antiretroviral; NRTI combination
Usual Dose: HLA-B*5701 negative patients—1 tablet (PO) daily
How Supplied: Oral tablet: (containing Abacavir Sulfate 600 mg + Lamivudine 300 mg)
Pharmacokinetic Parameters:
Peak serum level: 3/1.5 mcg/L
Bioavailability: 83/86%
Excreted unchanged (urine): 1.2/71%
Serum half-life (normal/ESRD): (1.5/8)/ (5–7/20) h
Plasma protein binding: 50/36%
Volume of distribution (V_d): 0.86/1.3 L/kg
Primary Mode of Elimination: Hepatic/ renal
Dosage Adjustments*

CrCl < 50 mL/min	Not recommended
Post-HD dose	Not recommended
Post-PD dose	Not recommended
CVVH dose	Not recommended
Mild hepatic insufficiency	Contraindicated
Moderate or severe hepatic insufficiency	Contraindicated

Drug Interactions: Methadone (↑methadone clearance with abacavir 600 mg bid); ethanol (↑abacavir serum levels/half-life; may ↑toxicity); didanosine, zalcitabine (↑risk of pancreatitis); TMP-SMX (↑lamivudine levels); zidovudine (↑zidovudine levels).
Adverse Effects: Abacavir may cause severe hypersensitivity reactions that may be fatal (see comments), usually during the first 4–6 weeks of therapy. Drug fever, rash, abdominal pain, diarrhea, nausea, vomiting, anorexia, anemia, leukopenia, photophobia, depression, insomnia, weakness, headache, cough, nasal complaints, dizziness, peripheral neuropathy, myalgias, ↑AST/ ALT, hyperglycemia, hypertriglyceridemia, pancreatitis, lactic acidosis with hepatic steatosis (rare, but potentially life-threatening toxicity with the NRTIs).
Allergic Potential: High (~ 5%)/Low
Safety in Pregnancy: C
Comments: May be taken with or without food. **HLA-B*5701 testing should precede the use of abacavir or an abacavir-containing regimen to reduce the risk of hypersensitivity reaction. Immediately and permanently discontinue if a hypersensitivity reaction occurs; never restart abacavir sulfate/lamivudine following a hypersensitivity reaction or if hypersensitivity cannot be ruled out, which may include fever, rash, fatigue, nausea, vomiting, diarrhea, abdominal pain, anorexia, respiratory symptoms. Potential cross-resistance with didanosine. Lamivudine prevents development of ZDV resistance and restores ZDV susceptibility. For patients co-infected with HIV and HBV, monitor hepatic function closely during therapy and for several months afterward. Cerebrospinal Fluid Penetration:** 27– 33/15%

REFERENCES:
Mallal S, Phillips E, Carosi G, et al. HLA-B*5701 screening for hypersensitivity to abacavir. N Engl J Med. 2008; 358:568–79.
Panel on Antiretroviral Guidelines for Adults and Adolescents. Guidelines for the use of antiretroviral agents in HIV-1-infected adults and adolescents, updated July 14, 2016. Department of Health and Human

"Usual dose" assumes normal renal/hepatic function. * For renal insufficiency, give usual dose × 1 followed by maintenance dose per CrCl. For dialysis patients, dose the same as for CrCl < 10 mL/min and give supplemental (post-HD/PD dose) immediately after dialysis. CrCl = creatinine clearance; CVVH = continuous venovenous hemofiltration; HD/PD = hemodialysis/peritoneal dialysis. See pp. 204–207 for explanations, pp. xi–xii for abbreviations.

Services; 1–288. Available at https://aidsinfo.nih.gov/contentfiles/lvguidelines/adultandadolescentgl.pdf.

Sosa N, Hill-Zabala C, Dejesus E, et al. Abacavir and lamivudine fixed-dose combination tablet once daily compared with abacavir and lamivudine twice daily in HIV-infected patients over 48 weeks. J Acquir Immune Defic Syndr. 2005;40:422–7.

Abacavir + Lamivudine + Zidovudine (Trizivir)

Drug Class: Antiretroviral; NRTI combination

Usual Dose: HLA-B*5701 negative patients—1 tablet (PO) bid with or without food.

How supplied: Oral tablet: (containing abacavir 300 mg + lamivudine 150 mg + zidovudine 300 mg)

Pharmacokinetic Parameters:
Peak serum level: 3/1.5/1.2 mcg/mL
Bioavailability: 86/86/64%
Excreted unchanged (urine): 1.2/90/16%
Serum half-life (normal/ESRD): [1.5/6/1.1]/8/20/2.2] h
Plasma protein binding: 30/36/20%
Volume of distribution (V_d): 0.86/1.3/1.6 L/kg

Primary Mode of Elimination: Hepatic/renal

Dosage Adjustments*

CrCl < 50 mL/min	Avoid
Post-HD or Post-PD	Avoid
CVVH dose	Avoid
Moderate or severe hepatic insufficiency	Not recommended

Drug Interactions: Amprenavir, atovaquone (↑zidovudine levels); clarithromycin (↓zidovudine levels); cidofovir (↑zidovudine levels, flu-like symptoms); doxorubicin (neutropenia); stavudine (antagonistic to zidovudine; avoid combination); TMP-SMX (↑ lamivudine and zidovudine levels); zalcitabine (↓lamivudine levels).

Adverse Effects: HLA-B*5701 testing should precede the use of abacavir or an abacavir-containing regimen to reduce the risk of hypersensitivity reaction. Immediately and permanently discontinue if a hypersensitivity reaction occurs; never restart abacavir sulfate/lamivudine/zidovudine following a hypersensitivity reaction or if hypersensitivity cannot be ruled out, which may include fever, rash, fatigue, nausea, vomiting, diarrhea, abdominal pain, anorexia, respiratory symptoms.

Most common (> 5%): Nausea, vomiting, diarrhea, anorexia, insomnia, fever/chills, headache, malaise/fatigue. Others (less common): peripheral neuropathy, myopathy, steatosis, pancreatitis. Lab abnormalities: mild hyperglycemia, anemia, LFT elevations, hypertriglyceridemia, leukopenia.

Allergic Potential: High (< 5%)

Safety in Pregnancy: C

Comments: Avoid in patients with CrCl < 50 mL/min. HBV hepatitis may relapse if lamivudine is discontinued.

REFERENCES:
Mallal S, Phillips E, Carosi G, et al. HLA-B*5701 screening for hypersensitivity to abacavir. N Engl J Med. 2008; 358:568–79.

McDowell JA, Lou Y, Symonds WS, et al. Multiple-dose pharmacokinetics and pharmacodynamics of abacavir alone and in combination with zidovudine in human immunodeficiency virus-infected adults. Antimicrob Agents Chemother. 2000;44:2061–7.

"Usual dose" assumes normal renal/hepatic function. * For renal insufficiency, give usual dose × 1 followed by maintenance dose per CrCl. For dialysis patients, dose the same as for CrCl < 10 mL/min and give supplemental (post-HD/PD dose) immediately after dialysis. CrCl = creatinine clearance; CVVH = continuous venovenous hemofiltration; HD/PD = hemodialysis/peritoneal dialysis. See pp. 204–207 for explanations, pp. xi–xii for abbreviations.

Panel on Antiretroviral Guidelines for Adults and Adolescents. Guidelines for the use of antiretroviral agents in HIV-1-infected adults and adolescents, updated July 14, 2016. Department of Health and Human Services; 1–28840. Available at https://aidsinfo.nih.gov/contentfiles/lvguidelines/adultandadolescentgl.pdf.

Adefovir dipivoxil (Hepsera)

Drug Class: Anti-hepatitis B agent (NRTI)
Usual Dose: 10 mg (PO) daily
How Supplied: Oral tablet: 10 mg
Pharmacokinetic Parameters:
Peak serum level: 18 ng/mL
Bioavailability: 59%
Excreted unchanged (urine): 45%
Serum half-life (normal/ESRD): 7.5/9 h
Plasma protein binding: 4%
Volume of distribution (V_d): 0.4 L/kg
Primary Mode of Elimination: Renal
Dosage Adjustments*

CrCl ≥ 50 mL/min	10 mg (PO) daily
CrCl 30–49 mL/min	10 mg (PO) q2d
CrCl 10–29 mL/min	10 mg (PO) q3d
Hemodialysis	10 mg (PO) q7d
Post-HD or PD dose	No information
CVVH dose	No information
Moderate or severe hepatic insufficiency	No change

Drug Interactions: No significant interaction with lamivudine, TMP-SMX, acetaminophen, ibuprofen.
Adverse Effects: Asthenia, headache, abdominal pain, nausea, flatulence, diarrhea, dyspepsia. Nephrotoxicity monitor for increased serum creatinine and decreased phosphorus. Avoid other nephrotoxic agents (see drug interactions above).
Allergic Potential: Low
Safety in Pregnancy: C
Comments: May be taken with or without food. Does not inhibit CYP450 isoenzymes. Do not discontinue abruptly to avoid exacerbation of HBV hepatitis.

REFERENCES:

Cundy KC, Burditch-Crovo P, Walker RE, et al. Clinical pharmacokinetics of adefovir in human HIV-1 infected patients. Antimicrob Agents Chemother. 1995;35:2401–2405.

Product Information: Hepsera oral tablets, adefovir dipivoxil oral tablets. Gilead Sciences, Inc., Foster City, CA; 2008.

Terrault, NA, Bzowej, NH, Chang, K-M, Hwang, JP, Jonas, MM, and Murad, MH. AASLD guidelines for treatment of chronic hepatitis B. Hepatology, 2016; 63:261–283.

Atazanavir (Reyataz) (ATV)

Drug Class: Antiretroviral; HIV-1 protease inhibitor (PI)
Usual Dose: 400 mg (PO) daily; 300 mg (PO) daily when given with ritonavir 100 mg (PO) daily
How Supplied: Oral capsule: 100 mg, 150 mg, 200 mg, 300 mg; oral powder packet (single): 50 mg
Pharmacokinetic Parameters:
Peak serum level: 3152 ng/mL
Bioavailability: No data
Excreted unchanged (urine/feces): 7%/20%
Serum half-life (normal/ESRD): 7 h/no data
Plasma protein binding: 86%
Volume of distribution (V_d): No data

"Usual dose" assumes normal renal/hepatic function. * For renal insufficiency, give usual dose × 1 followed by maintenance dose per CrCl. For dialysis patients, dose the same as for CrCl < 10 mL/min and give supplemental (post-HD/PD dose) immediately after dialysis. CrCl = creatinine clearance; CVVH = continuous venovenous hemofiltration; HD/PD = hemodialysis/peritoneal dialysis. See pp. 204–207 for explanations, pp. xi–xii for abbreviations.

Primary Mode of Elimination: Hepatic

Dosage Adjustments*

CrCl < 50 mL/min	No change
Post-HD or PD dose	See comment**
CVVH dose	No data
Mild-moderate hepatic insufficiency†	300 mg (PO) daily
Severe hepatic insufficiency	Avoid

** For ARV-naïve patients on HD: ATV 300 mg + RTV 100 mg PO daily. Not recommended for treatment-experienced patients.

† Boosting not recommended in patients with hepatic insufficiency

Antiretroviral Dosage Adjustments

Delavirdine	No information
Didanosine	Give atazanavir 2 hrs before or 1 hr after didanosine buffered formulations
Efavirenz	Do not coadminister with unboosted ATV. In treatment-naïve patients (ATV 400 mg + RTV 100 mg) once daily. Do not coadminister in treatment-experienced patients.
Indinavir	Avoid combination
Lopinavir/ ritonavir	ATV 300 mg once daily + LPV/r 400/100 mg bid
Nelfinavir	No information
Nevirapine	Do not coadminister with atazanavir +/– ritonavir

Ritonavir	Atazanavir 300 mg/d + ritonavir 100 mg/d as single daily dose with food
Saquinavir	↑ saquinavir (soft-gel) levels; no information
Rifampin	Avoid combination
Rifabutin	150 mg q2d or 3x/week
Etravirine	Do not coadminister with atazanavir +/– ritonavir
Maraviroc	MVC 150 mg bid with ATV +/– RTV
Raltegravir	No change

Drug Interactions: Antacids or buffered medications (↓ atazanavir levels; give atazanavir 2 hours before or 1 hour after); H$_2$-receptor blockers (↓ atazanavir levels. In <u>treatment-naïve</u> patients taking an H$_2$-receptor antagonist, give either atazanavir 400 mg once daily with food at least 2 hours before and at least 10 hours after the H$_2$-receptor antagonist, or give atazanavir 300 mg once daily with ritonavir 100 mg once daily with food, without the need for separation from the H$_2$-receptor antagonist. In <u>treatment-experienced</u> patients, give atazanavir 300 mg once daily with ritonavir 100 mg once daily with food at least 2 hours before and at least 10 hours after the H$_2$-receptor antagonist); antiarrhythmics (↑ amiodarone, systemic lidocaine, quinidine levels; prolongs PR interval; monitor antiarrhythmic levels); antidepressants (↑ tricyclic antidepressant levels; monitor levels); calcium channel blockers (↑ calcium channel blocker levels, ↑ PR interval; ↓ diltiazem dose by 50%; use with caution;

"Usual dose" assumes normal renal/hepatic function. * For renal insufficiency, give usual dose × 1 followed by maintenance dose per CrCl. For dialysis patients, dose the same as for CrCl < 10 mL/min and give supplemental (post-HD/PD dose) immediately after dialysis. CrCl = creatinine clearance; CVVH = continuous venovenous hemofiltration; HD/PD = hemodialysis/peritoneal dialysis. See pp. 204–207 for explanations, pp. xi–xii for abbreviations.

consider ECG monitoring); clarithromycin (↑ clarithromycin and atazanavir levels; consider 50% dose reduction; consider alternate agent for infections not caused by monoamine inhibitor [MAI]); cyclosporine, sirolimus, tacrolimus (↑ immunosuppressant levels; monitor levels); ethinyl estradiol, norethindrone (↑ oral contraceptive levels; use lowest effective oral contraceptive dose); lovastatin, simvastatin (↑ risk of myopathy, rhabdomyolysis; avoid combination); sildenafil (↑ sildenafil levels; do not give more than 25 mg q2h); tadalafil (max. 10 mg/72 hours); vardenafil (max. 2.5 mg/72 hours); St. John's wort (avoid combination); warfarin (↑ warfarin levels; monitor INR); rivaroxaban (↑ rivaroxaban); tenofovir (tenofovir reduces systemic exposure to atazanavir. Whenever the two are coadministered, the recommended dose of atazanavir is 300 mg once daily with ritonavir 100 mg once daily). *Drugs that should not be coadministered with atazanavir* include alfuzosin beta-blockers, cisapride, pimozide, rifampin, irinotecan, midazolam, triazolam, lovastatin, simvastatin, bepridil, some ergot derivatives, indinavir, proton pump inhibitors, St. John's wort.

Adverse Effects: Reversible, asymptomatic ↑ in indirect (unconjugated) bilirubin may occur. Asymptomatic, dose-dependent ↑ PR interval (~ 24 msec). Use with caution with drugs that ↑ PR interval (e.g., beta-blockers, verapamil, digoxin). May ↑ risk of hyperglycemia/diabetes. May ↑ risk of bleeding in hemophilia (types A + B). Rare cases of Stevens-Johnson syndrome, erythema multiforme, and toxic skin eruptions, including drug rash, eosinophilia and systemic symptoms (DRESS) syndrome, that have been reported. Nephrolithiasis and cholelithiasis.

Allergic Potential: Low
Cerebrospinal Fluid Penetration: Intermediate
Safety in Pregnancy: B
Comments: Monitor LFTs in patients with HBV, HCV. Take 400 mg (two 200-mg capsules) once daily with food.

REFERENCES:
Panel on Antiretroviral Guidelines for Adults and Adolescents. Guidelines for the use of antiretroviral agents in HIV-1-infected adults and adolescents, updated July 14, 2016. Department of Health and Human Services; 1–288. Available at https://aidsinfo.nih.gov/contentfiles/lvguidelines/adultandadolescentgl.pdf.

Product Information: Reyataz oral capsules, powder, atazanavir oral capsules, powder. Bristol-Myers Squibb (per FDA), Princeton, NJ; 2014.

Sanne I, Piliero P, Squires K, et al. Results of a phase 2 clinical trial at 48 weeks (AI424 007): a dose-ranging, safety, and efficacy comparative trial of atazanavir at three doses in combination with didanosine and stavudine in antiretroviral-naïve subjects. J Acquir Immune Defic Syndr. 2003;32:18–29.

Atazanavir/Cobicistat (Evotaz)

Drug Class: HIV-1 protease inhibitor/CYP3A inhibitor
Usual Dose: 1 tablet PO daily with food
How Supplied: Oral tablet: (containing 300 mg of atazanavir and 150 mg of cobicistat)
Pharmacokinetic Parameters:
Peak serum level: Atazanavir: 3.91 mcg/mL (with emtricitabine, tenofovir, & cobicistat)
Bioavailability: Increased with food (28%/24%)
Excreted unchanged (urine/feces): Atazanavir (7/20)%; Cobicistat (8.2/86.2)%
Serum half-life: 7.5 h/ 3–4h

Plasma protein binding: 86%/97–98%
Primary Mode of Elimination: Hepatic/hepatic
Dosage Adjustments:

CrCl < 70 mL/min	Avoid CrCl < 70 mL/min*
Post-HD or PD dose	Avoid
CVVH dose	Avoid
Moderate hepatic insufficiency	Avoid
Severe hepatic insufficiency	Avoid

*Not recommended if CrCl < 70 mL/min or in patients receiving a nephrotoxic agent.

Drug Interactions: *Coadministration with the following drugs are contraindicated: (1) highly dependent on CYP3A or UGT1A1 for clearance and elevated plasma concentrations are associated with serious adverse events and/or (2) drugs that strongly induce CYP3A, leading to reduced atazanavir concentrations.*
<u>Contraindicated:</u>
↑ alfuzosin, ↑ ranolazine, ↑ dronedarone, anticonvulsants ↓ atazanavir, ↑ colchicine, rifampin ↓ atazanavir, ↑ irinotecan, ↑ lurasidone, ↑ benzodiazepines, ↑ ergot derivatives, ↑ cisapride, St. John's wort ↓ atazanavir, ↑ simvastatin, ↑ lovastatin, ↑ pimozide, nevirapine ↓ atazanavir, ↑ PDE5 inhibitors, indinavir (hyperbilirubinemia)
<u>Other Significant Interactions:</u> *Please refer to individual drug monographs for more complete list of interactions.*
Adverse Effects: *Please refer to individual drug monographs/prescribing information for more complete details.*
> 10%: jaundice, ocular icterus, nausea

Other: Cardiac conduction abnormalities (PR prolongation), rash (including severe skin reactions), new onset/worsening renal impairment (with tenofovir), nephrolithiasis and cholelithiasis, transaminase elevations, indirect hyperbilirubinemia, hyperglycemia, fat maldistribution, hyperlipidemia.
Allergic Potential: Low (severe skin reactions)
Safety in Pregnancy: Category B

REFERENCES:
Panel on Antiretroviral Guidelines for Adults and Adolescents. Guidelines for the use of antiretroviral agents in HIV-1-infected adults and adolescents, updated July 14, 2016. Department of Health and Human Services; 1–288. Available at https://aidsinfo.nih.gov/contentfiles/lvguidelines/adultandadolescentgl.pdf.

Product Information: Evotaz oral tablets, atazanavir, cobicistat oral tablets. Bristol-Myers Squibb Company (per manufacturer), Princeton, NJ; 2015.

Cobicistat (Tybost)

Drug Class: CYP3A inhibitor
Indication: Pharmacokinetic enhancer (devoid of antiretroviral activity)
Usual Dose: 150 mg (PO) daily with food (to be administered at the same time as atazanavir or darunavir)

Cobicistat 150 mg	Atazanavir 300 mg once daily	Treatment-naïve or experienced
	Darunavir 800 mg once daily	Treatment-naïve or experienced <u>without</u> darunavir-associated mutations

---

"Usual dose" assumes normal renal/hepatic function. * For renal insufficiency, give usual dose × 1 followed by maintenance dose per CrCl. For dialysis patients, dose the same as for CrCl < 10 mL/min and give supplemental (post-HD/PD dose) immediately after dialysis. CrCl = creatinine clearance; CVVH = continuous venovenous hemofiltration; HD/PD = hemodialysis/peritoneal dialysis. See pp. 204–207 for explanations, pp. xi–xii for abbreviations.

How Supplied: Tablets, 150 mg of cobicistat

Pharmacokinetic Parameters:

Peak serum level: 0.9 mcg/mL
Excreted (urine/feces): 8.2/82%
Serum half-life: 3–4 h
Plasma protein binding: 97–98%

Primary Mode of Elimination: Hepatic

Dosage Adjustments:

Renal Dysfunction: No adjustments needed in renal impairment; however, see atazanavir and darunavir information regarding dose adjustments in this population. Do not use with tenofovir if CrCl < 70 mL/min before starting treatment. Note: Cobicistat inhibits tubular secretion of creatinine (increase serum creatinine) without affecting glomerular filtration.

Hepatic Dysfunction: No change in dose for mild-moderate hepatic impairment (Child-Pugh A or B); not studied in severe hepatic impairment (Child-Pugh C).

Drug Interactions: Cobicistat inhibits CYP3A and CYP 2D6 and transporters P-gp, BCRP, and OATP1B1/3. Cobicistat can increase the concentration of drugs metabolized by CYP3A or CYP2D6. Drugs that induce CYP3A can alter the concentrations of cobicistat, atazanavir, and darunavir.

Contraindicated: ↑ alfuzosin, ↑ ranolazine, ↑ dronedarone, ↑ colchicine, anticonvulsants ↓ darunavir/atazanavir, rifamycins ↓ darunavir/atazanavir, irinotecan ↑ (atazanavir only), ↑ lurasidone, ↑ pimozide, ↑ ergot derivatives, ↑ cisapride, St. John's wort ↓ darunavir, ↑ simvastatin, ↑ lovastatin, nevirapine (↓ atazanavir, ↑ nevirapine), ↑ PDE5 inhibitors (when dosed for PAH), indinavir (atazanavir only), ↑ benzodiazepines, ↑ antipsychotics

Other Interactions: Protease inhibitors other than atazanavir or darunavir, etravirine (with atazanavir), efavirenz (with atazanavir in treatment-experienced patients, darunavir dosed twice daily), ↑ antiarrhythmics, ↑ digoxin, ↑ macrolide or ketolide antibiotics, ↑ anticancer agents, ↑ anticoagulants, ↑ TCAs, ↑ trazodone, ↑ azole antifungals and cobicistat, atazanavir & darunavir, ↑ colchicine, ↑ rifabutin, ↑ beta blockers, ↑ calcium channel blockers, ↑ dexamethasone & ↓cobicistat, atazanavir, & darunavir, ↑fluticasone, ↑ bosentan & ↓ cobicistat, atazanavir, & darunavir, HCV protease inhibitors, ↑ immunosuppressants, ↑ fentanyl, ↑ tramadol, ↑ salmeterol

Adverse Effects:

When administered with atazanavir: jaundice (6%), rash (5%), ocular icterus (4%), nausea (2%), diarrhea (2%), headache (2%), increased serum creatinine without decrease in glomerular filtration. However, monitor for new onset or worsening renal impairment, particularly with tenofovir. Avoid other nephrotoxic agents.

Allergic Potential: Low

Safety in Pregnancy: No human data; inconclusive animal data (maternal toxicity, increased postimplantation loss, decreased fetal weight) to determine fetal risk.

Comments: Not interchangeable with ritonavir as a pharmacokinetic enhancer for darunavir 600 mg bid, fosamprenavir, saquinavir, or tipranavir. Different drug interactions may occur when cobicistat is given with atazanavir or darunavir compared to ritonavir.

Do not use when pharmacokinetic enhancer is needed for two or more antiretrovirals (example: protease inhibitor plus elvitegravir).

"Usual dose" assumes normal renal/hepatic function. * For renal insufficiency, give usual dose × 1 followed by maintenance dose per CrCl. For dialysis patients, dose the same as for CrCl < 10 mL/min and give supplemental (post-HD/PD dose) immediately after dialysis. CrCl = creatinine clearance; CVVH = continuous venovenous hemofiltration; HD/PD = hemodialysis/peritoneal dialysis. See pp. 204–207 for explanations, pp. xi–xii for abbreviations.

REFERENCES:

Panel on Antiretroviral Guidelines for Adults and Adolescents. Guidelines for the use of antiretroviral agents in HIV-1-infected adults and adolescents, updated July 14, 2016. Department of Health and Human Services; 1–288. Available at https://aidsinfo.nih.gov/contentfiles/lvguidelines/adultandadolescentgl.pdf.

Product Information: Tybost oral tablets, cobicistat oral tablets. Gilead Sciences, Inc. (per manufacturer), Foster City, CA; 2014.

Daclatasvir (Daklinza) (DCV)

Drug Class: Antihepatitis C agent; NS5A replication complex inhibitor

Indication: Hepatitis C virus genotypes 1 and 3; off-label use in genotype 2 patients in combination with sofosbuvir with or without ribavirin.

Usual Dose: Usual dose is daclatasvir 60 mg by mouth once daily with or without food. In the presence of strong CYP3A inhibitors or certain antiretrovirals (see interactions below), reduce the daclatasvir dose to 30 mg by mouth once daily. In the presence of moderate CYP3A inducers, increase the daclatasvir dose to 90 mg by mouth daily. Use with strong CYP3A inducers is contraindicated.

How Supplied: Tablets: 30 mg, 60 mg, and 90 mg

Treatment Duration: 12 weeks (see below):

Genotype 1※	Without cirrhosis	Daclatasvir + SOF x 12 weeks
	Compensated (Child-Pugh A) cirrhosis	
	Decompensated (Child-Pugh B or C) cirrhosis	Daclatasvir + SOF + RBV¶ x 12 weeks
	Post-transplant	

Genotype 2	Treatment-naïve without cirrhosis	Daclatasvir + SOF x 12 weeks*
Genotype 3	Without cirrhosis	Daclatasvir + SOF x 12 weeks
	Compensated (Child-Pugh) or decompensated (Child-Pugh B or C) cirrhosis	Daclatasvir + SOF + RBV¶ x 12 weeks
	Post-transplant	

RBV: ribavirin; SOF: sofosbuvir.

※Consider screening for NS5A resistance associated polymorphisms (at positions M28, Q30, L31, or Y93) in patients with genoype 1a prior to treatment.

*Off-label use; alternative regimen per AASLD/IDSA HCV guidelines.

¶Ribavirin dosing in compensated cirrhosis (Child-Pugh A) and normal renal function: If weight < 75 kg, administer ribavirin 1000 mg/d; if weight ≥ 75 kg: 1200 mg/d as two divided doses with food. Ribavirin dosing in decompensated cirrhosis (Child-Pugh B or C)/post-transplant and normal renal function: Ribavirin 600 mg daily in two divided doses with food. Increase as tolerated up to 1000 mg/day. (See ribavirin prescribing information for more details.)

Pharmacokinetic Parameters (following 60-mg dose):

Peak serum level: 1534 mcg/mL
Bioavailability: 67%
Excreted unchanged (urine/feces): 6.6/53%
Serum half-life: 12–15 h
Plasma protein binding: 99%
Volume of distribution (Vd): 47 L
Primary Mode of Elimination: Hepatic

"Usual dose" assumes normal renal/hepatic function. * For renal insufficiency, give usual dose × 1 followed by maintenance dose per CrCl. For dialysis patients, dose the same as for CrCl < 10 mL/min and give supplemental (post-HD/PD dose) immediately after dialysis. CrCl = creatinine clearance; CVVH = continuous venovenous hemofiltration; HD/PD = hemodialysis/peritoneal dialysis. See pp. 204–207 for explanations, pp. xi–xii for abbreviations.

Dosage Adjustments:

CrCl < 50 mL/min	Avoid (due to sofosbuvir)
Post-HD or PD dose	Avoid (due to sofosbuvir)
CVVH dose	Avoid (due to sofosbuvir)
Moderate hepatic insufficiency	No change
Severe hepatic insufficiency	No change

Renal Dysfunction: No dose adjustment is required for daclatasvir; however, refer to ribavirin and sofosbuvir sections and/or prescribing information regarding use in renal impairment. Unlikely to be dialyzable due high protein binding and molecular weight.

Hepatic Dysfunction: No dose adjustment required for daclatasvir in mild, moderate, or severe hepatic impairment. Refer to ribavirin and sofosbuvir sections and/or prescribing information regarding use in hepatic impairment.

Drug Interactions: Daclatasvir is a CYP3A substrate. Moderate or strong CYP3A inducers may reduce plasma concentrations and therapeutic effect; strong CYP3A inhibitors may increase plasma daclatasvir concentrations. In addition, daclatasvir inhibits P-gp, OATP-1B1/3, and BCRP and may prolong the effects of drugs that are substrates for these transporters.

Contraindicated: Strong CYP3A inducers, including, *but not limited to:*

Anticonvulsants (phenytoin, carbamazepine); antimycobacterials (rifampin), and St. John's wort.

Other Significant Interactions:

Antiretrovirals		
Protease inhibitors (atazanavir/r, indinavir, nelfinavir, saquinavir)	↑ Daclatasvir	Decrease daclatasvir to 30 mg once daily.
Cobicistat-containing regimens (atazanavir/ cobicistat, elvitegravir/ cobicistat/ emtricitabine/ tenofovir)	↑ Daclatasvir	Decrease daclatasvir to 30 mg once daily (except for darunavir/ cobicistat).
Non-nucleoside reverse transcriptase inhibitors (NNRTI): efavirenz, etravirine, nevirapine	↓ Daclatasvir	Increase daclatasvir to 90 mg once daily.
Strong CYP3A Inhibitors (see also Antiretrovirals)		
Clarithromycin, itraconazole, ketoconazole, nefazodone, posaconazole, telithromycin, voriconazole	↑ Daclatasvir	Decrease daclatasvir to 30 mg once daily.

"Usual dose" assumes normal renal/hepatic function. * For renal insufficiency, give usual dose × 1 followed by maintenance dose per CrCl. For dialysis patients, dose the same as for CrCl < 10 mL/min and give supplemental (post-HD/PD dose) immediately after dialysis. CrCl = creatinine clearance; CVVH = continuous venovenous hemofiltration; HD/PD = hemodialysis/peritoneal dialysis. See pp. 204–207 for explanations, pp. xi–xii for abbreviations.

Moderate CYP3A Inducers (see also Antiretrovirals)		
Bosentan, dexamethasone, modafinil, nafcillin, rifapentine	↓ Daclatasvir	Increase daclatasvir to 90 mg once daily.
Anticoagulants		
Dabigatran	↑ Dabigatran	Combination not recommended in some renal impairment groups (see prescribing information).
Cardiovascular Agents		
Amiodarone		Symptomatic bradycardia with SOF (See sofosbuvir information).
Digoxin	↑ Digoxin	May require 15–30% digoxin dose reduction; see prescribing information.
Lipid Lowering Agents		
HMG-CoA reductase inhibitors (atorvastatin, fluvastatin, pitavastatin, pravastatin, rosuvastatin, simvastatin)	↑ HMG CoA reductase inhibitors	Monitor for myopathy.

Narcotic Analgesic/Treatment of Opioid Dependence		
Buprenorphine Buprenorphine/ naloxone	↑ Buprenorphine ↑ Nor- buprenorphine	No dose adjustment needed; clinical monitoring required.

Adverse Effects: In combination with sofosbuvir with or without ribavirin: Headache (8–30%), nausea (6–15%), fatigue (14–17%), rash (2–8%), elevated lipase (2–4%), diarrhea (3–7%), insomnia (3–6%), somnolence (5%), increase bilirubin (5–8%), ALT increase (2%), AST increase (3%)

Other: See bradycardia warnings with sofosbuvir and amiodarone.

Allergic Potential: Low

Safety in Pregnancy: Insufficient human data. Maternal toxicity and fetal abnormalities were observed in animal studies at doses of up to 120 times the recommended human dose gestation days 6–19. In addition, fetal abnormalities and maternal toxicity were seen at doses of 3.6 fold the recommended human dose when given from gestation day 6 to lactation day 20. See prescribing information for details. *If used with ribavirin (contraindicated in pregnancy), pregnancy warnings for ribavirin apply to the combination. See ribavirin prescribing information for details.*

Comments: Poorer outcomes were observed among patients with cirrhosis, especially genotype 1a. See above regarding testing for resistance-associated polymorphisms in patients with genotype 1a prior to treatment.

"Usual dose" assumes normal renal/hepatic function. * For renal insufficiency, give usual dose × 1 followed by maintenance dose per CrCl. For dialysis patients, dose the same as for CrCl < 10 mL/min and give supplemental (post-HD/PD dose) immediately after dialysis. CrCl = creatinine clearance; CVVH = continuous venovenous hemofiltration; HD/PD = hemodialysis/peritoneal dialysis. See pp. 204–207 for explanations, pp. xi–xii for abbreviations.

REFERENCES:

AASLD-IDSA. Recommendations for testing, managing, and treating hepatitis C. http://www.hcvguidelines.org. Accessed on September 27, 2016.

Product Information: Daklinza oral tablets, daclatasvir oral tablets. Bristol-Myers Squibb Company (per manufacturer), Princeton, NJ; 2016.

Poordad F, Schiff ER, Vierling JM, et al. Daclatasvir with sofosbuvir and ribavirin for hepatitis C virus infection with advanced cirrhosis or post-liver transplantation recurrence. Hepatology. 2016 May;63(5):1493–505. doi: 10.1002/hep.28446. Epub 2016 Mar 7.

Sulkowski MS, Gardiner DF, Rodriguez-Torres M, et al. Daclatasvir plus sofosbuvir for previously treated or untreated chronic HCV infection. N Engl J Med. 2014a,16;370(3):211–21.

Welzel TM, Herzer K, Ferenci P, et al. Daclatasvir plus sofosbuvir with or without ribavirin for the treatment of HCV in patients with severe liver disease: interim results of a multicenter compassionate use program. [Abstract P0072.] 50th Annual Meeting of the European Association for the Study of the Liver (EASL). April 22–26, 2015;S619; Vienna, Austria.

Wyles DL, Ruane PJ, Sulkowski MS, et al. Daclatasvir plus Sofosbuvir for HCV in patients coinfected with HIV-1. N Engl J Med. 2015 August 20;373(8):714–25.

Darunavir Ethanolate (Prezista) (DRV)

Drug Class: Antiretroviral; HIV-1 protease inhibitor

Usual Dose: Treatment-naïve patients: Darunavir 800 mg (PO) daily plus ritonavir 100 mg (PO) daily with food. Treatment-experienced patients: Darunavir 600 mg (PO) bid plus ritonavir 100 mg (PO) bid with food

How Supplied: Oral tablet: 75 mg, 150 mg, 400 mg, 600 mg, 800 mg

Pharmacokinetic Parameters:
Peak serum level: 3578 ng/mL
Bioavailability: 37% (alone)/82% (with ritonavir)

Excreted unchanged (feces/urine): 41.2/7.7%
Serum half-life (normal/ESRD): 15/15 hrs
Plasma protein binding: 95%
Volume of distribution (V_d): not studied

Primary Mode of Elimination: Fecal/renal

Dosage Adjustments*

CrCl < 50 mL/min	No change
Post-HD or PD dose	No change
CVVH dose	No change
Moderate hepatic insufficiency	No change
Severe hepatic insufficiency	Avoid

Antiretroviral Dosage Adjustments

Efavirenz	No change
Nevirapine	No change
Didanosine	1 hour before or 1 hour after darunavir
Tenofovir	No change
Fosamprenavir	No change
Indinavir	No information
Lopinavir/ ritonavir	Avoid
Saquinavir	Avoid
Rifabutin	150 mg qid
Etravirine	No change
Maraviroc	150 mg bid
Raltegravir	No change

"Usual dose" assumes normal renal/hepatic function. * For renal insufficiency, give usual dose × 1 followed by maintenance dose per CrCl. For dialysis patients, dose the same as for CrCl < 10 mL/min and give supplemental (post-HD/PD dose) immediately after dialysis. CrCl = creatinine clearance; CVVH = continuous venovenous hemofiltration; HD/PD = hemodialysis/peritoneal dialysis. See pp. 204–207 for explanations, pp. xi–xii for abbreviations.

Drug Interactions: Alfuzosin indinavir, ketoconazole, nevirapine, tenofovir (↑ darunavir levels); lopinavir/ritonavir, saquinavir, efavirenz (↓ darunavir levels); concomitant administration of darunavir/ritonavir with agents highly dependent on CYP3A for clearance, astemizole, cisapride, dihydroergotamine, ergonovine, ergotamine, methylergonovine, midazolam, pimozide, terfenadine, midazolam, triazolam (may ↓ darunavir levels and ↓effectiveness); sildenafil, vardenafil, tadalafil (↑PDE-5 inhibitors; sildenafil do not exceed 25 mg in 48 hrs, vardenafil do not exceed 2.5 mg in 72 hrs, or tadalafil do not exceed 10 mg in 72 hrs); rivaroxaban (↑ rivaroxaban); warfarin (↑ warfarin, monitor INR).

Adverse Effects: Diarrhea, nausea, headache, nasopharyngitis.

Allergic Potential: High (see comments)

Safety in Pregnancy: C

Comments: Always take with food (increases AUC, C_{max} by approximately 30%). Must be given with ritonavir to boost bioavailability. Darunavir contains a sulfonamide moiety (as do fosamprenavir and tipranavir); use with caution in patients with sulfonamide allergies. A mild-to-moderate rash occurred in 7% of patients receiving the drug in clinical trial; it did not usually require drug cessation, but severe rashes (including Stevens-Johnson syndrome) have been reported.

Cerebrospinal Fluid Penetration: No data

REFERENCES:

Clotet B, Bellos N, Moloina JM, et al. Efficacy and safety of darunavir-ritonavir at week 48 in treatment-experienced patients with HIV-1 infection in POWER 1 and 2: a pooled subgroup analysis of data from two randomised trials. Lancet 2007;369:1169–78.

De Meyer SM, Spinosa-Guzman S, Vangeneugden TJ, et al. Efficacy of once-daily darunavir/ritonavir 800/100 mg in HIV-infected, treatment experienced patients with no baseline resistance-associated mutations to darunavir. J Acquir Immune Defic Syndr, 2008;49(2):179–82.

Madruga JV, Berger D, McMurchie M, et al. Efficacy and safety of darunavir-ritonavir compared with that of lopinavir-ritonavir at 48 weeks in treatment-experienced, HIV-infected patients in TITAN: a randomized controlled phase III trial. Lancet 2007;370:3–5.

Ortiz R, Dejesus E, Khanlou H, et al. Efficacy and safety of once-daily darunavir/ritonavir versus lopinavir/ritonavir in treatment-naive HIV-1-infected patients at week 48 (ARTMIS). AIDS 2008;22(12):1389–97.

Panel on Antiretroviral Guidelines for Adults and Adolescents. Guidelines for the use of antiretroviral agents in HIV-1-infected adults and adolescents, updated July 14, 2016. Department of Health and Human Services; 1–288. Available at https://aidsinfo.nih.gov/contentfiles/lvguidelines/adultandadolescentgl.pdf.

Product Information: Prezista oral tablets, darunavir oral tablets. Tibotec Therapeutics, Inc, Raritan, NJ; 2006.

Darunavir/Cobicistat (Prezcobix)

Drug Class: Antiretroviral; HIV-1 protease inhibitor/CYP3A inhibitor

Usual Dose: 1 tablet (PO) daily with food

How Supplied: Oral tablet: (containing darunavir 800 mg and cobicistat 150 mg)

Pharmacokinetic Parameters:

Bioavailability: Darunavir AUC increased 70% when administered with food

Excreted unchanged (urine): 7.7%/8.2%

Serum half-life: 7 h/4 h

Plasma protein binding: 95/97–98%

Primary Mode of Elimination: Hepatic/hepatic

"Usual dose" assumes normal renal/hepatic function. * For renal insufficiency, give usual dose × 1 followed by maintenance dose per CrCl. For dialysis patients, dose the same as for CrCl < 10 mL/min and give supplemental (post-HD/PD dose) immediately after dialysis. CrCl = creatinine clearance; CVVH = continuous venovenous hemofiltration; HD/PD = hemodialysis/peritoneal dialysis. See pp. 204–207 for explanations, pp. xi–xii for abbreviations.

Dosage Adjustments:

CrCl < 70 mL/min	Avoid CrCl < 70 mL/min
Post-HD or PD dose	Avoid
CVVH dose	Avoid
Mild-moderate hepatic insufficiency	No change
Severe hepatic insufficiency	Avoid

Drug Interactions: Darunavir and cobicistat inhibit CYP3A and 2D6. Cobicistat inhibits P-gp, BCRP, and OATP1B1/3. Increased plasma concentrations of CYP3A or 2D6 substrates or substrates of P-gp, BCRP, or OATP1B1/3 may result when coadministered with darunavir/cobicistat.

Darunavir is metabolized by CYP3A and cobicistat is metabolized by CYP3A (major) and CYP2D6 (minor). Drugs that induce CYP3A may result in loss of therapeutic effect.

Contraindicated drugs only listed below. Please refer to individual drug monographs for more complete list of interactions.

Contraindicated: ↑ alfuzosin, ↑ ranolazine, ↑ dronedarone, ↑ colchicine, rifampin ↓ darunavir, ↑ lurasidone, ↑ pimozide, ↑ ergot derivatives, ↑ cisapride, St. John's wort ↓ darunavir, ↑ simvastatin, ↑ lovastatin, ↑ PDE5 inhibitors, ↑midazolam, ↑triazolam

Adverse Effects:
Please refer to individual drug monographs for more complete details.
> 5%: Diarrhea, nausea, rash, abdominal pain, headache, vomiting
Other/severe: Drug-induced hepatitis, skin reactions (ranging from mild-severe), change in serum creatinine/new-onset or worsening renal impairment (particularly with tenofovir)
Allergic Potential: High (risk of severe skin reactions), monitor with sulfa allergy (darunavir contains sulfa moiety).
Safety in Pregnancy: C
Comments:
Monitor in patients with sulfonamide allergy. Do not use in combination with other darunavir or cobicistat-containing formulations.
Monitor hepatic and renal function.
High drug interaction potential; see prescribing information for details.

REFERENCES:
Panel on Antiretroviral Guidelines for Adults and Adolescents. Guidelines for the use of antiretroviral agents in HIV-1-infected adults and adolescents, updated July 14, 2016. Department of Health and Human Services; 1–288. Available at https://aidsinfo.nih.gov/contentfiles/lvguidelines/adultandadolescentgl.pdf.

Product Information: Prezcobix oral tablets, darunavir, cobicistat oral tablets. Janssen Pharmaceuticals, Inc., Titusville, NJ; 2015.

Delavirdine (Rescriptor) (DLV)

Drug Class: Antiretroviral; NNRTI (non-nucleoside reverse transcriptase inhibitor)
Usual Dose: 400 mg (PO) tid
How Supplied: Oral tablet: 100 mg, 200 mg
Pharmacokinetic Parameters:
Peak serum level: 35 mcg/mL
Bioavailability: 85%
Excreted unchanged (urine): 5%
Serum half-life (normal/ESRD): 5.8 h/no data
Plasma protein binding: 98%
Volume of distribution (V_d): 0.5 L/kg
Primary Mode of Elimination: Hepatic

Dosage Adjustments*

CrCl ≤ 50 mL/min	No change
Post-HD dose	None
Post-PD dose	None
CVVH dose	No change
Moderate hepatic insufficiency	No information
Severe hepatic insufficiency	No information/use caution

Antiretroviral Dosage Adjustments

Efavirenz	No information
Indinavir	Indinavir 600 mg tid
Lopinavir/ ritonavir	No information
Nelfinavir	No information (monitor for neutropenia)
Nevirapine	No information
Ritonavir	Delavirdine: no change; ritonavir: no information
Saquinavir soft-gel	Saquinavir soft-gel 800 mg tid (monitor transaminases)
Rifampin, rifabutin	Avoid combination
Statins	Not recommended

Drug Interactions: Antiretrovirals, rifabutin, rifampin (see dose adjustment grid above); astemizole, terfenadine, benzodiazepines, cisapride, H_2 blockers, proton pump inhibitors, ergot alkaloids, quinidine, statins (avoid if possible); carbamazepine, phenobarbital, phenytoin (may ↓ delavirdine levels, monitor anticonvulsant levels); clarithromycin, dapsone, nifedipine, warfarin (↑ interacting drug levels); sildenafil (do not exceed 25 mg in 48 hrs); tadalafil (max. 10 mg/72 hrs); vardenafil (max. 2.5 mg/72 hrs).
Adverse Effects: Drug fever/rash, Stevens-Johnson syndrome (rare), headache, nausea/vomiting, diarrhea, ↑ SGOT/SGPT.
Allergic Potential: High
Safety in Pregnancy: C
Comments: May be taken with or without food, but food decreases absorption by 20%. May disperse four 100-mg tablets in > 3 oz. water to produce slurry; 200-mg tablets should be taken as intact tablets and not used to make an oral solution. Separate dosing with ddI or antacids by 1 hour.
Cerebrospinal Fluid Penetration: 0.4%

REFERENCES:

Justesen US, Klitgaard NA, Brosen K, et al. Dose-dependent pharmacokinetics of delavirdine in combination with amprenavir in healthy volunteers. J Antimicrob Chemother. 2004;54:206–10.

Panel on Antiretroviral Guidelines for Adults and Adolescents. Guidelines for the use of antiretroviral agents in HIV-1-infected adults and adolescents, updated July 14, 2016. Department of Health and Human Services; 1–288. Available at https://aidsinfo.nih.gov/contentfiles/lvguidelines/adultandadolescentgl.pdf.

Product Information: Rescriptor oral tablets, delavirdine mesylate oral tablets. Pfizer, Inc., New York, NY; 2006.

Didanosine (Videx) (ddI)

Drug Class: Antiretroviral; NRTI (nucleoside reverse transcriptase inhibitor)
Usual Dose: 400 mg QD for weight > 60 kg; 250 QD for < 60 kg

"Usual dose" assumes normal renal/hepatic function. * For renal insufficiency, give usual dose × 1 followed by maintenance dose per CrCl. For dialysis patients, dose the same as for CrCl < 10 mL/min and give supplemental (post-HD/PD dose) immediately after dialysis. CrCl = creatinine clearance; CVVH = continuous venovenous hemofiltration; HD/PD = hemodialysis/peritoneal dialysis. See pp. 204–207 for explanations, pp. xi–xii for abbreviations.

How Supplied:
Generic—Oral capsule, delayed release: 125 mg, 200 mg, 250 mg, 400 mg
Videx EC—Oral capsule, delayed release: 125 mg, 200 mg, 250 mg, 400 mg
Videx—Oral tablet, chewable: 100 mg
Videx Pediatric—Oral powder for suspension: 10 mg/mL

Pharmacokinetic Parameters:
Peak serum level: 29 mcg/mL
Bioavailability: 42%
Excreted unchanged (urine): 60%
Serum half-life (normal/ESRD): 1.6/4.1 hrs
Plasma protein binding: ≤ 5%
Volume of distribution (V_d): 1.1 L/kg

Primary Mode of Elimination: Renal
Dosage Adjustments* 60 kg/[< 60 kg]:

CrCl 30–59 mL/min	200 mg (PO) QD (125 mg [PO] QD)
CrCl 10–29 mL/min	125 mg (PO) QD (125 mg [PO] QD)
CrCl < 10 mL/min	125 mg (PO) QD (not recommended)
Post-HD dose	No information
Post-PD dose	100 mg (PO)
CVVH dose	150 mg (PO) QD
Moderate hepatic insufficiency	No change
Severe hepatic insufficiency	No change

Drug Interactions: Alcohol, lamivudine, pentamidine, valproic acid (↑ risk of pancreatitis); dapsone, fluoroquinolones, ketoconazole, itraconazole, tetracyclines (↓ absorption of interacting drug; give 2 hours after didanosine); dapsone, INH, metronidazole, nitrofurantoin, stavudine, vincristine, zalcitabine, neurotoxic drugs or history of neuropathy (↑ risk of neuropathy); dapsone (↓ dapsone absorption, which increases risk of PCP); tenofovir (if possible, avoid concomitant tenofovir due to impaired CD4 response and increased risk of virologic failure). Avoid ribavirin in HIV patients.

Adverse Effects: Headache, depression, nausea, vomiting, GI upset/abdominal pain, diarrhea, drug fever/rash, anemia, leukopenia, thrombocytopenia, hepatotoxicity/hepatic necrosis, pancreatitis (may be fatal; ↑ risk in patients on concomitant tenofovir), hypertriglyceridemia, hyperuricemia, lactic acidosis, lipoatrophy, wasting, dose dependent (≥ 0.06 mg/kg/d) peripheral neuropathy, hyperglycemia, reports of noncirrhotic portal hypertension lactic acidosis with hepatic steatosis (rare, but potentially life-threatening toxicity with use of NRTIs; *pregnant women taking didanosine + stavudine may be at increased risk*).

Allergic Potential: Low
Safety in Pregnancy: B; should be avoided in pregnancy as it may cause fatal pancreatitis.

Comments: Available as buffered powder for oral solution and enteric-coated extended-release capsules (Videx EC 400 mg PO QD). Take 30 minutes before or 2 hours after meal (food decreases serum concentrations by 49%). Avoid in patients with alcoholic cirrhosis/history of pancreatitis. Use with caution with ribavirin. Na^+ content = 11.5 mEq/g. Buffered tablets discontinued by US manufacturer in February 2006.

Cerebrospinal Fluid Penetration: 20%

"Usual dose" assumes normal renal/hepatic function. * For renal insufficiency, give usual dose × 1 followed by maintenance dose per CrCl. For dialysis patients, dose the same as for CrCl < 10 mL/min and give supplemental (post-HD/PD dose) immediately after dialysis. CrCl = creatinine clearance; CVVH = continuous venovenous hemofiltration; HD/PD = hemodialysis/peritoneal dialysis. See pp. 204–207 for explanations, pp. xi–xii for abbreviations.

REFERENCES:

Panel on Antiretroviral Guidelines for Adults and Adolescents. Guidelines for the use of antiretroviral agents in HIV-1-infected adults and adolescents, updated July 14, 2016. Department of Health and Human Services; 1–288. Available at https://aidsinfo.nih.gov/contentfiles/lvguidelines/adultandadolescentgl.pdf.

Perry CM, Balfour JA. Didanosine: An update on its antiviral activity, pharmacokinetic properties, and therapeutic efficacy in the management of HIV disease. Drugs 1996;52:928–62.

Product Information: Videx EC delayed-release oral capsules, enteric-coated beadlets, didanosine delayed-release oral capsules, enteric-coated beadlets. Bristol-Myers Squibb Company, Princeton, NJ; 2009.

Dolutegravir (Tivicay) (DTG)

Drug Class: Antiretroviral; HIV-1 integrase strand transfer inhibitor (INSTI)

Usual Dose: Treatment-naïve or treatment experienced-INSTI naïve: 50 mg once daily. Treatment-naïve or treatment-experienced INSTI naïve when coadministered with the following potent UGT1A/CYP3A inducers: efavirenz, fosamprenavir/ritonavir, tipranavir/ritonavir, or rifampin: 50 mg twice daily. INSTI experienced with certain INSTI-associated resistance mutations or clinically suspected INSTI resistance: 50 mg twice daily. Can be taken with or without food.

How Supplied: Oral tablet, 50 mg

Pharmacokinetic Parameters (50 mg once daily dose):

Peak serum level: 3.67 mcg/mL
Bioavailability: Not established
Excreted unchanged: 53% (feces), 31% (urine)
Serum half-life: 14 hours
Plasma protein binding: 98.9%
Volume of Distribution: 17.4 L

Primary Mode of Elimination: Hepatic

Dosage Adjustments for Renal and Hepatic Insufficiency

CrCl < 50 mL/min	No change
Post-HD dose	No information
Post-PD dose	No information
Mild-moderate hepatic insufficiency	No change
Severe hepatic insufficiency	Do not use

Antiretroviral Dosage Adjustments: Increase dose to 50 mg twice daily when coadministered with the following potent UGT1A/CYP3A inducers: efavirenz, fosamprenavir/ritonavir, tipranavir/ritonavir, or rifampin. Also increase to 50 mg twice daily when given to a patient with certain INSTI-inhibitor resistance mutations or suspected INSTI resistance.

Drug Interactions: In vivo, dolutegravir inhibits tubular secretion of creatinine by inhibiting OCT2. Dolutegravir may increase plasma concentrations of drugs eliminated via OCT2 (dofetilide and metformin). Coadministration of dolutegravir and dofetilide should be avoided; close monitoring is recommended when starting or stopping dolutegravir and metformin together. A dose adjustment of metformin may be necessary. Dolutegravir should not be used with etravirine without coadministration of atazanavir/ritonavir, darunavir/ritonavir, or lopinavir/ritonavir. Rifampin, efavirenz, fosamprenavir/ritonavir, and tipranavir/ritonavir induce metabolism of dolutegravir, requiring a dolutegravir dose increase to 50 mg twice daily. Coadministration of dolutegravir with phenytoin, phenobarbital, carbamazepine, or St. John's wort will lower dolutegravir levels and should not be given together. Medications containing polyvalent cations (e.g., MG, Al, Fe, or Ca) decrease absorption of dolutegravir; dolutegravir should be administered 2 hours before or 6 hours after taking medications containing polyvalent cations.

Adverse Effects: Hypersensitivity reactions characterized by rash, constitutional findings, and sometimes organ dysfunction, including liver injury, have been reported. Discontinue dolutegravir and other suspect agents immediately if signs or symptoms of hypersensitivity reactions develop, as a delay in stopping treatment may result in a life-threatening reaction. The most common adverse reactions of moderate to severe intensity and incidence > 2% were insomnia and headache.

Allergic Potential: Low **(note: risk of hypersensitivity reactions)**

Safety in Pregnancy: Category B. Experience in pregnancy is limited, and should be used during pregnancy only if clearly needed.

Cerebrospinal Fluid: In 11 treatment-naïve subjects on dolutegravir 50 mg daily plus abacavir/lamivudine, the median dolutegravir concentration in cerebrospinal fluid (CSF) was 18 ng/mL (range: 4 ng/mL to 232 ng/mL) 2 to 6 hours postdose after 2 weeks of treatment.

REFERENCES:

Cahn, P, Pozniak AL, Mingrone H, et al. Once-daily dolutegravir versus raltegravir in antiretroviral-experienced, integrase-inhibitor-naive adults with HIV: week 48 results from the randomised, double-blind, non-inferiority SAILING study. Lancet 2013; 382:700–708.

Raffi F, Rachlis A, Stellbrink HJ, et al. Once-daily dolutegravir versus raltegravir in antiretroviral-naive adults with HIV-1 infection: 48 week results from the randomised, double-blind, non-inferiority SPRING-2 study, Lancet 2013;381:735–743.

Walmsley SL, Antela A, Clumeck N, et al. Dolutegravir plus abacavir–lamivudine for the treatment of HIV-1 infection. N Engl J Med. 2013;369:1807–1818.

Product Information. Tivicay (dolutegravir) oral tablets. ViiV Healthcare, Middlesex, United Kingdom; 2013.

Efavirenz (Sustiva) (EFV)

Drug Class: Antiretroviral; NNRTI (non-nucleoside reverse transcriptase inhibitor)
Usual Dose: 600 mg (PO) daily (at bedtime)
How Supplied: Oral capsule: 50 mg, 200 mg; oral tablet: 600 mg
Pharmacokinetic Parameters:
Peak serum level: 12.9 mcg/mL
Bioavailability: Increased with food
Excreted unchanged (urine): 14–34%
Serum half-life (normal/ESRD): 40–55 h/ no data
Plasma protein binding: 99%
Volume of distribution (V_d): No data
Primary Mode of Elimination: Hepatic
Dosage Adjustments*

CrCl < 60 mL/min	No change
Post-HD or PD dose	None
CVVH dose	No change
Moderate or severe hepatic insufficiency	No information

Antiretroviral Dosage Adjustments

Delavirdine	No information
Indinavir	Indinavir 1000 mg tid
Lopinavir/ ritonavir (l/r)	Consider l/r 533/133 mg bid in PI-experienced patients
Nelfinavir	No changes
Nevirapine	Do not coadminister

"Usual dose" assumes normal renal/hepatic function. * For renal insufficiency, give usual dose × 1 followed by maintenance dose per CrCl. For dialysis patients, dose the same as for CrCl < 10 mL/min and give supplemental (post-HD/PD dose) immediately after dialysis. CrCl = creatinine clearance; CVVH = continuous venovenous hemofiltration; HD/PD = hemodialysis/peritoneal dialysis. See pp. 204–207 for explanations, pp. xi–xii for abbreviations.

Ritonavir	Ritonavir 600 mg bid (500 mg bid for intolerance)
Saquinavir	Avoid use as sole PI
Rifampin	No changes
Rifabutin	Rifabutin 450–600 mg QD or 600 mg 2–3×/week if not on protease inhibitor
Etravirine	Do not coadminister
Maraviroc	600 mg bid
Raltegravir	No change

Drug Interactions: Antiretrovirals, rifabutin, rifampin (see dose adjustment grid above); astemizole, terfenadine, cisapride, ergotamine, midazolam, triazolam (avoid); carbamazepine, phenobarbital, phenytoin (monitor anticonvulsant levels; use with caution); caspofungin (↓caspofungin levels, may ↓caspofungin effect); methadone, clarithromycin (↓interacting drug levels; titrate methadone dose to effect; consider using azithromycin instead of clarithromycin).
Adverse Effects: Drug fever/rash, central nervous system (CNS) effects (nightmares, dizziness, neuropsychiatric symptoms, difficulty concentrating, somnolence), ↑SGOT/SGPT, Erythema multiforme/Stevens-Johnson syndrome (rare), false positive cannabinoid test.
Allergic Potential: High
Safety in Pregnancy: Teratogenic in animal studies and potentially teratogenic in first trimester of human pregnancy (neural tube defects). Perform pregnancy test prior to initiating EFV in women of child bearing age. Consider alternate regimen in women with potential for pregnancy. See perinatal guidelines for continuing efavirenz-based therapy in women who present for antenatal care in the first trimester of pregnancy.

Comments: Rash/CNS effects usually resolve spontaneously over 2–4 weeks. Take at bedtime and avoid taking after high-fat meals (levels ↑50%).
Cerebrospinal Fluid Penetration: 0.26%–1.19%

REFERENCES:
Gallant JE, DeJesus D, Arribas JR, et al. Tenofovir DF, emtricitabine, and efavirenz vs. zidovudine, lamivudine, and efavirenz for HIV. N Engl J Med. 2006;354:251–60.
la Porte CJ, de Graaff-Teulen MJ, Colbers EP, et al. Effect of efavirenz treatment on the pharmacokinetics of nelfinavir boosted by ritonavir in healthy volunteers. Br J Clin Pharmacol. 2004;58:632–40.
Marzolini C, Telenti A, Decosterd LA, et al. Efavirenz plasma levels can predict treatment failure and central nervous system side effects in HIV-1-infected patients. AIDS. 2001;15:71–5.
Panel on Antiretroviral Guidelines for Adults and Adolescents. Guidelines for the use of antiretroviral agents in HIV-1-infected adults and adolescents, updated July 14, 2016. Department of Health and Human Services; 1–288. Available at https://aidsinfo.nih.gov/contentfiles/lvguidelines/adultandadolescentgl.pdf.
Panel on Treatment of HIV-Infected Pregnant Women and prevention of perinatal Transmission. Recommendations for use of antiretroviral drugs in Pregnant HIV-1-infected women for maternal health and interventions to reduce Perinatal HIV transmission in the United States, updated June 7, 2016. Accessed September 27, 2016. Department of Health and Human Services. Available from: https://aidsinfo.nih.gov/guidelines/html/3/perinatal-guidelines.
Product Information: Sustiva oral capsules, tablets, efavirenz oral capsules, tablets. Bristol-Myers Squibb Company, Princeton, NJ; 2013.

Efavirenz + Emtricitabine + Tenofovir disoproxil fumarate (Atripla)

Drug Class: Antiretroviral combination (NRTI and NNRTI)

"Usual dose" assumes normal renal/hepatic function. * For renal insufficiency, give usual dose × 1 followed by maintenance dose per CrCl. For dialysis patients, dose the same as for CrCl < 10 mL/min and give supplemental (post-HD/PD dose) immediately after dialysis. CrCl = creatinine clearance; CVVH = continuous venovenous hemofiltration; HD/PD = hemodialysis/peritoneal dialysis. See pp. 204–207 for explanations, pp. xi–xii for abbreviations.

Usual Dose: 1 tablet (efavirenz 600 mg/ emtricitabine 200 mg/tenofovir 300 mg) (PO) daily (at bedtime) on an empty stomach

How Supplied: Oral tablet: Contains 600 mg efavirenz + 200 mg emtricitabine + 300 mg tenofovir disoproxil fumarate

Pharmacokinetic Parameters:
Peak serum level: 4.0/1.8 mcg/mL/296 ng/mL
Bioavailability: NR/93%/25%
Excreted unchanged: < 1% unchanged and 14–30% as metabolites/86%/32%
Serum half-life (normal/ESRD): (40–55 h/~ 10 h on HD)/(10 h/extended)/(17 h/no data)
Plasma protein binding: 99/< 4/< 0.7%
Volume of distribution (V_d): NR/NR/1.2 L/kg

Primary Mode of Elimination: Hepatic/ renal/renal

Dosage Adjustments*

CrCl 50–80 mL/min	No change
CrCl 10–50 mL/min	Avoid
CrCl < 10 mL/min	Avoid
Post-HD dose	Avoid
Post-PD dose	Avoid
CVVH dose	Avoid
Mild hepatic insufficiency	No information
Moderate or severe hepatic insufficiency	No information

Antiretroviral Dosage Adjustments

Fosamprenavir/ ritonavir	An additional 100 mg/day (300 mg total) of ritonavir is recommended when Atripla is administered with fosamprenavir/ ritonavir QD. No change in ritonavir dose when Atripla is administered with fosamprenavir/ ritonavir bid.

Atazanavir	Avoid
Indinavir	Indinavir 1000 mg tid
Lopinavir/ ritonavir	Increase lopinavir/ritonavir to 600/150 mg (3 tablets) bid
Ritonavir	No information
Saquinavir	Avoid
Didanosine	Avoid
Rifabutin	Rifabutin 450–600 mg QD or 600 mg 2–3x/week if not on protease inhibitor
Rifampin	No change

Drug Interactions: Antiretrovirals, rifabutin (see dose adjustment grid above); astemizole, cisapride, ergotamine, methylergonovine, midazolam, triazolam, St John's wort (↓ efavirenz levels), voriconazole (↓ voriconazole levels; avoid); caspofungin (↓ caspofungin levels); carbamazepine, phenytoin, phenobarbital (monitor anticonvulsant levels; use with caution; potential for ↓ efavirenz levels); statins (may ↓ statin levels); methadone, (↓ methadone levels); clarithromycin (may ↓ clarithromycin effectiveness, consider using azithromycin).

Adverse Effects: Headache, diarrhea, nausea, vomiting, GI upset, lactic acidosis, osteopenia, rash, dizziness, fatigue, lactic acidosis with hepatic steatosis (rare but potentially life threatening with NRTIs), relapsing type B viral hepatitis, depression, vivid dreams, renal impairment.

Allergic Potential: High

Safety in Pregnancy: Efavirenz is teratogenic in animal studies and potentially teratogenic in first trimester of human

---

"Usual dose" assumes normal renal/hepatic function. * For renal insufficiency, give usual dose × 1 followed by maintenance dose per CrCl. For dialysis patients, dose the same as for CrCl < 10 mL/min and give supplemental (post-HD/PD dose) immediately after dialysis. CrCl = creatinine clearance; CVVH = continuous venovenous hemofiltration; HD/PD = hemodialysis/peritoneal dialysis. See pp. 204–207 for explanations, pp. xi–xii for abbreviations.

pregnancy (neural tube defects). Perform pregnancy test prior to initiating EFV in women of child bearing age. Consider alternate regimen in women with potential for pregnancy. See DHHS perinatal guidelines for continuing efavirenz-based therapy in women who present for antenatal care in the first trimester of pregnancy. *See emtricitabine/tenofovir monograph for more details on safety in pregnancy.*

Comments: Rash/CNS symptoms usually resolve spontaneously over 2–4 weeks. Take at bedtime. Avoid taking after high-fat meals (levels ↑ 50%).

Cerebrospinal Fluid Penetration: See individual agents for details.

REFERENCES:

Gallant JE, DeJesus D, Arribas JR, et al. Tenofovir DF, emtricitabine, and efavirenz vs. zidovudine, lamivu-dine, and efavirenz for HIV. N Engl J Med. 2006; 354:251–60.

la Porte CJ, de Graaff-Teulen MJ, Colbers EP, et al. Effect of efavirenz treatment on the pharmacokinetics of nelfinavir boosted by ritonavir in healthy volunteers. Br J Clin Pharmacol. 2004;58:632–40.

Marzolini C, Telenti A, Decosterd LA, et al. Efavirenz plasma levels can predict treatment failure and cen-tral nervous system side effects in HIV-1-infected patients. AIDS. 2001;15:71–5.

Panel on Antiretroviral Guidelines for Adults and Adoles-cents. Guidelines for the use of antiretroviral agents in HIV-1-infected adults and adolescents, updated July 14, 2016. Department of Health and Human Services; 1–288. Available at https://aidsinfo.nih.gov/contentfiles/lvguidelines/adultandadolescentgl.pdf.

Elbasvir/Grazoprevir (Zepatier) (EBR/GZR)

Drug Class: Anti-hepatitis C agents; elbasvir (NS5A replication complex inhibitor) and grazoprevir (NS3/4A protease inhibitor)

Indication: HCV genotypes (GT) 1 and 4 and <u>without</u> decompensated cirrhosis *(contraindicated in patients with Child-Pugh B or C cirrhosis CTP ≥ 7; MELD ≥ 15, and/or clinical manifestations due to elevated GZR concentrations and risk of ALT elevations).*

Usual Dose: 1 tablet (PO) daily with or without food

How Supplied: Oral tablet (containing elbasvir 50 mg and grazoprevir 100 mg)

Treatment Duration: 12 or 16 weeks with or without ribavirin

Genotype 1a: Treatment-naïve or PegIFN/RBV-experienced* and **without** baseline NS5A polymorphisms§	EBR/GZR	12 weeks
Genotype 1a: Treatment-naïve or PegIFN/RBV-experienced* and **with** baseline NS5A polymorphisms§	EBR/GZR + RBV¶	16 weeks
Genotype 1b: Treatment-naïve or PegIFN/RBV-experienced*	EBR/GZR	12 weeks
Genotype 1 (a or b): PegIFN/RBV/PI-experienced⌘	EBR/GZR + RBV¶	12 weeks
Genotype 4: Treatment-naive	EBR/GZR	12 weeks
Genotype 4: PegIFN/RBV-experienced^	EBR/GZR + RBV¶	16 weeks

"Usual dose" assumes normal renal/hepatic function. * For renal insufficiency, give usual dose × 1 fol-lowed by maintenance dose per CrCl. For dialysis patients, dose the same as for CrCl < 10 mL/min and give supplemental (post-HD/PD dose) immediately after dialysis. CrCl = creatinine clearance; CVVH = continuous venovenous hemofiltration; HD/PD = hemodialysis/peritoneal dialysis. See pp. 204–207 for explanations, pp. xi–xii for abbreviations.

Abbreviations: EBR/GZR: elbasvir/grazoprevir; RBV: ribavirin; PegIFN: Peginterferon alfa; PI: NS3/4A protease inhibitor.

* Patients who have failed previous treatment with PegIFN and RBV.

§ NS5A resistance-associated polymorphisms at positions M28, Q30, L31, or Y93.

¶ Weight-based ribavirin dosing when CrCl > 50 mL/min: < 66 kg: 800 mg/d; 66–80 kg: 1000 mg/d; 81–105 kg: 1200 mg/d, given in two divided doses with food. *See Ribavirin prescribing information for more information.*

✖ The optimal dose and duration of EBR/GZR has not been established in PegIFN/RBV/PI-experienced, genotype 1a patients with baseline NS5A polymorphisms.

^ Patients who have failed treatment with PegIFN, RBV, and NS3/4a protease inhibitor (boceprevir, telaprevir or simeprevir).

Pharmacokinetic Parameters:
Peak serum level: 121 ng/mL (EBR); 165 ng/mL (GZR)
Excreted unchanged: Feces > 90% (EBR/GZR)
Serum half-life (normal/ESRD): 24 h (EBR); 31 h (GZR)
Plasma protein binding: 99% (EBR); 98.8% (GZR)
Volume of distribution (Vd): 680 L (EBR); 1250 L (GZR)
Primary Mode of Elimination: Fecal
Dosage Adjustments:

CrCl < 60 mL/min and HD	No change
Post-HD/PD dose*	None/none likely
CVVH dose	No information
Mild (Child-Pugh A) hepatic insufficiency	No change
Moderate or severe (Child-Pugh B or C) hepatic insufficiency	Contraindicated

* No adjustments required in patients with renal dysfunction or requiring hemodialysis. Due to high protein binding, need for dose adjustments in peritoneal dialysis are unlikely.

Drug Interactions: Both elbasvir and grazoprevir are CYP3A substrates. Moderate-strong CYP3A inducers may reduce EBR/GRZ concentrations and are contraindicated; strong CYP3A inhibitors may increase EBR/GRZ concentrations. In addition, GZR is a substrate of OATP1B1/3; drugs that inhibit the transporters may increase GZR concentrations and are contraindicated. Both elbasvir and grazoprevir inhibit the transporter BCRP and may increase concentrations of BCRP substrates.

Contraindicated with EBR/GZR: Anticonvulsants (phenytoin, carbamazepine) ↓ EBR/GRZ, antimycobacterials (rifampin) ↓ EBR/GRZ, St. John's wort ↓ EBR/GRZ, efavirenz ↓ EBR/GRZ, other antiretrovirals (atazanavir, darunavir, lopinavir, saquinavir, tipranavir) ↑ GRZ (and risk of ALT elevations), cyclosporine ↑ EBR/GRZ (and risk of ALT elevations)

Other Significant Interactions: Naficllin ↓ EBR/GRZ, ketoconazole ↑ EBR/GRZ, bosentan ↓ EBR/GRZ, EBR/GRZ ↑ tacrolimus, etravirine ↓ EBR/GRZ (use not recommended), cobicistat-containing regimens ↑ EBR/GRZ (not recommended), EBR/GRZ ↑ atorvastatin (max. 20 mg/d), ↑ rosuvastatin (max. 10 mg/d), ↑ fluvastatin, lovastatin, & simvastatin (use lowest possible dose/monitor), modafinil ↓ EBR/GRZ (not recommended)

"Usual dose" assumes normal renal/hepatic function. * For renal insufficiency, give usual dose × 1 followed by maintenance dose per CrCl. For dialysis patients, dose the same as for CrCl < 10 mL/min and give supplemental (post-HD/PD dose) immediately after dialysis. CrCl = creatinine clearance; CVVH = continuous venovenous hemofiltration; HD/PD = hemodialysis/peritoneal dialysis. See pp. 204–207 for explanations, pp. xi–xii for abbreviations.

Adverse Effects: *Warning: Increased risk of ALT elevation (GZR) up to 5x ULN, at or after week 8 of treatment (1%) and (more common in females, age > 65 and Asian race).*
Common: ≥ 5%: Nausea, diarrhea, headache, fatigue, insomnia
Less Common/with ribavirin: Serum bilirubin increase, depression, irritability
Allergic Potential: Low
Safety in Pregnancy: No human pregnancy data for EBR or GZR. Both EBR and GZR cross placenta. No evidence of adverse developmental outcomes in animal studies. *If used with ribavirin (contraindicated in pregnancy), pregnancy warnings for ribavirin apply to the combination. See ribavirin prescribing information for details.*
Comments: Available only as a combination. Contraindicated in patients with decompensated cirrhosis Child-Pugh score ≥ 7, Model for End-Stage Liver Disease (MELD) ≥ 15, and/or clinical manifestations of decompensation. Presence of NS5A polymorphisms (positions M28, Q30, L31, and/or Y93) at baseline associated with poorer response to treatment. Prior to starting EBR/GZR, test for presence of NS5A polymorphisms in patients with genotype 1 infection in select situations to guide treatment regimen and duration. Close monitoring of liver function (ALT) with GZR.

REFERENCES:

AASLD-IDSA. Recommendations for testing, managing, and treating hepatitis C. http://www.hcvguidelines.org. Accessed on September 27, 2016.

Lawitz E., et al. Efficacy and safety of 12 weeks versus 18 weeks of treatment with grazoprevir (MK-5172) and elbasvir (MK-8742) with or without ribavirin for hepatitis C virus genotype 1 infection in previously untreated patients with cirrhosis and patients with previous null response with or without cirrhosis (C-WORTHY): a randomised, open-label phase 2 trial. Lancet 2015;385(9973):1075–86.

Roth D, Nelson DR, Bruchfeld A, et al. Grazoprevir plus elbasvir in treatment-naive and treatment-experienced patients with hepatitis C virus genotype 1 infection and stage 4-5 chronic kidney disease (the C-SURFER study): a combination phase 3 study. Lancet. 2015 Oct 17;386(10003):1537–1545. Published online 2015 Oct 5.

Product Information: Zepatier oral tablets, elbasvir, grazoprevir oral tablets. Merck Sharp & Dohme Corp. (per manufacturer), Whitehouse Station, NJ; 2016.

Zeuzem S, et al. Grazoprevir-elbasvir combination therapy for treatment-naive cirrhotic and noncirrhotic patients with chronic hepatitis C virus genotype 1, 4, or 6 infection: A randomized trial. Ann Intern Med. 2015;163(1):1–13.

Elvitegravir, Cobicistat, Emtricitabine, Tenofovir Alafenamide (Genvoya) (EVG/c/FTC/TAF)

Drug Class: HIV combination antiretroviral agent
Usual Dose: 1 tablet (PO) daily with food
How Supplied: Oral tablet: (containing emtricitabine 200 mg, tenofovir alafenamide 10 mg, elvitegravir 150 mg, and cobicistat 150 mg)
Pharmacokinetic Parameters:
Peak serum level (mcg/mL):
2.1/0.16/2.1/1.5 mcg/mL
Bioavailability: 18–87% increased with food (high-fat meal)
Excreted unchanged (urine):
70%/<1%/6.7%/8.2%
Serum half-life: 10 h/0.51 h (150–180 h in PBMC)/12.9h/3.5 h

"Usual dose" assumes normal renal/hepatic function. * For renal insufficiency, give usual dose × 1 followed by maintenance dose per CrCl. For dialysis patients, dose the same as for CrCl < 10 mL/min and give supplemental (post-HD/PD dose) immediately after dialysis. CrCl = creatinine clearance; CVVH = continuous venovenous hemofiltration; HD/PD = hemodialysis/peritoneal dialysis. See pp. 204–207 for explanations, pp. xi–xii for abbreviations.

Plasma protein binding: < 4%/80%/99%/98%
Primary Mode of Elimination: Renal/renal/fecal/fecal
Dosage Adjustments:

CrCl 30–50 mL/min	No change
CrCl < 30 mL/min	Avoid
Post-HD/PD dose*	Avoid
CVVH dose	Avoid
Mild-moderate (Child-Pugh A or B) hepatic insufficiency	No change
Severe (Child-Pugh C) hepatic insufficiency	Avoid

Drug Interactions: *Coadministration with the following drugs are contraindicated: (1) Highly dependent on CYP3A for clearance and elevated plasma concentrations are associated with serious adverse events and/or (2) Drugs that strongly induce CYP3A* antacids (↓ EVG), ↑ antiarrhythmics, ↑ digoxin, ↑ alfuzosin, anticonvulsants (↓ TAF/EVG/c), ↑ ethosuximide), rifamycins (↓ TAF/EVG/c), ↑ lurasidone, ↑ pimozide, ↑ergot derivatives, ↑ cisapride, St. John's wort (↓ TAF/EVG/c), ↑ HMG-CoA reductase inhibitors, ↑ PDE5 inhibitors, ↑ oral midazolam, ↑ triazolam, ↑ diazepam, ↑ sedative hypnotics, ↑ clarithromycin/telithromycin (↑ cobicistat), ↑ warfarin (monitor INR), ↑ salmeterol, ↑ TCAs/trazodone/SSRIs (except sertraline), ↑ azole antifungals, ↑ colchicine, ↑ antipsychotics, ↑ beta blockers, ↑ calcium channel blockers, dexamethasone ↓ EVG/c, ↑ fluticasone, ↑ bosentan, ↑ norgestimate, ↓ ethinyl estradiol, ↑ immunosuppressants
Adverse Effects: *Please refer to individual drug monographs for more complete details.*

Nausea (10%), renal effects (renal insufficiency, Fanconi syndrome, and proximal renal tubulopathy), and decreased bone mineral density effects less with TAF than TDF. Rare: lactic acidosis with hepatic steatosis
Allergic Potential: Low
Safety in Pregnancy: B
Cerebrospinal Fluid Penetration: See individual drug monographs for details.

REFERENCES:
Panel on Antiretroviral Guidelines for Adults and Adolescents. Guidelines for the use of antiretroviral agents in HIV-1-infected adults and adolescents, updated July 14, 2016. Department of Health and Human Services; 1–288. Available at https://aidsinfo.nih.gov/contentfiles/lvguidelines/adultandadolescentgl.pdf.
Product Information: Genvoya oral tablets, elvitegravir, cobicistat, emtricitabine, tenofovir alafenamide oral tablets. Gilead Sciences, Inc. (per manufacturer), Foster City, CA; 2015.

Elvitegravir, Cobicistat, Emtricitabine, Tenofovir disoproxil fumarate (Stribild) (EVG/c/FTC/TDF)

Drug Class: Combination antiretroviral agent
Usual Dose: 1 tablet (PO) daily with a meal (preferably high fat)
How Supplied: Oral tablet: (containing elvitegravir 150 mg, cobicistat 150 mg, emtricitabine 200 mg, and tenofovir disoproxil fumarate 300 mg)
Pharmacokinetic Parameters:
Peak serum level: 1.7 mcg/mL/1.1 mcg/mL/1.9 mcg/mL/0.45 mcg/mL
Bioavailability: 23% to 87% increased with food (high-fat meals)

Excreted unchanged: 6.7% (urine)/8.2% (urine)/extensive (urine)/extensive (urine)
Serum half-life (normal/ESRD):
12.9/3.5/10/17(hrs)/no data
Plasma protein binding:
99%/98%/4%/0.7%
Volume of distribution (V_d): not data/no data/no data/1.2 L/kg
Primary Mode of Elimination: Hepatic & fecal/Hepatic & fecal/renal/renal
Dosage Adjustments*

CrCl > 70 mL/min	No change
CrCl 30–70 mL/min	*Not recommended
CrCl < 30 mL/min	*Not recommended
ESRD	*Not recommended
Post-HD dose	*Not recommended
Post-PD dose	*Not recommended
CVVH dose	*Not recommended
Mild-moderate hepatic insufficiency	No change
Severe hepatic insufficiency	Not studied

* The fixed dose tablet is not recommended for patients with CrCl < 70 mL/min, however therapy with one or more of the individual components might be possible. Please refer agent specific drug monographs.

Antiretroviral Dosage Adjustments:
Please refer to individual drug monographs.
Drug Interactions: *Co administration with drugs that are highly dependent on CYP3A for clearance and for which elevated plasma concentrations are associated with serious and/or life-threatening events:* antacids (↓ elvitegravir), ↑ alfuzosin, ↑ midazolam, pimozide, triazolam, rifampin (↓ elvitegravir),

↑ simvastatin, ↑ atrovastatin, ↑ fluticasone, ↑ colchicine, avanafil (do not coadminister), ↑ sildenafil (max. 25 mg in 48 hrs), ↑ tadalafil, ↑ vardenafil, ↑ beta-blockers, ↑ SSRIs, ↑ TCAs, ↑ digoxin, ↑↓ voriconazole, ketoconazole, itraconazole, (↑ elvitegravir), rivaroxaban (↑ rivaroxaban), warfarin (↑ warfarin, monitor INR)
Adverse Effects: *Please refer to individual drug monographs for more complete details.*
Most common adverse drug reactions to elvitegravir/cobicistat are ≥ 10% all grades: gastrointestinal (diarrhea and nausea) and renal (proteinuria)
Most common adverse drug reactions to emtricitabine and tenofovir disoproxil fumarate are: diarrhea, nausea, fatigue, headache, dizziness, depression, insomnia, abnormal dreams, lacticacidosis, myalgia, decreased bone mineral density, and rash.
Allergic Potential: Low
Safety in Pregnancy: B
Comments: Must be taken with food. Concomitant use with other antiretrovirals, including ritonavir, is not recommended. Avoid administering with concurrent or recent use of nephrotoxic drugs. In patients coinfected with HIV-1 and HBV, abrupt withdrawal of emtricitabine or tenofovir DF have caused severe acute exacerbations of hepatitis B virus infection. Patients who fail elvitegravir can develop cross-resistance to raltegravir.
Cerebrospinal Fluid Penetration: See individual drug monographs for details.

REFERENCES:
DeJesus E, Rockstroh JK, Henry K, et al: Co-formulated elvitegravir, cobicistat, emtricitabine, and tenofovir disoproxil fumarate versus ritonavir-boosted atazanavir

plus co-formulated emtricitabine and tenofovir disoproxil fumarate for initial treatment of HIV 1 infection: a randomised, double-blind, phase 3, non-inferiority trial. Lancet 2012;379(9835):2429–38.

Panel on Antiretroviral Guidelines for Adults and Adolescents. Guidelines for the use of antiretroviral agents in HIV-1-infected adults and adolescents, updated July 14, 2016. Department of Health and Human Services; 1–288. Available at https://aidsinfo.nih.gov/contentfiles/lvguidelines/adultandadolescentgl.pdf.

Product Information: Stribild oral tablets, elvitegravir, cobicistat, emtricitabine, tenofovir disoproxil fumarate oral tablets. Gilead Sciences, Inc., Foster City, CA; 2012.

Ramanathan S, Mathias AA, German P, Kearney BP. Clinical pharmacokinetic and pharmacodynamic profile of the HIV integrase inhibitor elvitegravir. Clinical Pharmacokinetics. Apr 2011;50(4):229–244.

Sax PE, DeJesus E, Mills A, et al: Co-formulated elvitegravir, cobicistat, emtricitabine, and tenofovir versus co-formulated efavirenz, emtricitabine, and tenofovir for initial treatment of HIV-1 infection: a randomised, double-blind, phase 3 trial, analysis of results after 48 weeks. Lancet 2012;379(9835):2439–48.

Emtricitabine (Emtriva) (FTC)

Drug Class: Antiretroviral; NRTI (nucleoside reverse transcriptase inhibitor)
Usual Dose: 200 mg (PO) daily
How Supplied: Oral capsule: 200 mg, oral solution: 10 mg/mL
Pharmacokinetic Parameters:
Peak serum level: 1.8 mcg/mL
Bioavailability: 93%
Excreted unchanged (urine): 86%
Serum half-life (normal/ESRD): 10 h/ extended
Plasma protein binding: 4%

Primary Mode of Elimination: Renal
Dosage Adjustments*

CrCl ≥ 30 mL/min	200 mg (PO) daily
CrCl 15–29 mL/min	200 mg (PO) q3d
CrCl < 15 mL/min	200 mg (PO) q4d
Post-HD dose	200 mg (PO) q4d
Post-PD dose	No information
CVVH dose	No information
Moderate or severe hepatic insufficiency	No change

Drug Interactions: No significant interactions with indinavir, stavudine, zidovudine, famciclovir, tenofovir.
Adverse Effects: Headache, diarrhea, nausea, rash, lactic acidosis with hepatic steatosis (rare, but potentially life-threatening with NRTIs).
Allergic Potential: Low
Safety in Pregnancy: B
Comments: May be taken with or without food. Does not inhibit CYP450 enzymes. Mean intracellular half-life of 39 hours. Potential cross-resistance to lamivudine and zalcitabine. Low affinity for DNA polymerase-gamma.
Cerebrospinal Fluid Penetration: See emtricitabine/tenofovir for details.

REFERENCES:
Anderson PL. Pharmacologic perspectives for once-daily antiretroviral therapy. Ann Pharmacother. 2004; 38:1924–34.

"Usual dose" assumes normal renal/hepatic function. * For renal insufficiency, give usual dose × 1 followed by maintenance dose per CrCl. For dialysis patients, dose the same as for CrCl < 10 mL/min and give supplemental (post-HD/PD dose) immediately after dialysis. CrCl = creatinine clearance; CVVH = continuous venovenous hemofiltration; HD/PD = hemodialysis/peritoneal dialysis. See pp. 204–207 for explanations, pp. xi–xii for abbreviations.

Gallant JE, DeJesus D, Arribas JR, et al. Tenofovir DF, emtricitabine, and efavirenz vs. zidovudine, lamivudine, and efavirenz for HIV. N Engl J Med. 2006;354:251–60.

Lim SG, Ng TN, Kung N, et al. A double-blind placebo-controlled study of emtricitabine in chronic hepatitis B. Arch Intern Med. 2006;166:49–56.

Panel on Antiretroviral Guidelines for Adults and Adolescents. Guidelines for the use of antiretroviral agents in HIV-1-infected adults and adolescents, updated July 14, 2016. Department of Health and Human Services; 1–288. Available at https://aidsinfo.nih.gov/contentfiles/lvguidelines/adultandadolescentgl.pdf.

Product Information: Emtriva oral capsules solution, emtricitabine oral capsules solution. Gilead Sciences, Inc., Foster City, CA; 2011.

Emtricitabine/Tenofovir Alafenamide (Descovy) (FTC/TAF)

Drug Class: Combination antiretroviral; NRTI (nucleoside reverse transcriptase inhibitor)
Usual Dose: One tablet (PO) daily with or without food
How Supplied: Oral tablet (containing emtricitabine 200 mg + tenofovir alafenamide 25 mg)
Pharmacokinetic Parameters:
Peak serum level: 2.1/0.16 mcg/mL
Excreted unchanged: 70% urine/13% feces (FTC); < 1% urine/31.7% feces (TAF)
Serum half-life: 10 h (FTC); 0.51 h (TAF;150–180 h in PBMC)
Plasma protein binding: < 4%/80%
Primary Mode of Elimination: Renal/fecal
Dosage Adjustments:

CrCl > 30 mL/min	No change
CrCl ≤ 30 mL/min or HD*	Not recommended
CVVH dose	Not recommended

| Mild-moderate (Child-Pugh A/B) hepatic insufficiency | No change |
| Severe (Child-Pugh C) hepatic insufficiency | Not studied |

*Removed by HD: [30% (FTC); 54% (TAF)].

Drug Interactions: TAF is a P-gp, BCRP, and OATPB1/3 substrate. Strong P-gp inhibitors or inducers may affect TAF absorption. FTC and TDF also undergo elimination via glomerular filtration and tubular secretion. Drugs that reduce renal function or compete for tubular secretion may increase FTC and tenofovir concentrations.
The following ↓ TAF and are not recommended: tipranavir/ritonavir, anticonvulsants (carbamazepine, oxcarbazepine, phenobarbital, phenytoin), antimycobacterials (rifampin, rifabutin, rifapentine), St. John's wort.
Adverse Effects: Diarrhea, nausea, headache, renal effects (renal insufficiency, Fanconi syndrome, and proximal renal tubulopathy), and decreased bone mineral density effects less than tenofovir disoproxil fumarate. Rare: lactic acidosis with hepatic steatosis.
Allergic Potential: Low
Safety in Pregnancy: No data on TAF in human pregnancy. FTC use during human pregnancy showed no difference in overall birth defects.
Cerebrospinal Fluid Penetration: See FTC/TDF monograph; no data (TAF).
Comments: TAF only available in fixed dose combinations, although TAF for hepatitis B treatment expected soon. HIV/HBV co-infected patients may experience exacerbation of hepatitis with discontinuation FTC/TAF.

Pending ongoing studies, should not be used for pre-exposure prophylaxis (PrEP).

REFERENCES:

Panel on Antiretroviral Guidelines for Adults and Adolescents. Guidelines for the use of antiretroviral agents in HIV-1-infected adults and adolescents, updated July 14, 2016. Department of Health and Human Services; 1–288. Available at https://aidsinfo.nih.gov/contentfiles/lvguidelines/adultandadolescentgl.pdf.

Product Information: Descovy oral tablets, emtricitabine, tenofovir alafenamide oral tablets. Gilead Sciences, Inc. (per manufacturer), Foster City, CA; 2016.

Emtricitabine + Tenofovir disoproxil fumarate (Truvada)

Drug Class: Antiretroviral combination; NRTI (nucleoside reverse transcriptase inhibitor) + nucleotide analog
Usual Dose: One tablet (PO) daily
How Supplied: Oral tablet: (containing emtricitabine 200 mg + tenofovir disoproxil 300 mg)
Pharmacokinetic Parameters:
Peak serum level: 1.8/0.3 mcg/L
Bioavailability: 93%/27% if fasting (39% with high-fat meal)
Excreted unchanged (urine): 86/32%
Serum half-life (normal/ESRD): (10 h/extended)/(17 h/no data)
Plasma protein binding: 4/0.7–7.2%
Volume of distribution (V_d): no data/1.3 L/kg
Primary Mode of Elimination: Renal/renal
Dosage Adjustments*

CrCl ≥ 50 mL/min	No change
CrCl 30–49 mL/min	One capsule (PO) q2d
CrCl 15–29 mL/min	Avoid
CrCl < 15 mL/min	Avoid
Post-HD dose	Avoid
Post-PD dose	Avoid
CVVH dose	Avoid
Moderate or severe hepatic insufficiency	No change

Drug Interactions: No significant interactions with indinavir, stavudine, zidovudine, famciclovir, lamivudine, lopinavir/ritonavir, efavirenz, methadone, oral contraceptives.
Tenofovir ↑ didanosine levels. Tenofovir reduces systemic exposure to atazanavir; whenever the two are coadministered, the recommended dose of atazanavir is 300 mg once daily with ritonavir 100 mg once daily.
Adverse Effects: Headache, diarrhea, nausea, vomiting, GI upset, rash, lactic acidosis with hepatic steatosis (rare but potentially life-threatening with NRTIs).
Allergic Potential: Low
Safety in Pregnancy: B
Comments: May be taken with or without food. Does not inhibit CYP450 enzymes. Mean intracellular half-life with emtricitabine is 39 hours. Potential cross-resistance to lamivudine, zalcitabine, abacavir, didanosine. Low affinity for DNA polymerase-gamma. Avoid coadministration with didanosine.
Cerebrospinal Fluid Penetration: Variable/low; below quantification limit: 6 mcg/mL (TDF); 32.2–212 mcg/mL (FTC)

REFERENCES:

Gallant JE, DeJesus D, Arribas JR, et al. Tenofovir DF, emtricitabine, and efavirenz vs. zidovudine, lamivudine, and efavirenz for HIV. N Engl J Med. 2006;354:251–60.

Panel on Antiretroviral Guidelines for Adults and Adolescents. Guidelines for the use of antiretroviral agents in HIV-1-infected adults and adolescents, updated July 14, 2016. Department of Health and Human Services; 1–288. Available at https://aidsinfo.nih.gov/contentfiles/lvguidelines/adultandadolescentgl.pdf.

Lahri CD, Reed-Walker K, Sheth et al. Cerebrospinal fluid concentrations of tenofovir and emtricitabine in the setting of HIV-1 protease inhibitor-based regimens. J Clin Pharmacol. 2016;56:492–6.

Best BM, Letendre SL, Koopmans P, et al. Low cerebrospinal fluid concentrations of the nucleotide HIV reverse transcriptase inhibitor, tenofovir. Journal of Acquired Immune Deficiency Syndromes. 2012 Apr 1;59(4):376–381.

Calcagno A, Bonora S, Simiele M, et al. Tenofovir and emtricitabine cerebrospinal fluid-to-plasma ratios correlate to the extent of blood-brainbarrier damage. AIDS. 2011 Jul 17;25(11):1437–1439.

Enfuvirtide (Fuzeon) (ENF) (T-20)

Drug Class: Antiretroviral; fusion inhibitor
Usual Dose: 90 mg (SC) bid
How Supplied: Subcutaneous powder for solution: 90 mg
Pharmacokinetic Parameters:
Peak serum level: 4.9 mcg/mL
Bioavailability: 84.3%
Serum half-life (normal/ESRD): 3.8 h/no data
Plasma protein binding: 92%
Volume of distribution (V_d): 5.5 L
Primary Mode of Elimination: Metabolized
Dosage Adjustments*

CrCl > 35 mL/min	No change
CrCl < 35 mL/min	No data
Post-HD dose	No data
Post-PD dose	No data
CVVH dose	No data
Moderate or severe hepatic insufficiency	No data

Drug Interactions: No clinically significant interactions with other antiretrovirals. Does not inhibit CYP450 enzymes.
Adverse Effects: Local injection site reactions are common. Diarrhea, nausea, fatigue may occur. Laboratory abnormalities include mild/transient eosinophilia. Pneumonia may occur, but cause is unclear and may not be due to drug therapy. Pancreatitis, myalgia, conjunctivitis (rare).
Allergic Potential: Hypersensitivity reactions may occur, including fever, chills, hypotension, rash, ↑ serum transaminases. Do not rechallenge following a hypersensitivity reaction.
Safety in Pregnancy: B
Comments: Reconstitute in 1.1 mL of sterile water. SC injection should be given into upper arm, anterior thigh, or abdomen. Rotate injection sites; do not inject into moles, scars, bruises. After reconstitution, use immediately or refrigerate and use within 24 hours (no preservatives added).

REFERENCES:
Kilby JM, Lalezari JP, Eron JJ, et al. The safety, plasma pharmacokinetics, and antiviral activity of subcutaneous enfuvirtide (T-20), a peptide inhibitor of gp41-mediated virus fusion, in HIV-infected adults. AIDS Res Hum Retroviruses. 2002;18:685–93.

Lalezari JP, Henry K, O'Hearn M, et al. TORO 1 Study Group. Enfuvirtide, an HIV-1 fusion inhibitor, for drug-resistant HIV infection in North and South America. N Engl J Med. 2003;348:2175–85.

Lazzarin A, Clotet B, Cooper D, et al. TORO 2 Study Group. Efficacy of enfuvirtide in patients infected with drug-resistant HIV-1 in Europe and Australia. N Engl J Med. 2003;348:2186–95.

Leen C, Wat C, Nieforth K. Pharmacokinetics of enfuvirtide in a patient with impaired renal function. Clin Infect Dis. 2004;4:339–55.

Panel on Antiretroviral Guidelines for Adults and Adolescents. Guidelines for the use of antiretroviral agents in HIV-1-infected adults and adolescents, updated July 14, 2016. Department of Health and Human Services; 1–288. Available at https://aidsinfo.nih.gov/contentfiles/lvguidelines/adultandadolescentgl.pdf

Entecavir (Baraclude) (ETV)

Drug Class: Anti-hepatitis B agent—guanosine nucleoside analog

Usual Dose: Compensated Liver Disease: (1) Nucleoside-treatment-naïve patients: Entecavir 0.5 mg (PO) daily without food; (2) History of hepatitis B viremia while receiving lamivudine or known lamivudine-resistant mutations: Entecavir 1 mg (PO) daily, without food.

Decompensated Liver Disease: Entecavir 1 mg (PO) daily without food

How Supplied: Oral solution: 0.05 mg/mL; oral tablet: 0.5 mg, 1 mg

Pharmacokinetic Parameters:
Peak serum level: 4.2 ng/mL (0.5 mg), 8.2 ng/mL (1 mg)
Bioavailability: ~ 100%
Excreted unchanged (urine): 62–73% (urine)
Serum half-life (normal/ESRD): 128–149 h/ no data
Plasma protein binding: 13%
Volume of distribution (V_d): Extensively distributed into tissues

Primary Mode of Elimination: Renal

Dosage Adjustments*

	Treatment-naïve (0.5 mg)	Lamivudine-refractory (1 mg)
CrCl > 50 mL/min	0.5 mg QD	1 mg QD
CrCl 30–50 mL/min	0.25 mg QD or 0.5 mg q2d	0.5 mg QD or 1 mg q2d
CrCl 10–30 mL/min	0.15 mg QD or 0.5 mg q3d	0.3 mg QD or 1 mg q3d
CrCl < 10 mL/min	0.05 mg QD or 0.5 mg q7d	0.1 mg QD or 1 mg q7d
Post-HD dose[†]	0.05 mg QD or 0.5 mg q7d	0.1 mg QD or 1 mg q7d
Post-PD dose[†]	0.05 mg QD or 0.5 mg q7d	0.1 mg QD or 1 mg q7d
CVVH dose	No data	No data
Mild-moderate hepatic insufficiency	No change	No change
Severe hepatic insufficiency	No change	No change

[†] On dialysis days, give dose after dialysis.

Drug Interactions: Since entecavir is primarily eliminated by the kidneys, coadministration of entecavir with drugs that reduce renal function or compete for active tubular secretion may increase serum concentrations of either entecavir or the coadministered drug. Coadministration of entecavir with lamivudine, adefovir dipivoxil,

---

"Usual dose" assumes normal renal/hepatic function. * For renal insufficiency, give usual dose × 1 followed by maintenance dose per CrCl. For dialysis patients, dose the same as for CrCl < 10 mL/min and give supplemental (post-HD/PD dose) immediately after dialysis. CrCl = creatinine clearance; CVVH = continuous venovenous hemofiltration; HD/PD = hemodialysis/peritoneal dialysis. See pp. 204–207 for explanations, pp. xi–xii for abbreviations.

or tenofovir disoproxil fumarate did not result in significant drug interactions.

Adverse Effects: Rash has been reported with entecavir therapy during postmarketing surveillance. Lactic acidosis and severe hepatomegaly with steatosis have been reported, predominantly in women, with the use of nucleoside analogs alone or in combination with antiretrovirals, including entecavir. Obesity and prolonged exposure may be risk factors.

GI effects: nausea/vomiting/diarrhea/indigestion (< 1%); neurologic effects: dizziness (3%), headache (3%), insomnia (< 1%), somnolence (< 1%); renal effects: hematuria (9%); fatigue (3%).

Allergic Potential: Low; anaphylactoid reaction has been reported with entecavir during postmarketing surveillance.

Safety in Pregnancy: C

Comments: Entecavir should be taken on an empty stomach (at least 2 hours after a meal and 2 hours before the next meal). Oral solution: Do not dilute or mix with water or any other liquid. HIV coinfection: Entecavir is not recommended in patients who are not receiving concurrent HIV treatment (i.e., highly active antiretroviral therapy) due to the risk of HIV nucleoside reverse transcriptase inhibitor resistance. Lactic acidosis and severe hepatomegaly with steatosis, including fatalities, have been reported with nucleoside analogs. Patients with obesity, female gender, prolonged nucleoside exposure, or known risk factors for liver disease may be at increased risk; suspend treatment if signs or symptoms of lactic acidosis or hepatotoxicity occur. Entecavir is potent and well tolerated and has extremely low resistance rates in nucleoside/nucleotide analogue-naïve patients.

Comments: Entecavir may select for the M184V mutation in HIV. As a result, it is contraindicated in patients with HIV who are not on suppressive ART.

REFERENCES:

Chang TT, Gish RG, deMan R, et al. A comparison of entecavir and lamivudine for HBeAg-positive chronic hepatitis B. N Engl J Med. 2006;354(10):1001–10.

Lai CL, Rosmawati M, Lao J. Entecavir is superior to lamivudine in reducing hepatitis B virus DNA in patients with chronic hepatitis B infection. Gastroenterology. 2002;123:1831–38.

Lai CL, Shouval D, Lok AS, et al. Entecavir versus lamivudine for patients with HBeAg-negative chronic hepatitis B. N Engl J Med. 2006;354(10):1011–20.

Product Information: Baraclude oral tablets, solution, entecavir oral tablets, solution. Bristol-Myers Squibb Company (per manufacturer), Princeton, NJ; 2014.

Sherman M, Yurdaydin C, Sollano J, et al. Entecavir for treatment of lamivudine refractory, HBeAg-positive chronic hepatitis B. Gastroenterology. 2006;130(7):2039–49.

Tenney DJ, Levine SM, Rose RE, et al. Clinical emergence of entecavir-resistant hepatitis B virus requires additional substitutions in virus already resistant to lamivudine. Antimicrob Agents Chemother. 2004;48(9):3498–3507.

Etravirine (Intelence) (ETR)

Drug Class: Antiretroviral; NNRTI (non-nucleoside reverse transcriptase inhibitor)

Usual Dose: 200 mg (PO) bid following a meal. Half-life supports dose of 400 mg once daily, but this is not listed in package insert.

How Supplied: Oral tablet: 100 mg, 200 mg

Pharmacokinetic Parameters:
Peak serum level: 296 ng/mL
Bioavailability: Unknown (food increases systemic exposure)

"Usual dose" assumes normal renal/hepatic function. * For renal insufficiency, give usual dose × 1 followed by maintenance dose per CrCl. For dialysis patients, dose the same as for CrCl < 10 mL/min and give supplemental (post-HD/PD dose) immediately after dialysis. CrCl = creatinine clearance; CVVH = continuous venovenous hemofiltration; HD/PD = hemodialysis/peritoneal dialysis. See pp. 204–207 for explanations, pp. xi–xii for abbreviations.

Excreted unchanged: 81–86% (feces); 0% (urine)
Serum half-life (normal/ESRD): 41 h/not studied
Plasma protein binding: 99.9%
Volume of distribution (V_d): Not studied
Primary Mode of Elimination: Fecal 93.7%/renal 1.2%
Dosage Adjustments*

CrCl 50–80 mL/min	No change
CrCl 30–50 mL/min	No change
CrCl < 30 mL/min	No change*
Post-HD dose	None*
Post-PD dose	None*
CVVH dose	Not studied
Mild or moderate hepatic insufficiency	No change
Severe hepatic insufficiency	Not studied

* Renal elimination is negligible; unlikely to accumulate in renal dysfunction. Highly bound to plasma proteins—unlikely to be removed by HD or PD.

Antiretroviral Dosage Adjustments

Atazanavir/ritonavir	Avoid
Delavirdine	Avoid (↑ etravirine)
Efavirenz/nevirapine	Avoid (↓ etravirine)
Fosamprenavir/ritonavir	Use with caution (↑ amprenavir)
Lopinavir/ritonavir	Use with caution (↑ etravirine)
Ritonavir (600 mg bid)	Avoid (↓ etravirine)
Darunavir/ritonavir	No change
Rifabutin, rifampin	Avoid (↓ etravirine)
Tipranavir/ritonavir	Avoid (↓ etravirine)
Saquinavir/ritonavir	No change
Maraviroc	600 mg bid
Raltegravir	No change

Drug Interactions: Etravirine is a substrate for the liver enzymes CYP3A4, CYP2C9, and CYP2C19. Coadministration with drugs that inhibit or induce these enzymes may alter the therapeutic effect or adverse reaction profile of etravirine or concomitant drug. Amiodarone, bepridil, disopyramide, flecainide, lidocaine (systemic), mexiletine, propafenone, quinidine (↓ antiarrhythmic levels); warfarin (↑ warfarin levels); carbamazepine, phenobarbital, phenytoin (↓ etravirine levels); antifungals (↑ etravirine levels)—also etravirine decreases itraconazole and ketoconazole levels and increases voriconazole levels but has no effect on fluconazole or posaconazole levels; clarithromycin (↑ etravirine levels, ↓ clarithromycin levels), atorvastatin (↓ atorvastatin levels), sildenafil (↓ sildenafil levels), tadalafil (↓ tadalafil levels), vardenafil (↓ vardenafil levels); etravirine has no effect on methadone levels.
Adverse Effects: Hypertension, rash, abdominal pain, nausea, diarrhea, ↑ liver enzymes AST(SGOT)/ALT(SGPT), myocardial infarction, hypersensitivity reaction.
Allergic Potential: Low (< 2%)
Safety in Pregnancy: B

"Usual dose" assumes normal renal/hepatic function. * For renal insufficiency, give usual dose × 1 followed by maintenance dose per CrCl. For dialysis patients, dose the same as for CrCl < 10 mL/min and give supplemental (post-HD/PD dose) immediately after dialysis. CrCl = creatinine clearance; CVVH = continuous venovenous hemofiltration; HD/PD = hemodialysis/peritoneal dialysis. See pp. 204–207 for explanations, pp. xi–xii for abbreviations.

Cerebrospinal Fluid Penetration: 9.24 ng/mL (median). Unbound ETR may not reach optimal concentrations in CNS.

Comments: Severe and potentially life-threatening skin reactions have been reported, including Stevens-Johnson syndrome, hypersensitivity reaction, and erythema multiforme. Discontinue treatment if severe rash develops. Efficacy in treatment-naïve patients has not been established. Take with meals; food increases systemic exposure by 50%.

REFERENCES:

Panel on Antiretroviral Guidelines for Adults and Adolescents. Guidelines for the use of antiretroviral agents in HIV-1-infected adults and adolescents, updated July 14, 2016. Department of Health and Human Services; 1–288. Available at https://aidsinfo.nih.gov/contentfiles/lvguidelines/adultandadolescentgl.pdf.

Product Information: Intelence oral tablets, etravirine oral tablets. Tibotec Therapeutics, Inc., Raritan, NJ; 2008.

Tiraboschi JM, Vila NA, Perez-Pujol S, et al. Etravirine concentrations in CSF in HIV-infected patients. J Antimicrob Chemother. 2012;67:1446–8.

Nguyen A, Rossi S, Croteau D, et al. Etravirine in CSF is highly protein bound. J Antimicrob Chemother. 2013;1161–8.

Fosamprenavir (Lexiva) (FPV)

Drug Class: Antiretroviral; protease inhibitor
Usual Dose: Treatment-naïve patients: 1400 mg bid or 1400 mg + ritonavir 100–200 mg QD or 700 mg + ritonavir 100 mg bid
Treatment-experienced patients: (once daily dosing not recommended) 700 mg + ritonavir 100 mg bid

Pharmacokinetic Parameters:
Peak serum level: 4.8 mcg/mL
Bioavailability: No data

Excreted unchanged (urine): 1%
Serum half-life (normal/ESRD): 7 h/no data
Plasma protein binding: 90%
Volume of distribution (V_d): 6.1 L/kg
Primary Mode of Elimination: Hepatic
Dosage Adjustments*

CrCl 50–80 mL/min	No change
CrCl 10–50 mL/min	No change
CrCl < 10 mL/min	No change
Post-HD or PD dose	No change
CVVH dose	No change
Mild-moderate hepatic insufficiency (Child-Pugh score 5–8)	700 mg (PO) bid if given without ritonavir; no data with ritonavir
Severe hepatic insufficiency (Child-Pugh score 9–12)	Avoid

Antiretroviral Dosage Adjustments:

Didanosine	Administer didanosine 1 hour apart
Delavirdine	Avoid combination
Efavirenz	Fosamprenavir 700 mg bid + ritonavir 100 mg bid + efavirenz; fosamprenavir 1400 mg QD + ritonavir 200 mg QD + efavirenz; no data for fosamprenavir 1400 mg bid + efavirenz
Indinavir	No information
Lopinavir/ritonavir	Avoid
Nelfinavir	No information

"Usual dose" assumes normal renal/hepatic function. * For renal insufficiency, give usual dose × 1 followed by maintenance dose per CrCl. For dialysis patients, dose the same as for CrCl < 10 mL/min and give supplemental (post-HD/PD dose) immediately after dialysis. CrCl = creatinine clearance; CVVH = continuous venovenous hemofiltration; HD/PD = hemodialysis/peritoneal dialysis. See pp. 204–207 for explanations, pp. xi–xii for abbreviations.

Nevirapine	(FPV 700 mg + RTV 100 mg) bid NVP standard
Saquinavir	No information
Rifampin	Avoid combination
Rifabutin	Reduce usual rifabutin dose by 50% (or 75% if given with fosamprenavir plus ritonavir; max. 150 mg q2d)
Etravirine	Avoid combination
Maraviroc	150 mg bid
Raltegravir	No data

Drug Interactions: Antiretrovirals (see dose adjustment grid above). Contraindicated with: ergot derivatives, cisapride, midazolam, triazolam, pimozide, flecainide, and propafenone (if administered with ritonavir). Do not coadminister with: rifampin, lovastatin, simvastatin, St. John's wort, delavirdine. Dose reduction (of other drug): atorvastatin, rifabutin, sildenafil, vardenafil, ketoconazole, itraconazole. Concentration monitoring (of other drug): amiodarone, systemic lidocaine, quinidine, warfarin (INR), rivaroxaban ($\uparrow$rivaroxaban), tricyclic antidepressants, cyclosporin, tacrolimus, sirolimus. H_2 blockers, and proton pump inhibitors interfere with absorption. Sildenafil (do not give > 25 mg/48 hrs); tadalafil (max. 10 mg/72 hrs); vardenafil (max. 2.5 mg/72 hrs).
Adverse Effects: Rash, Stevens-Johnson syndrome (rare), GI upset, headache, depression, diarrhea, hyperglycemia (including worsening diabetes, new-onset diabetes, diabetic ketoacidosis [DKA]), $\uparrow$ cholesterol/ triglycerides (evaluate risk for coronary disease/pancreatitis), fat redistribution, $\uparrow$ SGOT/ SGPT, possible increased bleeding in hemophilia; potential increased risk of myocardial infarction has been reported.
Allergic Potential: High. Fosamprenavir contains a sulfonamide moiety; use with caution in patients with sulfonamide allergies.
Safety in Pregnancy: C
Comments: Usually given in conjunction with ritonavir. May be taken with or without food. Fosamprenavir is a prodrug that is rapidly hydrolyzed to amprenavir by gut epithelium during absorption. Amprenavir inhibits CYP3A4. Fosamprenavir contains a sulfonamide moiety (as do darunavir and tipranavir).

REFERENCES:

Product Information: Lexiva oral tablets, suspension, fosamprenavir calcium oral tablets, suspension. ViiV Healthcare (per FDA), Research Triangle Park, NC; 2012.

Panel on Antiretroviral Guidelines for Adults and Adolescents. Guidelines for the use of antiretroviral agents in HIV-1-infected adults and adolescents, updated July 14, 2016. Department of Health and Human Services; 1–288. Available at https://aidsinfo.nih.gov/contentfiles/lvguidelines/adultandadolescentgl.pdf.

Indinavir (Crixivan) (IDV)

Drug Class: Antiretroviral; protease inhibitor
Usual Dose: 800 mg (PO) tid on empty stomach or 800 mg with ritonavir 100–200 mg (PO) bid with or without food
How Supplied: Oral capsule: 100 mg, 200 mg, 400 mg
Pharmacokinetic Parameters:
Peak serum level: 252 mcg/mL
Bioavailability: 65% (77% with food)

Excreted unchanged (urine): < 20%
Serum half-life (normal/ESRD): 2 h/no data
Plasma protein binding: 60%
Volume of distribution (V_d): No data
Primary Mode of Elimination: Hepatic
Dosage Adjustments*

CrCl 50–80 mL/min	No change
CrCl 10–50 mL/min	No change
CrCl < 10 mL/min	No change
Post-HD dose	None
Post-PD dose	None
CVVH dose	No change
Moderate hepatic insufficiency	600 mg (PO) tid
Severe hepatic insufficiency	400 mg (PO) tid

Antiretroviral Dosage Adjustments

Didanosine	Administer didanosine 1 hour apart
Delavirdine	Indinavir 600 mg tid
Efavirenz	Indinavir 1000 mg tid or IDV 800 mg + RTV 100–200 mg bid
Lopinavir/ ritonavir	Indinavir 600 mg bid
Nelfinavir	Limited data for indinavir 1200 mg bid + nelfinavir 1250 mg bid
Nevirapine	Indinavir 1000 mg tid or IDV 800 mg + RTV 100–200 mg bid
Ritonavir	Indinavir 800 mg bid + ritonavir 100–200 mg bid, or 400 mg bid of each drug

Saquinavir	No information
Rifampin	Avoid combination
Rifabutin	Indinavir 1000 mg tid; rifabutin 150 mg QD or 300 mg 2–3x/ week
Etravirine	Avoid combination
Maraviroc	150 mg bid
Raltegravir	No information

Drug Interactions: Antiretrovirals, rifabutin, rifampin (see dose adjustment grid above); astemizole, terfenadine, benzodiazepines, cisapride, ergot alkaloids, statins, St. John's wort (avoid if possible); calcium channel blockers (↑ calcium channel blocker levels); carbamazepine, phenobarbital, phenytoin (↓ indinavir levels, ↑ anticonvulsant levels; monitor); tenofovir (↓ indinavir levels, ↑ tenofovir levels); clarithromycin, erythromycin, telithromycin (↑ indinavir and macrolide levels); didanosine (administer indinavir on empty stomach 1 hour apart); ethinyl estradiol, norethindrone (↑ interacting drug levels; no dosage adjustment); grapefruit juice (↓ indinavir levels); itraconazole, ketoconazole (↑ indinavir levels); sildenafil (↑ or ↓ sildenafil levels; do not exceed 25 mg in 48 hrs), tadalafil (max. 10 mg/72 hrs), vardenafil (max. 2.5 mg/72 hrs); theophylline (↓ theophylline levels); rivaroxaban (↑ rivaroxaban); warfarin (↑ warfarin, monitor INR); fluticasone nasal spray (avoid concomitant use).
Adverse Effects: Nephrolithiasis, nausea, vomiting, diarrhea, anemia, leukopenia, headache, insomnia, hyperglycemia (including worsening diabetes, new-onset diabetes, DKA), ↑ SGOT/SGPT,

---

"Usual dose" assumes normal renal/hepatic function. * For renal insufficiency, give usual dose × 1 followed by maintenance dose per CrCl. For dialysis patients, dose the same as for CrCl < 10 mL/min and give supplemental (post-HD/PD dose) immediately after dialysis. CrCl = creatinine clearance; CVVH = continuous venovenous hemofiltration; HD/PD = hemodialysis/peritoneal dialysis. See pp. 204–207 for explanations, pp. xi–xii for abbreviations.

↑ indirect bilirubin (2° to drug-induced Gilbert's syndrome; inconsequential), fat redistribution, lipid abnormalities (evaluate risk of coronary disease/pancreatitis), abdominal pain, possible ↑ bleeding in hemophilia, dry skin, chelitis, paronychiae.

Allergic Potential: Low

Safety in Pregnancy: C

Comments: Renal stone formation may be prevented/minimized by adequate hydration (1–3 liters water daily); ↑risk of nephrolithiasis with alcohol. Take 1 hour before or 2 hours after meals (may take with skim milk or low-fat meal). Separate dosing with ddI by 1 hour.

Cerebrospinal Fluid Penetration: 16%

REFERENCES:

Antinori A, Giancola MI, Griserri S, et al. Factors influencing virological response to antiretroviral drugs in cerebrospinal fluid of advanced HIV-1-infected patients. AIDS. 2002;16:1867–76.

DiCenzo R, Forrest A, Fischl MA, et al. Pharmacokinetics of indinavir and nelfinavir in treatment-naïve, human immunodeficiency virus-infected subjects. Antimicrob Agents Chemother. 2004;48:918–23.

Meraviglia P, Angeli E, Del Sorbo F, et al. Risk factors for indinavir-related renal colic in HIV patients: predicative value of indinavir dose-body mass index. AIDS. 2002;16:2089–93.

Panel on Antiretroviral Guidelines for Adults and Adolescents. Guidelines for the use of antiretroviral agents in HIV-1-infected adults and adolescents, updated July 14, 2016. Department of Health and Human Services; 1–288. Available at https://aidsinfo.nih.gov/contentfiles/lvguidelines/adultandadolescentgl.pdf.

Product Information: Crixivan oral capsules, indinavir sulfate oral capsules. Merck & Co, Inc, Whitehouse Station, NJ; 2008.

Lamivudine (Epivir) (3TC)

Drug Class: Antiretroviral NRTI (nucleoside reverse transcriptase inhibitor); antiviral (hepatitis B virus)

Usual Dose: 150 mg (PO) bid or 300 mg (PO) QD (HIV); 100 mg (PO) QD (HBV)

How Supplied:
Epivir A/F—Oral solution: 10 mg/mL
Epivir HBV—Oral solution: 5 mg/mL; tablets: 100 mg
Epivir—Oral solution: 10 mg/mL; tablets: 150 mg, 300 mg
Generic—Oral tablet: 100, 150, 300 mg; oral solution: 10 mg/mL

Pharmacokinetic Parameters:
Peak serum level: 1.5 mcg/mL
Bioavailability: 86%
Excreted unchanged (urine): 71%
Serum half-life (normal/ESRD): 5–7/20 h
Plasma protein binding: 36%
Volume of distribution (V_d): 1.3 L/kg

Primary Mode of Elimination: Renal

Dosage Adjustments*

CrCl 30–49 mL/min	150 mg (PO) Q24h
CrCl 15–29 mL/min	150 mg × 1; then, 100 mg (PO) Q24h
CrCl 5–14 mL/min	150 mg × 1, then 50 mg (PO) Q24h
CrCl < 5 mL/min or HD	50 mg × 1, then 25 mg (PO) Q24h
Post-HD dose	None; dose after HD on HD days

"Usual dose" assumes normal renal/hepatic function. * For renal insufficiency, give usual dose × 1 followed by maintenance dose per CrCl. For dialysis patients, dose the same as for CrCl < 10 mL/min and give supplemental (post-HD/PD dose) immediately after dialysis. CrCl = creatinine clearance; CVVH = continuous venovenous hemofiltration; HD/PD = hemodialysis/peritoneal dialysis. See pp. 204–207 for explanations, pp. xi–xii for abbreviations.

Post-PD dose	No information
CVVH dose	No information
Moderate hepatic insufficiency	No change
Severe hepatic insufficiency	No change

Drug Interactions: Didanosine, zalcitabine (↑ risk of pancreatitis); TMP-SMX (↑ lamivudine levels); zidovudine (↑ zidovudine levels).
Adverse Effects: Drug fever/rash, abdominal pain/diarrhea, nausea, vomiting, anemia, leukopenia, photophobia, depression, cough, nasal complaints, headache, dizziness, peripheral neuropathy, pancreatitis, myalgias, lactic acidosis with hepatic steatosis (rare, but potentially life-threatening toxicity with NRTIs).
Allergic Potential: Low
Safety in Pregnancy: C
Comments: Potential cross-resistance with didanosine. Prevents development of AZT resistance and restores AZT susceptibility. May be taken with or without food. Effective against HBV, but HBV may reactivate after lamivudine therapy is stopped. Also a component of Combivir, Trizivir, and Epzicom.
Cerebrospinal Fluid Penetration: 15%

REFERENCES:

Liaw YF, Sung JY, Chow WC, et al. Lamivudine for patients with chronic hepatitis B and advanced liver disease. N Engl J Med. 2004;351:1521–31.

Panel on Antiretroviral Guidelines for Adults and Adolescents. Guidelines for the use of antiretroviral agents in HIV-1-infected adults and adolescents, updated July 14, 2016. Department of Health and Human Services; 1–288.

Available at https://aidsinfo.nih.gov/contentfiles/lvguidelines/adultandadolescentgl.pdf.

Perry CM, Faulds D. Lamivudine. A review of its antiviral activity, pharmacokinetic properties and therapeutic efficacy in the management of HIV infection. Drugs. 1997;53:657–80.

Product Information: Epivir oral tablets, oral solution, lamivudine oral tablets, oral solution. ViiV Healthcare (per FDA), Research Triangle Park, NC; 2015.

Lamivudine + Zidovudine (Combivir)

Drug Class: Antiretroviral; NRTI combination
Usual Dose: 1 tablet (PO) bid
How Supplied: Oral tablet: (containing lamivudine 150 mg + zidovudine 300 mg)
Pharmacokinetic Parameters:
Peak serum level: 2.6/1.2 mcg/mL
Bioavailability: 82/60%
Excreted unchanged (urine): 86/64%
Serum half-life (normal/ESRD): (6/1.1)/ (20/2.2) h
Plasma protein binding: < 36/< 38%
Volume of distribution (V_d): 1.3/1.6 L/kg
Primary Mode of Elimination: Renal
Dosage Adjustments*

CrCl 50–80 mL/min	No change
CrCl 10–50 mL/min	Avoid
CrCl < 10 mL/min	Avoid
Post-HD dose	Avoid
Post-PD dose	Avoid
CVVH dose	Avoid
Moderate hepatic insufficiency	Avoid
Severe hepatic insufficiency	Avoid

- -
"Usual dose" assumes normal renal/hepatic function. * For renal insufficiency, give usual dose × 1 followed by maintenance dose per CrCl. For dialysis patients, dose the same as for CrCl < 10 mL/min and give supplemental (post-HD/PD dose) immediately after dialysis. CrCl = creatinine clearance; CVVH = continuous venovenous hemofiltration; HD/PD = hemodialysis/peritoneal dialysis. See pp. 204–207 for explanations, pp. xi–xii for abbreviations.

Drug Interactions: Atovaquone ($\uparrow$zidovudine levels); stavudine (antagonist to stavudine; avoid combination); ganciclovir, doxorubicin (neutropenia); tipranavir ($\downarrow$zidovudine levels); TMP-SMX ($\uparrow$lamivudine and zidovudine levels); vinca alkaloids (neutropenia).

Adverse Effects: Most common (> 5%): nausea, vomiting, diarrhea, anorexia, insomnia, fever/chills, headache, malaise/fatigue. Others (less common): peripheral neuropathy, myopathy, steatosis, pancreatitis. Lab abnormalities: mild hyperglycemia, anemia, LFT elevations, hypertriglyceridemia, leukopenia.

Allergic Potential: Low

Safety in Pregnancy: C

Cerebrospinal Fluid Penetration: Lamivudine = 12%; zidovudine = 60%

REFERENCES:

Panel on Antiretroviral Guidelines for Adults and Adolescents. Guidelines for the use of antiretroviral agents in HIV-1-infected adults and adolescents, updated July 14, 2016. Department of Health and Human Services; 1–288. Available at https://aidsinfo.nih.gov/contentfiles/lvguidelines/adultandadolescentgl.pdf.

Product Information: Combivir oral tablets, lamivudine zidovudine oral tablets. ViiV Healthcare (per FDA), Research Triangle Park, NC; 2015.

Staszewski S, Morales-Ramirez J, Trashima KT, et al. Efavirenz plus zidovudine and lamivudine, efavirenz plus indinavir, and indinavir plus zidovudine and lamivudine in the treatment of HIV-1 infection in adults. N Engl J Med. 1999;341:1865–1873.

Ledipasvir/Sofosbuvir (Harvoni) (LDV/SOF)

Drug Class: anti-hepatitis C agents; ledipasvir (NS5A replication complex inhibitor) and sofosbuvir (nucleotide NS5B polymerase inhibitor)

Indication: Active against HCV genotypes (GT) 1, 4, 5, and 6

Usual Dose: 1 tablet by mouth once daily with or without food

How Supplied: Oral tablet (containing ledipasvir 90 mg and sofosbuvir 400 < mg

Treatment Duration: 12 or 24 weeks (see below):

Genotype 1	Treatment-naïve without cirrhosis or with compensated cirrhosis (Child-Pugh A)	LDV/SOF × 12 weeks*
	Treatment-experienced※ without cirrhosis	LDV/SOF × 12 weeks
	Treatment-experienced※ with compensated cirrhosis (Child-Pugh A)	LDV/SOF × 24 weeks
	Treatment-naïve and experienced※ with decompensated cirrhosis (Child-Pugh B or C)	LDV/SOF + RBV¶ × 12 weeks

"Usual dose" assumes normal renal/hepatic function. * For renal insufficiency, give usual dose × 1 followed by maintenance dose per CrCl. For dialysis patients, dose the same as for CrCl < 10 mL/min and give supplemental (post-HD/PD dose) immediately after dialysis. CrCl = creatinine clearance; CVVH = continuous venovenous hemofiltration; HD/PD = hemodialysis/peritoneal dialysis. See pp. 204–207 for explanations, pp. xi–xii for abbreviations.

Genotype 1 or 4	Treatment-naïve and experienced※ liver transplant recipients without cirrhosis, or with compensated cirrhosis (Child-Pugh A)	LDV/SOF + RBV¶ × 12 weeks
Genotype 4, 5, or 6	Treatment-naïve and experienced※ without cirrhosis or with compensated cirrhosis (Child-Pugh A)	LDV/SOF × 12 weeks

LDV/SOF: ledipasvir/sofosbuvir; RBV: ribavirin.

*May consider shortening duration to 8 weeks for naïve patients without cirrhosis and pre-treatment HCV viral load < 6 million IU/mL. Do not shorten duration if: African-American, IL-28B CT/ TT, or HIV positive.

※Treatment-experienced is defined as failure of a previous regimen containing PegIFN/RBV with or without a HCV protease inhibitor.

¶ Ribavirin dosing in eligible patients with normal renal function: (1) Compensated cirrhosis (Child-Pugh A): ribavirin 1000 mg/day (if weight ≤ 75 kg) or 1200 mg/day (if weight > 75 kg) in 2 divided doses with food; (2): Decompensated cirrhosis (Child-Pugh B or C): initiate ribavirin at 600 mg/day and titrate if/as tolerated to 1000 mg/day (weight < 75 kg) or 1200 mg/day (weight > 75 kg) in 2 divided doses with food. If unable to tolerate at the initial dose, further dose reductions can be made.

Pharmacokinetic Parameters:
Peak serum level: 323/618 ng/mL
Excreted unchanged: 70% feces (LDV), 80% (urine), 14% (feces) (SOF)

Serum half-life: 47 h (LDV); 0.5 h (SOF); 27 h (GS-331007)
Plasma protein binding: > 99.8/61–65%
Primary Mode of Elimination: Fecal/renal
Dosage Adjustments:

CrCl > 30 mL/min	No change
CrCl < 30 mL/min or HD*	Not recommended
CVVH dose	Not recommended
Mild-moderate (Child-Pugh A/B) hepatic insufficiency	No change
Severe (Child-Pugh C) hepatic insufficiency	No change

*Renal dysfunction: Not recommended due to high exposure of sofosbuvir metabolite, GS-331007.

Drug Interactions: Both LDV and SOF are substrates of P-gp and BCRP; GS-331007 is not. P-gp inducers may decrease concentrations of LDV/SOF and are not recommended. Coadministration with drugs that inhibit P-gp and/or BCRP may increase LDV/SOF, but not GS-331007. Inhibitors of P-gp and/or BCRP may be coadministered with LDV/SOF.

Warnings: Amiordarone: Not recommended due to risk of serious symptomatic bradycardia, particularly when taken in combination with beta blockers or in patients with underlying cardiac disease and/or advanced liver disease. P-gp inducers may decrease LDV/SOF concentrations and reduce effectiveness; coadministration is not recommended.

Acid-reducing agents (↓ solubility and plasma LDV concentrations): Separate antacids and LDV/SOF by 4 hours; administer H_2-receptor antagonists (dose not

---

"Usual dose" assumes normal renal/hepatic function. * For renal insufficiency, give usual dose × 1 followed by maintenance dose per CrCl. For dialysis patients, dose the same as for CrCl < 10 mL/min and give supplemental (post-HD/PD dose) immediately after dialysis. CrCl = creatinine clearance; CVVH = continuous venovenous hemofiltration; HD/PD = hemodialysis/peritoneal dialysis. See pp. 204–207 for explanations, pp. xi–xii for abbreviations.

to exceed comparable to famotidine 40 mg twice daily) simultaneously or 12 hours apart from LDV/SOF. Proton pump inhibitors (NTE doses comparable to omeprazole 20 mg) may be administered simultaneously with LDV/SOF on empty stomach.

LDV/SOF ↑ digoxin (monitor levels); anticonvulsants (carbamazepine, phenytoin, phenobarbital, oxcarbazepine) ↓ LDV/SOF and are not recommended. Antimycobacterials (rifampin, rifabutin, rifapentene) ↓ LDV/SOF and are not recommended.

LDV/SOF ↑ tenofovir concentrations. If given without HIV protease inhibitor or cobicistat, monitor renal function. If administered with HIV protease inhibitor (atazanavir, darunavir, lopinavir) and/or cobicistat-containing regimen, consider alternative treatments. LVD/SOF not recommended with the following: tipranavir/ritonavir (↓ LDV/SOF); simeprevir (↑ LDV & ↑ simeprevir), St. John's wort (↓ LDV/SOF), and rosuvastatin (↑ rosuvastatin).

Adverse Effects: Common (≥ 5%): asthenia (31–36%), fatigue (4–18%), headache (11–29%), diarrhea (3–7%), nausea (6–9%), dyspnea (3–9%), cough (5–11%), irritability (7–8%), skin rash (2–8%), dizziness (1–5%)

Allergic Potential: Low

Safety in Pregnancy: No human pregnancy data for LDV or SOF. No evidence of adverse developmental outcomes in animal studies.

If used with ribavirin (contraindicated in pregnancy), pregnancy warnings for ribavirin apply to the combination. See ribavirin prescribing information for details.

REFERENCES:

AASLD-IDSA. Recommendations for testing, managing, and treating hepatitis C. http://www.hcvguidelines.org. Accessed on September 27, 2016.

Afdhal N, Zeuzem S, Kwo P, et al. Ledipasvir and sofosbuvir for untreated HCV genotype 1 infection. N Engl J Med. 2014;370(20):1889–1898.

O'Brien TR, Lang Kuhs KA, Pfeiffer RM. Subgroup differences in response to 8 weeks of ledipasvir/sofosbuvir for chronic hepatitis C. Open Forum Infect Dis. 2014.

Product Information: Harvoni oral tablets, ledipasvir, sofosbuvir oral tablets. Gilead Sciences Inc., Foster City, CA; 2016.

Wilder JM, Jeffers LJ, Ravendhran N, et al. Safety and efficacy of ledipasvir-sofosbuvir in black patients with hepatitis C virus infection: A retrospective analysis of phase 3 data. Hepatology 2016;63(2):437–444.

Lopinavir + Ritonavir (Kaletra) (LPV/r)

Drug Class: Antiretroviral; protease inhibitor combination

Usual Dose: 400/100 mg (PO) bid or 800/200 mg (PO) daily.

Do not use once-daily dosing in the following groups: > 3 LPV-associated mutations, pregnancy, or concomitant EFV, NVP, FPV, NFV, or anticonvulsants. PI-experienced patients or when used with EFV or NVP: 500/125 mg (PO) bid (tablet dosing) or 520/130 mg (PO) bid (solution dosing). Tablets may be given with or without food; administer solution with food.

How Supplied: Oral solution: Contains 80 mg/mL lopinavir +20 mg/mL ritonavir; oral tablet: Available as 100 mg lopinavir + 25 mg ritonavir, or 200 mg lopinavir + 50 mg ritonavir

---

"Usual dose" assumes normal renal/hepatic function. * For renal insufficiency, give usual dose × 1 followed by maintenance dose per CrCl. For dialysis patients, dose the same as for CrCl < 10 mL/min and give supplemental (post-HD/PD dose) immediately after dialysis. CrCl = creatinine clearance; CVVH = continuous venovenous hemofiltration; HD/PD = hemodialysis/peritoneal dialysis. See pp. 204–207 for explanations, pp. xi–xii for abbreviations.

Pharmacokinetic Parameters:
Peak serum level: 9.6/≤ 1 mcg/mL
Bioavailability: No data
Excreted unchanged (urine): 3%
Serum half-life (normal/ESRD): 5–6/5–6 hrs
Plasma protein binding: 99%
Volume of distribution (V$_d$): No data/0.44 L/kg
Primary Mode of Elimination: Hepatic
Dosage Adjustments*

CrCl 50–80 mL/min	No change
CrCl 10–50 mL/min	No change
CrCl < 10 mL/min	No change
Post-HD dose*	None
Post-PD dose	None
CVVH dose	No change
Moderate hepatic insufficiency	No recommendation; use with caution
Severe hepatic insufficiency	No recommendation; use with caution

* Avoid once-daily dosing in patients on HD.

Antiretroviral Dosage Adjustments

Fosamprenavir	Avoid
Delavirdine	No information
Efavirenz	LPV/r tablets 500/125 mg‡ bid; LPV/r oral solution 533/133 mg bid
Indinavir	Indinavir 600 mg bid
Nelfinavir	Same as for efavirenz
Nevirapine	Same as for efavirenz
Rifabutin	Max. dose of rifabutin 150 mg qod (every other day) or 3 times per week

Saquinavir	Saquinavir 1000 mg bid
Etravirine	No change
Maraviroc	150 mg bid
Raltegravir	No information

Drug Interactions: Antiretrovirals, rifabutin, (see dose adjustment grid above); astemizole, terfenadine, benzodiazepines, cisapride, ergotamine, flecainide, pimozide, propafenone, rifampin, statins, St. John's wort (avoid); tenofovir (↓ lopinavir levels, ↑ tenofovir levels). ↓ effectiveness of oral contraceptives. Insufficient data on other drug interactions listed for ritonavir alone; rivaroxaban (↑ rivaroxaban), warfarin (↑ warfarin, monitor INR).

Adverse Effects: Diarrhea (very common), headache, nausea, vomiting, asthenia, ↑ SGOT/SGPT, hepatotoxicity, abdominal pain, pancreatitis, paresthesias, hyperglycemia (including worsening diabetes, new-onset diabetes, DKA), ↑ cholesterol/triglycerides (evaluate risk for coronary disease, pancreatitis), ↑ CPK, ↑ uric acid, fat redistribution, possible increased bleeding in hemophilia. May prolong PR and QT interval; use with caution in patients with underlying structural heart disease, preexisting conduction system abnormalities, ischemic heart disease, or cardiomyopathies.

Allergic Potential: Low
Safety in Pregnancy: C
Comments: Tablet formulation does not require refrigeration and may be taken with or without food. Oral solution contains 42.4% alcohol. Stable until date on label if in refrigerator or 2 months at room temperature.

"Usual dose" assumes normal renal/hepatic function. * For renal insufficiency, give usual dose × 1 followed by maintenance dose per CrCl. For dialysis patients, dose the same as for CrCl < 10 mL/min and give supplemental (post-HD/PD dose) immediately after dialysis. CrCl = creatinine clearance; CVVH = continuous venovenous hemofiltration; HD/PD = hemodialysis/peritoneal dialysis. See pp. 204–207 for explanations, pp. xi–xii for abbreviations.

Lopinavir serum concentrations with moderately fatty meals are increased 54%.

REFERENCES:

Benson CA, Deeks SG, Brun SC, et al. Safety and antiviral activity at 48 weeks of lopinavir/ritonavir plus nevi-rapine and 2 nucleoside reverse-transcriptase inhibi-tors in human immunodeficiency virus type 1-infected protease inhibitor-experienced patients. J Infect Dis. 2002;185:599–60.

Manfredi R, Calza L, Chiodo F. First-line efavirenz versus lopi-navir-ritonavir-based highly active antiretroviral therapy for naïve patients. AIDS. 2004;18:2331–2333.

Panel on Antiretroviral Guidelines for Adults and Adoles-cents. Guidelines for the use of antiretroviral agents in HIV-1-infected adults and adolescents, updated July 14, 2016. Department of Health and Human Services; 1–288. Available at https://aidsinfo.nih.gov/contentfiles/lvguidelines/adultandadolescentgl.pdf.

Riddler S, et al. Initial treatment for HIV infection—an embar-rassment of riches. N Engl J Med. May 15 2008; 358(20): 2095–2106.

Walmsley S, Bernstein B, King M, et al. Lopinavir-ritonavir versus nelfinavir for the initial treatment of HIV infec-tion. N Engl J Med. 2002;346:2039–46.

Maraviroc (Selzentry) (MVC)

Drug Class: Antiretroviral; HIV-1 chemokine receptor 5 (CCR5) antagonist
Usual Dose: 150 mg, 300 mg, or 600 mg (PO) bid, depending on concomitant medications (see below), in CCR5-tropic HIV-1 isolates.
How Supplied: Oral tablet: 150 mg, 300 mg
Pharmacokinetic Parameters:
Peak serum level: 266–618 mcg/mL
Bioavailability: 23–33%
Excreted unchanged: 20% (urine); 76% (feces)
Serum half-life (normal/ESRD): 14–18 h/not studied

Plasma protein binding: 76%
Volume of distribution (V_d): 194 L
Primary Mode of Elimination: Fecal/renal
Dosage Adjustments*

CrCl 50–80 mL/min	No change
CrCl 10–25 mL/min	Use caution
CrCl < 10 mL/min	Use caution
Post-HD dose	No information
Post-PD dose	No information
CVVH dose	No information
Mild hepatic insufficiency	No information
Moderate or severe hepatic insufficiency	No information

Drug Interaction Dosage Adjustments

Strong CYP3A inhibitors (with or without CYP3A inducers) including protease inhibitors (except tipranavir/ritonavir)	150 mg (PO) bid
Tipranavir/ritonavir, nevirapine, raltegravir, all NRTIs and enfuvirtide and other drugs that are not strong inducers or inhibitors of CYP3A	300 mg (PO) bid
CYP inducers- such as efavirenz, etravirine, rifampin, carbamazepine, phenobarbital, phenytoin when given without a CYP 3A inhibitor	600 mg (PO) bid

Drug Interactions: Maraviroc is a substrate of CYP3A and P-glycoprotein and is likely to

---

be modulated by inhibitors and inducers of these enzymes/transporters.

Adverse Effects: Hepatotoxicity has been reported. A systemic allergic reaction (e.g., pruritic rash, eosinophilia, or elevated IgE) prior to the development of hepatotoxicity may occur. Other adverse effects: cough, infection, upper respiratory tract infection, rash, pyrexia, dizziness, abdominal pain, musculoskeletal symptoms (joint/muscle pain). Myocardial infarction/ischemia reported in < 2% in clinical trials. Orthostatic hypotension, especially in patients with severe renal insufficiency.

Allergic Potential: Low

Safety in Pregnancy: B

Comments: Indicated for treatment-experienced adult patients infected with only cellular chemokine receptor (CCR) 5-tropic HIV-1 virus detectable who have evidence of viral replication and HIV-1 strains resistant to multiple antiretroviral agents. Used in combination with other antiretroviral agents. Trofile phenotype test is needed to confirm infection with CCR5-tropic HIV-1 (also known as "R5 virus").

Cerebrospinal Fluid Penetration: MVC CSF: Plasma was 0.022; 0.094 (free MVC) [Tiraboschi et al, 2010]; median MVC CSF: Plasma was 0.03 [Yilmaz et al, 2009].

REFERENCES:

Gulick R. Maraviroc for previously treated patients with R5 HIV-1 infection, N Engl J Med. Oct. 2, 2008; 359(14):1429–41.

Panel on Antiretroviral Guidelines for Adults and Adolescents. Guidelines for the use of antiretroviral agents in HIV-1-infected adults and adolescents, updated July 14, 2016. Department of Health and Human Services; 1–288. Available at https://aidsinfo.nih.gov/contentfiles/lvguidelines/adultandadolescentgl.pdf.

Product Information: Selzentry oral tablets, maraviroc oral tablets. Pfizer Labs, New York, NY; 2007.

Tiraboschi JM, Niubo J, Curto J, et al. Maraviroc concentrations in cerebrospinal fluid in HIV-infected patients. J Acquir Immune Defic Syndr. 2010;55:606–9.

Yilmaz A, Watson V, Else L, et al. Cerebrospinal fluid maraviroc concentrations in HIV-1 infected patients. AIDS 2009;23:2537–40.

Nelfinavir (Viracept) (NFV)

Drug Class: Antiretroviral; protease inhibitor

Usual Dose: 1250 mg (PO) bid or 750 mg (PO) tid; take with food

How Supplied: Oral powder for suspension: 50 mg/g, oral tablet: 250 mg, 625 mg

Pharmacokinetic Parameters:
Peak serum level: 35 mcg/mL
Bioavailability: 20–80%
Excreted unchanged (urine): 1–2%
Serum half-life (normal/ESRD): 4 h/no data
Plasma protein binding: 98%
Volume of distribution (V_d): 5 L/kg

Primary Mode of Elimination: Hepatic

Dosage Adjustments*

CrCl 50–80 mL/min	No change
CrCl 10–50 mL/min	No change
CrCl < 10 mL/min	No change
Post-HD dose	None
Post-PD dose	None
CVVH dose	No change
Mild hepatic insufficiency	No change
Moderate-severe hepatic insufficiency	Avoid

"Usual dose" assumes normal renal/hepatic function. * For renal insufficiency, give usual dose × 1 followed by maintenance dose per CrCl. For dialysis patients, dose the same as for CrCl < 10 mL/min and give supplemental (post-HD/PD dose) immediately after dialysis. CrCl = creatinine clearance; CVVH = continuous venovenous hemofiltration; HD/PD = hemodialysis/peritoneal dialysis. See pp. 204–207 for explanations, pp. xi–xii for abbreviations.

Antiretroviral Dosage Adjustments

Delavirdine	No information (monitor for neutropenia)
Efavirenz	No changes
Indinavir	Limited data for nelfinavir 1250 mg bid + indinavir 1200 mg bid
Lopinavir/ ritonavir	Nelfinavir 1000 mg bid or lopinavir/r 600/150 mg bid
Nevirapine	No changes
Ritonavir	No recommendation
Saquinavir	Saquinavir 1200 mg bid
Rifampin	Avoid combination
Rifabutin	Nelfinavir 1250 mg bid; rifabutin 150 mg QD or 300 mg 2–3×/week
Etravirine	Avoid
Maraviroc	150 mg bid
Raltegravir	No data

Drug Interactions: Antiretrovirals, rifabutin, rifampin (see dose adjustment grid above); amiodarone, quinidine, astemizole, terfenadine, benzodiazepines, cisapride, ergot alkaloids, statins, St. John's wort (avoid); carbamazepine, phenytoin, phenobarbital (↓ nelfinavir levels, ↑ anticonvulsant levels; monitor); caspofungin (↓ caspofungin levels, may ↓ caspofungin effect); clarithromycin, erythromycin, telithromycin (↑ nelfinavir and macrolide levels); didanosine (dosing conflict with food; give nelfinavir with food 2 hours before or 1 hour after didanosine); itraconazole, voriconazole, ketoconazole (↑ nelfinavir levels); lamivudine (↑ lamivudine levels); methadone (may require ↑ methadone dose); oral contraceptives, zidovudine (↓zidovudine levels); sildenafil (↑ or ↓ sildenafil levels; do not exceed 25 mg in 48 hrs), tadalafil (max. 10 mg/72 hrs, vardenafil (max. 2.5 mg/72 hrs); rivaroxaban (↑ rivaroxaban); warfarin (↑ warfarin, monitor INR).

Adverse Effects: Impaired concentration, nausea, abdominal pain, secretory diarrhea, ↑ SGOT/SGPT, rash, ↑ cholesterol/ triglycerides (evaluate risk for coronary disease/pancreatitis), fat redistribution, hyperglycemia (including worsening diabetes, new-onset diabetes, DKA), possible increased bleeding in hemophilia.

Allergic Potential: Low

Safety in Pregnancy: B

Comments: Take with food (absorption increased 300%)

Cerebrospinal Fluid Penetration: Undetectable

REFERENCES:

DiCenzo R, Forrest A, Fischl MA, et al. Pharmacokinetics of indinavir and nelfinavir in treatment-naïve, human immunodeficiency virus-infected subjects. Antimicrob Agents Chemother. 2004;48:918–23.

Kaul DR, Cinti SK, Carver PL, et al. HIV protease inhibitors: Advances in therapy and adverse reactions, including metabolic complications. Pharmacotherapy. 1999;19:281–98.

Panel on Antiretroviral Guidelines for Adults and Adolescents, updated July 14, 2016. Guidelines for the use of antiretroviral agents in HIV-1-infected adults and adolescents, updated July 14,2016. Department of Health and Human Services; 1–288. Available at https://aidsinfo.nih.gov/contentfiles/lvguidelines/adultandadolescentgl.pdf.

Walmsley S, Bernstein B, King M, et al. Lopinavir-ritonavir versus nelfinavir for the initial treatment of HIV infection. N Engl J Med. 2002;346:2039–46.

"Usual dose" assumes normal renal/hepatic function. * For renal insufficiency, give usual dose × 1 followed by maintenance dose per CrCl. For dialysis patients, dose the same as for CrCl < 10 mL/min and give supplemental (post-HD/PD dose) immediately after dialysis. CrCl = creatinine clearance; CVVH = continuous venovenous hemofiltration; HD/PD = hemodialysis/peritoneal dialysis. See pp. 204–207 for explanations, pp. xi–xii for abbreviations.

Nevirapine (Viramune) (NVP)

Drug Class: Antiretroviral; NNRTI (non-nucleoside reverse transcriptase inhibitor).
Usual Dose: Initiate with 200 mg (PO) daily × 2 weeks, then 200 mg (PO) bid thereafter; after initial dose escalation, extended release formulation is 400 mg QD.
How Supplied: Oral suspension: 50 mg/5 mL; oral tablet: 200 mg; oral tablet, extended release: 400 mg.
Pharmacokinetic Parameters:
Peak serum level: 0.9–3.6 mcg/mL
Bioavailability: 90%
Excreted unchanged (urine): 5%
Serum half-life (normal): 40 h
Plasma protein binding: 60%
Volume of distribution (V_d): 1.4 L/kg
Primary Mode of Elimination: Hepatic
Dosage Adjustments*

CrCl > 20 mL/min	No change
CrCl < 20 mL/min	No change; use caution
Post-HD dose	Limited data/no recommendation
Post-PD dose	None
CVVH dose	No change
Mild hepatic insufficiency	No change
Moderate-severe hepatic insufficiency	Avoid

Antiretroviral Dosage Adjustments

Delavirdine	No information
Efavirenz	Avoid combination
Indinavir	Indinavir 1000 mg tid
Lopinavir/ ritonavir (l/r)	Consider l/r 600/150 mg bid in PI-experienced patients
Nelfinavir	No information
Ritonavir	No change
Saquinavir	No information
Rifampin	Not recommended
Rifabutin	Use caution
Etravirine	Avoid combination
Maraviroc	Without PI: MVC 300 mg bid; with PI (except TPV/r): MVC 150 mg bid
Raltegravir	No data

Drug Interactions: Antiretrovirals, rifabutin, rifampin (see dose adjustment grid above); carbamazepine, phenobarbital, phenytoin (monitor anticonvulsant levels); caspofungin (↓ caspofungin levels, may ↓ caspofungin effect); ethinyl estradiol (↓ ethinyl estradiol levels; use additional/alternative method); ketoconazole (avoid); voriconazole (↑ nevirapine levels); methadone (↓ methadone levels; titrate methadone dose to effect); tacrolimus (↓ tacrolimus levels).
Adverse Effects: Drug fever/rash (may be severe; usually occurs within 6 weeks), Stevens-Johnson syndrome, ↑SGOT/SGPT, *fatal hepatitis*, headache, diarrhea, leukopenia, stomatitis, peripheral neuropathy, paresthesias. Greater risk of fatal hepatitis and Stevens-Johnson syndrome when CD4 > 400/mm³ (males) or > 250/mm³ (females) (monitor patients intensely for first 18 weeks of therapy).
Allergic Potential: High
Safety in Pregnancy: B
Comments: Absorption not affected by food. Not to be used for post exposure prophylaxis because of potential for fatal hepatitis.

"Usual dose" assumes normal renal/hepatic function. * For renal insufficiency, give usual dose × 1 followed by maintenance dose per CrCl. For dialysis patients, dose the same as for CrCl < 10 mL/min and give supplemental (post-HD/PD dose) immediately after dialysis. CrCl = creatinine clearance; CVVH = continuous venovenous hemofiltration; HD/PD = hemodialysis/peritoneal dialysis. See pp. 204–207 for explanations, pp. xi–xii for abbreviations.

Cerebrospinal Fluid Penetration: 45%

REFERENCES:

Johnson S, Chan J, Bennett CL. Hepatotoxicity after prophylaxis with a nevirapine containing antiretroviral regimen. Ann Intern Med. 2002;137:146–7.

Negredo E, Ribalta J, Paredes R, et al. Reversal of atherogenic lipoprotein profile in HIV 1 infected patients with lipodystrophy after replacing protease inhibitors by nevirapine. AIDS. 2002;16:1383–9.

Panel on Antiretroviral Guidelines for Adults and Adolescents. Guidelines for the use of antiretroviral agents in HIV-1-infected adults and adolescents, updated July 14, 2016. Department of Health and Human Services; 1–288. Available at https://aidsinfo.nih.gov/contentfiles/lvguidelines/adultandadolescentgl.pdf.

Product Information: Viramune oral tablets, oral suspension, nevirapine oral tablets, oral suspension. Boehringer Ingelheim Pharmaceuticals, Inc., Ridgefield, CT; 2014.

Paritaprevir/Ritonavir/Ombitasvir (Technivie) (OBV/PTV/r, PrO)

Drug Class: Anti-hepatitis C agents; paritaprevir (NS3/4A protease inhibitor), ritonavir (CYP3A inhibitor), ombitasvir (NS5A replication complex inhibitor)
Indication: Hepatitis C virus, genotype 4 without cirrhosis
Usual Dose: 2 tablets (paritaprevir 75 mg, ritonavir 50 mg, ombitasvir 12.5 mg) once daily in the morning with food.
How Supplied: Tablets (containing paritaprevir 75 mg, ritonavir 50 mg, and ombitasvir 12.5 mg
Treatment Duration: 12 weeks

Genotype 4 without cirrhosis*	Paritaprevir/ritonavir/ombitasvir + RBV	12 weeks

RBV: ribavirin

* See HCV guidelines for off-label use in genotype 4 patients with compensated cirrhosis.

Pharmacokinetic Parameters:
Peak serum level: 194/543/82 ng/mL
Bioavailability: When given with ritonavir 100 mg: 52.6% (PTV); 48.1% (OMB)
Excreted unchanged(urine/feces): 0.05/1.1% (PTV); 0.03/87.3% (OMB)
Serum half-life (normal): 5.5/4/21–25 h
Plasma protein binding: 97/ > 99/99.9%
Volume of distribution (Vd): 16.7/ 21.5/50.1 L
Primary Mode of Elimination: Fecal/fecal/fecal
Dosage Adjustments:

CrCl > 30 mL/min	No change
CrCl < 30 mL/min (not on dialysis)	No change
Post-HD dose	Not studied
Post-PD dose	Not studied
CVVH dose	Not studied
Mild hepatic insufficiency (Child-Pugh A)	No change
Moderate-severe hepatic insufficiency (Child-Pugh B or C)	Contraindicated

Drug Interactions:
Paritaprevir: CYP3A substrate, P-gp substrate, BCRP substrate, OATP-1B1/3 substrate
Ritonavir: CYP3A substrate, P-gp substrate
Ombitasvir: Undergoes hydrolysis (primary); P-gp substrate, BCRP substrate

----

"Usual dose" assumes normal renal/hepatic function. * For renal insufficiency, give usual dose × 1 followed by maintenance dose per CrCl. For dialysis patients, dose the same as for CrCl < 10 mL/min and give supplemental (post-HD/PD dose) immediately after dialysis. CrCl = creatinine clearance; CVVH = continuous venovenous hemofiltration; HD/PD = hemodialysis/peritoneal dialysis. See pp. 204–207 for explanations, pp. xi–xii for abbreviations.

Contraindicated: Drugs highly dependent on CYP3A for clearance and moderate-to-strong CYP3A inducers.

Paritaprevir/ritonavir/ombitasvir increases the plasma concentrations of: alfuzosin, colchicine, estradiol-containing agents, efavirenz (resulting in ↑liver enzymes), lovastatin, simvastatin, pimozide, sildenafil (dosed for PAH), triazolam, oral midazolam.

Plasma concentrations of paritaprevir/ritonavir/ombitasvir reduced by: Anticonvulsants (carbamazepine, phenytoin, phenobarbital), rifampin, ergot derivatives (ergotamine, dhydroergotamine, methylergonovine), St. John's wort

Other Significant Interactions:

The following are ↑ by paritaprevir/ritonavir/ombitasvir: digoxin, antiarrhythmics (amiodarone, bepridil, disopyramide, flecainide, lidocaine [systemic], mexilteine, propafenone, quinidine), ketoconazole, quetiapine, calcium channel blockers, inhaled fluticasone, furosemide, rilpivirine (QT risk), rosuvastatin (max. 10 mg/d), pravastatin (max. 40 mg/d), cyclosporine, tacrolimus, salmeterol (QT risk), alprazolam

The following are ↓ by paritaprevir/ritonavir/ombitasvir: voriconazole, darunavir, carisprodol, cyclobenzaprine (& metabolite), omeprazole, diazepam (& metabolite)

The following ↑ paritaprevir concentrations: atazanavir, lopinavir

Other: metformin (increased risk of lactic acidosis with paritaprevir)

Adverse Effects:
Contraindicated in patients with moderate-to-severe hepatic impairment (due to risk of hepatic decompensation, with outcomes such as liver transplant or fatality).
Asthenia (25–29%), fatigue (7–15%), nausea (9–14%), pruritis (5–7%), rash (5–7%), hyperbilirubinemia (5%), ALT elevations (1%)

Allergic Potential: *Hypersensitivity reactions reported (including angioedema).*

Safety in Pregnancy: No human pregnancy data for paritaprevir/ritonavir, and ombitasvir. No evidence of adverse developmental outcomes in animal studies.

If used with ribavirin (contraindicated in pregnancy), the pregnancy warnings apply to the combination regimen.

Comments:
Contraindicated in patients with moderate-to-severe hepatic impairment.

Close monitoring of hepatic function is required (at baseline, every 4 weeks, and as clinically indicated). Do not administer to patients who are HIV positive not on antiretrovirals.

High drug interaction potential.

REFERENCES:

AASLD-IDSA. Recommendations for testing, managing, and treating hepatitis C. http://www.hcvguidelines.org. Accessed on September 27, 2016.

Asselah T, Hassanien T, Qaqish RB, et al. P1345: A randomized, open-label study to evaluate efficacy and safety of ombitasvir/paritaprevir/ritonavir co-administered with ribavirin in adults with genotype 4 chronic hepatitis C infection and cirrhosis. Journal of Hepatology, April 2015;62:S861.

Product Information: Technivie oral tablets, ombitasvir, paritaprevir, ritonavir oral tablets. AbbVie Inc. (per manufacturer), North Chicago, IL: 2015.

Paritaprevir/Ritonavir/Ombitasvir/Dasabuvir (Viekira Pak, Viekira XR) (PrOD)

Drug Class: Anti-hepatitis C agents; paritaprevir (NS3/4A protease inhibitor),

---

"Usual dose" assumes normal renal/hepatic function. * For renal insufficiency, give usual dose × 1 followed by maintenance dose per CrCl. For dialysis patients, dose the same as for CrCl < 10 mL/min and give supplemental (post-HD/PD dose) immediately after dialysis. CrCl = creatinine clearance; CVVH = continuous venovenous hemofiltration; HD/PD = hemodialysis/peritoneal dialysis. See pp. 204–207 for explanations, pp. xi–xii for abbreviations.

ritonavir (CYP3A inhibitor), ombitasvir (NS5A replication complex inhibitor), dasabuvir (NS5B non-nucleoside polymerase inhibitor)

Indication: Hepatitis C virus, genotype 1a and 1b in patients without cirrhosis or with compensated cirrhosis only

Usual Dose:

Immediate-release formulation: 2 tablets (paritaprevir 75 mg, ritonavir 50 mg, ombitasvir 12.5 mg) once daily plus dasabuvir 250 mg 1 tablet twice daily with food.

Extended-release formulation: 3 tablets (paritaprevir 50 mg, ritonavir 33.3 mg, ombitasvir 8.33 mg, and dasabuvir 200 mg) once daily with food.

How Supplied:

Immediate release formulation (Viekira Pak): Available as a kit containing:

- Combination tablet of paritaprevir 75 mg, ritonavir 50 mg, and ombitasvir 12.5 mg

- Dasabuvir 250 mg tablets

Extended-release (Viekira XR): Tablets containing paritaprevir 50 mg, ritonavir 33.3 mg, ombitasvir 8.33 mg, and dasabuvir 200 mg

Treatment Duration: 12–24 weeks (see below)

Genotype 1a without cirrhosis	Paritaprevir, ritonavir, ombitasvir, and dasabuvir + RBV*	12 weeks
Genotype 1a with compensated cirrhosis (Child-Pugh A)	Paritaprevir, ritonavir, ombitasvir, and dasabuvir + RBV*	24 weeks
Genotype 1b with or without compensated cirrhosis (Child-Pugh A)	Paritaprevir, ritonavir, ombitasvir, and dasabuvir	12 weeks

RBV: ribavirin.

*Ribavirin dose in normal renal function is weight based: < 75 kg = 1000 mg/day; > 75 kg = 1200 mg/day. Give in 2 divided doses with food.

Pharmacokinetic Parameters:

Bioavailability: 70% (dasabuvir); others unknown

Serum half-life (normal): 5.5/4/21–25/5.5–6 h

Plasma protein binding: 97/ > 99/99.9/ > 99.5%

Volume of distribution (Vd): 16.7/21.5/ 50.1/396 L

Primary Mode of Elimination: Fecal/fecal/fecal/fecal

Dosage Adjustments:

CrCl > 30 mL/min	No change
CrCl < 30 mL/min (not on dialysis)	No change
Post-HD dose*	Not studied
Post-PD dose	Not studied
CVVH dose	Not studied
Mild hepatic insufficiency (Child-Pugh A)	No change
Moderate-severe hepatic insufficiency (Child-Pugh B or C)	Contraindicated

*No adjustment needed at any level of renal impairment, including dialysis.

"Usual dose" assumes normal renal/hepatic function. * For renal insufficiency, give usual dose × 1 followed by maintenance dose per CrCl. For dialysis patients, dose the same as for CrCl < 10 mL/min and give supplemental (post-HD/PD dose) immediately after dialysis. CrCl = creatinine clearance; CVVH = continuous venovenous hemofiltration; HD/PD = hemodialysis/peritoneal dialysis. See pp. 204–207 for explanations, pp. xi–xii for abbreviations.

Contraindicated in patients with moderate-severe hepatic impairment (due to risk of hepatic decompensation, with outcomes requiring liver transplant or fatality).

Drug Interactions: Factors affecting potential for drug interactions are outlined for each agent below:

Paritaprevir: CYP3A substrate, P-gp substrate, BCRP substrate, OATP-1B1/3 substrate

Ritonavir: CYP3A substrate, P-gp substrate

Ombitasvir: Undergoes hydrolysis (primary); P-gp substrate, BCRP substrate

Dasabuvir: CYP2C8 substrate, P-gp substrate, BCRP substrate

Contraindicated: Estradiol-containing medications, CYP3A substrates, moderate to strong CYP3A inducers, strong inducers and inhibitors of CYP2C8

The following are ↑ by paritaprevir/ritonavir/ombitasvir/dasabuvir: alfuzosin, ranolazine, dronedarone, colchicine, lurasidone, pimozide, ergot derivatives (ergotamine, dihydroergotamine, methylergonovine), ethinyl estradiol-containing products, cisapride, simvastatin, lovastatin, efavirenz (resulting in ↑liver enzymes), sildenafil (when dosed for PAH), triazolam, oral midazolam

The following ↓ paritaprevir/ritonavir/ombitasvir/dasabuvir concentrations: Anticonvulsants (carbamazepine, phenytoin, phenobarbital), rifampin, St. John's wort

The following ↑ paritaprevir/ritonavir/ombitasvir/dasabuvir concentrations: gemfibrozil (↑ dasabuvir, increasing risk of prolonging QT), buprenorphine (& metabolite), hydrocodone

Other Significant Interactions:

The following are ↑ by paritaprevir/ritonavir/ombitasvir/dasabuvir: digoxin (reduce dose by 30–50%), antiarrhythmics (amiodarone, bepridil, disopyramide, flecainide, lidocaine [systemic], mexilteine, propafenone, quinidine), ketoconazole, quetiapine, amlodipine, inhaled fluticasone, furosemide, rilpivirine (QT risk), pravastatin (max. 40 mg/d), cyclosporine, tacrolimus, salmeterol (QT risk), alprazolam, buprenorphine/naloxone

The following are ↓ by paritaprevir/ritonavir/ombitasvir/dasabuvir: voriconazole, darunavir, omeprazole

The following ↑ paritaprevir concentrations: atazanavir, lopinavir

Adverse Effects:

Contraindicated in patients with moderate-severe hepatic impairment (due to risk of hepatic decompensation, with outcomes requiring liver transplant or fatality).

Other: Nausea (8% without ribavirin, 16–24% with ribavirin), fatigue (34–50% with ribavirin), skin reactions (7% without ribavirin, 10–24% with ribavirin) pruritis, insomnia (5% without ribavirin, 12–26% with ribavirin), asthenia, ALT increase (1%)

Allergic Potential: *Hypersensitivity reactions reported (including angioedema).*

Safety in Pregnancy: No human pregnancy data for paritaprevir/ritonavir, ombitasvir, and dasabuvir. No evidence of adverse developmental outcomes on animal studies. *If used with ribavirin, the pregnancy warnings apply to the combination regimen.*

Comments: Do not use in moderate-to-severe hepatic impairment.

"Usual dose" assumes normal renal/hepatic function. * For renal insufficiency, give usual dose × 1 followed by maintenance dose per CrCl. For dialysis patients, dose the same as for CrCl < 10 mL/min and give supplemental (post-HD/PD dose) immediately after dialysis. CrCl = creatinine clearance; CVVH = continuous venovenous hemofiltration; HD/PD = hemodialysis/peritoneal dialysis. See pp. 204–207 for explanations, pp. xi–xii for abbreviations.

Do not administer to patients who are HIV positive not on antiretrovirals.

Close monitoring of hepatic function is required (at baseline, every 4 weeks, and as clinically indicated).

High drug interaction potential.

REFERENCES:

AASLD-IDSA. Recommendations for testing, managing, and treating hepatitis C. http://www.hcvguidelines.org. Accessed on September 27, 2016.

Feld JJ, Kowdley KV, Coakley E, et al. Treatment of HCV with ABT-450/r-ombitasvir and dasabuvir with ribavirin. N Engl J Med. 2014;370(17):1594–1603.

Ferenci P, Bernstein D, Lalezari J, et al. ABT-450/r-ombitasvir and dasabuvir with or without ribavirin for HCV. N Engl J Med. 2014;370(21):1983–92.

Poordad F, Hezode C, Trinh R, et al. ABT-450/r-ombitasvir and dasabuvir with ribavirin for hepatitis C with cirrhosis. N Engl J Med. 2014;370:1973–82.

Product Information: Viekira Pak oral tablets, ombitasvir, paritaprevir, ritonavir oral tablets and dasabuvir oral tablets. AbbVie Inc. (per manufacturer), North Chicago, IL; 2014.

Product Information: Viekira XR oral extended-release tablets, dasabuvir, ombitasvir, paritaprevir, ritonavir oral extended-release tablets. AbbVie Inc. (per FDA), North Chicago, IL; 2016.

Raltegravir (Isentress) (RAL)

Drug Class: Antiretroviral; HIV-1 integrase inhibitor
Usual Dose: 400 mg (PO) bid
How Supplied: Oral tablet: 400 mg
Pharmacokinetic Parameters:
Peak serum level: 6.5 μM
Bioavailability: ~ 32% (20–43%)
Excreted unchanged: 51% (feces); 9% (urine)
Serum half-life: 9–12 h
Plasma protein binding: 83%

Volume of distribution (V_d): Not studied
Primary Mode of Elimination: Fecal/renal
Dosage Adjustments*

CrCl 50–80 mL/min	No change
CrCl 10–50 mL/min	No change
CrCl < 10 mL/min	No information
Post-HD dose	No information
Post-PD dose	No information
CVVH dose	No information
Mild/moderate hepatic insufficiency	No change
Severe hepatic insufficiency	No information

Antiretroviral Dosage Adjustments

Atazanavir	No change
Atazanavir/ritonavir	No change
Efavirenz	No change
Rifampin	Raltegravir 800 mg bid
Ritonavir	No change
Tenofovir	No change
Tipranavir/ritonavir	No change
Etravirine	No change
Nevirapine	No data
Maraviroc	No change

Drug Interactions: rifampin (↓ raltegravir levels, double dose to 800 mg BID). Omeprazole (↑ raltegravir levels, no adjustment needed). In vitro, raltegravir

---

"Usual dose" assumes normal renal/hepatic function. * For renal insufficiency, give usual dose × 1 followed by maintenance dose per CrCl. For dialysis patients, dose the same as for CrCl < 10 mL/min and give supplemental (post-HD/PD dose) immediately after dialysis. CrCl = creatinine clearance; CVVH = continuous venovenous hemofiltration; HD/PD = hemodialysis/peritoneal dialysis. See pp. 204–207 for explanations, pp. xi–xii for abbreviations.

does not inhibit CYP1A2, CYP2B6, CYP2C8, CYP2C9, CYP2C19, CYP2D6, or CYP3A and does not induce CYP3A4. In addition, raltegravir does not inhibit P-glycoprotein-mediated transport. Raltegravir is therefore not expected to affect the pharmacokinetics of drugs that are substrates of these enzymes or P-glycoprotein (e.g., protease inhibitors, NNRTIs, methadone, opioid analgesics, statins, azole antifungals, proton pump inhibitors, oral contraceptives, anti-erectile dysfunction agents).

Adverse Effects: Nausea, headache, diarrhea, pyrexia. CPK elevations, myopathy, and rhabdomyolysis have been reported—use with caution in patients at increased risk for myopathy or rhabdomyolysis, such as those receiving concomitant medications known to cause these conditions (e.g., statins).

Allergic Potential: Low

Safety in Pregnancy: C

Comments: May be taken with or without food. Raltegravir is indicated for treatment-naïve and treatment-experienced adult patients who have evidence of viral replication and HIV-1 strains resistant to multiple antiretroviral agents. Treatment-experienced patients who switch to raltegravir must have a least two other fully active agents in their regimen.

Cerebrospinal Fluid Penetration: Median total RAL concentration: 14.5–31 ng/mL

REFERENCES:

Iwamoto M, Wenning LA, Nguyen BY, et al. Effects of omeprazole on plasma levels of raltegravir. Clin Infect Dis. Feb 15 2009;48(4):489–492.

Iwamoto M, Wenning LA, Petry AS, et al. Safety, tolerability, and pharmacokinetics of raltegravir after single and multiple doses in healthy subjects. Clin Pharmacol Ther. 2007;83:293–9.

Product Information. Isentress oral tablets, raltegravir oral tablets. Merck & Co, Inc, Whitehouse Station, NJ; 2007.

Wenning LA, Hanley WD, Brainard DM, et al. Effect of rifampin, a potent inducer of drug-metabolizing enzymes, on the pharmacokinetics of raltegravir. Antimicrob Agents Chemother. July 2009;53(7):2852–56.

Panel on Antiretroviral Guidelines for Adults and Adolescents. Guidelines for the use of antiretroviral agents in HIV-1-infected adults and adolescents, updated July 14, 2016. Department of Health and Human Services; 1–288. Available at https://aidsinfo.nih.gov/contentfiles/lvguidelines/adultandadolescentgl.pdf.

Croteau D, Letendre S, Best BM, et al. Total raltegravir concentrations in cerebrospinal fluid exceed the 50-percent inhibitory concentration for wild-type HIV-1. Antimicrob Agents Chemother. 2010;54;5156–60.

Yilmaz A, Gisslén M, Spudich S, et al. Raltegravir cerebrospinal fluid concentrations in HIV-1 infection. PLoS ONE. 2009;4(9):e6877. doi: 10.1371/journal.pone.0006877

Calgano A, Cusato J, Simiele M, et al. High interpatient variability of raltegravir CSF concentrations in HIV positive patients: A pharmacogenetics analysis. J Antimicrob Chemother. 2014;69:241–5.

Rilpivirine (Edurant) (RPV)

Drug Class: Antiretroviral; NNRTI (non-nucleoside reverse transcriptase inhibitor)

Usual Dose: 25 mg (PO) daily with food (treatment-naïve with baseline HIV viral load VL) < 100,000 copies/mL)

How Supplied: Oral tablet: 25 mg

Pharmacokinetic Parameters:

Peak serum level: Not reported
Bioavailability: Not reported
Excreted unchanged: 25% (feces)/6.1% (urine)
Serum half-life (normal/ESRD): 50 h/no data
Plasma protein binding: 99.7% (primarily albumin)
Volume of distribution (Vd): Not studied

Primary Mode of Elimination: Fecal

Dosage Adjustments*

CrCl 50–80 mL/min	No change
CrCl 30–49 mL/min	No change
CrCl < 30 mL/min	No change
ESRD	No change
Post-HD dose	No change
Post-PD dose	No change
CVVH dose	No change
Mild-moderate hepatic insufficiency	No change
Severe hepatic insufficiency	No data, use caution

Antiretroviral Dosage Adjustments: It is not recommended to coadminister rilpivirine with other NNRTIs. No dose adjustment is needed when rilpivirine is coadministered with boosted and unboosted protease inhibitors.

Drug Interactions: Rilpivirine is primarily metabolized by cytochrome P450 CYP3A. Drugs that can induce or inhibit CYP3A can affect plasma concentrations of rilpivirine. Coadministration of rilpivirine with drugs that increase gastric pH may result in decreased plasma concentrations of rilpivirine. Drugs that may reduce rilpivirine plasma concentrations: Antacids, cimetidine, famotidine, ranitidine, esomeprazole, omeprazole, pantoparazole, lansoprazole, rabeprazole, nizatidine, rifampin, rifapentine, rifabutin, phenytoin, phenobarbital, oxcarbazepine. Drugs that may increase rilpivirine plasma concentrations: ketoconazole, itraconazole, voriconazole, posaconazole, clarithromycin, erythromycin.

Rilpivirine may decrease methadone concentrations.

Adverse Effects: Rash 3%, lipodystrophy, serum cholesterol raised, serum triglycerides raised, nausea/vomiting < 1%, elevated ALT/AST/serum bilirubin < 2%, membranous glomerulonephritis < 2%, mesangial proliferative glomerulonephritis < 2%, ↑ serum creatinine < 1%, dizziness/headache/insomnia < 2%, depression and suicidal thoughts: rare, vivid dreams: rare.

Allergic Potential: Low

Safety in Pregnancy: B

Comments: Must be taken with a meal (preferably high fat); rilpivirine exposure was about 40% lower when administered in the fasted state. Use with caution in patients with severe depressive disorders as depression, dysphoria, major depression, mood alteration, negative thoughts, suicide attempt, and suicidal ideation have been reported with rilpivirine. In clinical trials patients with HIV-1 RNA > 100,000 copies/mL at therapy initiation experienced virologic failure more often than patients with HIV-1 RNA < 100,000 copies/mL at the start of therapy. Patients who experience virological failure on rilpivirine may be at risk for cross-resistance to other NNRTIs and to emtricitabine/lamivudine.

Cerebrospinal Fluid Penetration: (mean RPV CSF): 0.8 ng/mL

Alias: TMC-278

REFERENCES:

Cohen CJ, Andrade-Villanueva J, Clotet B, et al: Rilpivirine versus efavirenz with two background nucleoside or nucleotide reverse transcriptase inhibitors in treatment-naïve adults infected with HIV-1 (THRIVE): A phase 3, randomized, non-inferiority trial. Lancet 2011;378(9787):229–37.

Molina JM, Cahn P, Grinsztejn B, et al. Rilpivirine versus efavirenz with tenofovir and emtricitabine in treatment-naive adults infected with HIV-1 (ECHO): A phase 3 randomized double-blind active-controlled trial. Lancet 2011;378(9787):238–46.

Mora-Peris B, Watson V, Vera JH, et al. Rilpivirine exposure in plasma and sanctuary site compartments after switching from nevirapine-containing combined antiretroviral therapy. J Antimicrob Chemother. 2014;69:1642–7.

Panel on Antiretroviral Guidelines for Adults and Adolescents. Guidelines for the use of antiretroviral agents in HIV-1-infected adults and adolescents, updated July 14, 2016. Department of Health and Human Services; 1–288. Available at https://aidsinfo.nih.gov/contentfiles/lvguidelines/adultandadolescentgl.pdf.

Product Information: Edurant oral tablets, rilpivirine oral tablets. Tibotec Therapeutics, Raritan, NJ, 2011.

Rilpivirine hydrochloride + Emtricitabine + Tenofovir disoproxil fumarate (Complera) or Tenofovir alafenamide (TAF)

Drug Class: HIV combination antiretroviral agent

Usual Dose: 1 tablet PO daily with a high-fat meal

How Supplied: Oral tablet: (containing emtricitabine 200 mg, rilpivirine 25 mg, and tenofovir disoproxil fumarate 300 mg or tenofovir alafenamide 25 mg)

Pharmacokinetic Parameters:

Peak serum level: 1.8 mcg/mL/NR/0.29 mcg/mL

Bioavailability: 93%/no data/25–39%

Excreted unchanged: 14%/25%/No data (feces); 86%/6.1%/32% (urine)

Serum half-life (normal/ESRD): 10/50/17(h)/no data

Plasma protein binding: 4%/99.7%/0.7%

Volume of distribution (Vd): No data/no data/1.3 L/kg

Primary Mode of Elimination: Renal/renal & fecal/renal

Dosage Adjustments*

CrCl 50–80 mL/min	No change
CrCl 30–49 mL/min	*Not recommended
CrCl < 30 mL/min	*Not recommended
ESRD	*Not recommended
Post-HD dose	*Not recommended
Post-PD dose	*Not recommended
CVVH dose	*Not recommended
Mild-moderate hepatic insufficiency	No change
Severe hepatic insufficiency	Not studied

*The fixed dose tablet is not recommended for patients with CrCl < 50 mL/min; however therapy with one or more of the individual components might be possible. Please refer agent-specific drug monographs.

Antiretroviral Dosage Adjustments: *Please refer to individual drug monographs.*

Drug Interactions: *Please refer to individual drug monographs.*

Adverse Effects: *Please refer to individual drug monographs for more complete details.*

Most common adverse drug reactions to rilpivirine (> 2%, Grades 2–4) are insomnia and headache.

Most common adverse drug reactions to emtricitabine and tenofovir disoproxil fumarate (≥ 10%) are diarrhea, nausea, fatigue,

---

"Usual dose" assumes normal renal/hepatic function. * For renal insufficiency, give usual dose × 1 followed by maintenance dose per CrCl. For dialysis patients, dose the same as for CrCl < 10 mL/min and give supplemental (post-HD/PD dose) immediately after dialysis. CrCl = creatinine clearance; CVVH = continuous venovenous hemofiltration; HD/PD = hemodialysis/peritoneal dialysis. See pp. 204–207 for explanations, pp. xi–xii for abbreviations.

headache, dizziness, depression, insomnia, abnormal dreams, and rash.

Allergic Potential: Low

Safety in Pregnancy: B

Comments: Must be taken with a full meal (preferably high fat); rilpivirine exposure was about 40% lower when administered in the fasted state. Use with caution in patients with severe depressive disorders as depression, dysphoria, major depression, mood alteration, negative thoughts, suicide attempt, and suicidal ideation have been reported with rilpivirine. In clinical trials, patients with HIV-1 RNA > 100,000 copies/mL at therapy initiation experienced virologic failure more often than patients with HIV-1 RNA < 100,000 copies/mL at the start of therapy. Patients who experience virological failure on rilpivirine may be at risk for cross-resistance to other NNRTIs and to emtricitabine/lamivudine.

Cerebrospinal Fluid Penetration: See individual drug monographs.

REFERENCES:

Cohen CJ, Andrade-Villanueva J, Clotet B, et al: Rilpivirine versus efavirenz with two background nucleoside or nucleotide reverse transcriptase inhibitors in treatment-naïve adults infected with HIV-1 (THRIVE): A phase 3, randomized, non-inferiority trial. Lancet 2011;378(9787):229–37.

Molina JM, Cahn P, Grinsztejn B, et al: Rilpivirine versus efavirenz with tenofovir and emtricitabine in treatment-naïve adults infected with HIV-1 (ECHO): A phase 3 randomized double-blind active-controlled trial. Lancet 2011;378(9787):238–46.

Panel on Antiretroviral Guidelines for Adults and Adolescents. Guidelines for the use of antiretroviral agents in HIV-1-infected adults and adolescents, updated July 14, 2016. Department of Health and Human Services; 1–288. Available at https://aidsinfo.nih.gov/contentfiles/lvguidelines/adultandadolescentgl.pdf.

Product Information: Complera oral tablets, emtricitabine/rilpivirine/tenofovir disoproxil fumarate oral tablets. Gilead Sciences, Inc. (per manufacturer), Foster City, CA; 2011.

Ritonavir (Norvir) (RTV)

Drug Class: Antiretroviral; protease inhibitor

Usual Dose: Ritonavir 100–200 mg per dose (total 100–200 mg/d) to be administered as pharmacokinetic booster (or enhancer) with other protease inhibitors.

How Supplied: Oral capsule, liquid filled: 100 mg; oral solution: 80 mg/mL; oral tablet (heat stable): 100 mg

Pharmacokinetic Parameters:
Peak serum level: 11 mcg/mL
Bioavailability: No data
Excreted unchanged (urine): 3.5%
Serum half-life (normal/ESRD): 4 h/no data
Plasma protein binding: 99%
Volume of distribution (V_d): 0.41 L/kg

Primary Mode of Elimination: Hepatic

Dosage Adjustments*

CrCl 50–80 mL/min	No change
CrCl 10–50 mL/min	No change
CrCl < 10 mL/min	No change
Post-HD dose	None
Post-PD dose	None
CVVH dose	None
Moderate hepatic insufficiency	No change
Severe hepatic insufficiency	No change; use caution

"Usual dose" assumes normal renal/hepatic function. * For renal insufficiency, give usual dose × 1 followed by maintenance dose per CrCl. For dialysis patients, dose the same as for CrCl < 10 mL/min and give supplemental (post-HD/PD dose) immediately after dialysis. CrCl = creatinine clearance; CVVH = continuous venovenous hemofiltration; HD/PD = hemodialysis/peritoneal dialysis. See pp. 204–207 for explanations, pp. xi–xii for abbreviations.

Antiretroviral Dosage Adjustments

Atazanavir	Ritonavir 100 mg QD + atazanavir 300 mg QD with food
Delavirdine	Delavirdine: no change; ritonavir: no information
Efavirenz	Ritonavir 600 mg bid (500 mg bid for intolerance)
Indinavir	Ritonavir 100–200 mg bid + indinavir 800 mg bid, or 400 mg bid of each drug
Nelfinavir	Ritonavir 400 mg bid + nelfinavir 500–750 mg bid
Nevirapine	No changes
Saquinavir	Ritonavir 400 mg bid + saquinavir 400 mg bid
Ketoconazole	Caution; do not exceed ketoconazole 200 mg QD
Rifampin	Avoid
Rifabutin	150 mg q2d or 3x/week

Drug Interactions: Antiretrovirals, rifabutin, rifampin (see dose adjustment grid above); alprazolam, diazepam, estazolam, flurazepam, midazolam, triazolam, zolpidem, meperidine, propoxyphene, piroxicam, quinidine, amiodarone, encainide, flecainide, propafenone, astemizole, bepridil, bupropion, cisapride, clorazepate, clozapine, pimozide, St. John's wort, terfenadine (avoid); alfentanil, fentanyl, hydrocodone, tramadol, disopyramide, lidocaine, mexiletine, erythromycin, clarithromycin, rivaroxaban (↑ rivaroxaban), warfarin (↑ warfarin, monitor INR); dronabinol, ondansetron, metoprolol, pindolol, propranolol, timolol, amlodipine, diltiazem, felodipine, isradipine, nicardipine, nifedipine, nimodipine, nisoldipine, nitrendipine, verapamil, etoposide, paclitaxel, tamoxifen, vinblastine, vincristine, loratadine, tricyclic antidepressants, paroxetine, nefazodone, sertraline, trazodone, fluoxetine, venlafaxine, fluvoxamine, cyclosporine, tacrolimus, chlorpromazine, haloperidol, perphenazine, risperidone, thioridazine, clozapine, pimozide, methamphetamine (↑ interacting drug levels); voriconazole (↓ voriconazole levels); telithromycin (↑ ritonavir levels); codeine, hydromorphone, methadone, morphine, ketoprofen, ketorolac, naproxen, diphenoxylate, oral contraceptives, theophylline (↓ interacting drug levels); carbamazepine, phenytoin, phenobarbital, clonazepam, dexamethasone, prednisone (↓ ritonavir levels, ↑ interacting drug levels; monitor anticonvulsant levels); metronidazole (disulfiram-like reaction); tenofovir, tobacco (↓ ritonavir levels); avanafil (do not coadminster); sildenafil (do not exceed 25 mg in 48 hrs); tadalafil (max. 10 mg/72 hrs); vardenafil (max. 2.5 mg/72 hrs); fluticasone and budesonide (inhaled) coadministration can result in adrenal insufficiency, including Cushing's syndrome.

Adverse Effects: Anorexia, anemia, leukopenia, hyperglycemia (including worsening diabetes, new-onset diabetes, DKA), ↑cholesterol/triglycerides (evaluate risk for coronary disease/pancreatitis), fat redistribution, ↑CPK, nausea, vomiting, diarrhea, abdominal pain, circumoral/extremity paresthesias, ↑SGOT/SGPT, pancreatitis, taste perversion, possible increased bleeding in hemophilia.

Allergic Potential: Low

Safety in Pregnancy: B

"Usual dose" assumes normal renal/hepatic function. * For renal insufficiency, give usual dose × 1 followed by maintenance dose per CrCl. For dialysis patients, dose the same as for CrCl < 10 mL/min and give supplemental (post-HD/PD dose) immediately after dialysis. CrCl = creatinine clearance; CVVH = continuous venovenous hemofiltration; HD/PD = hemodialysis/peritoneal dialysis. See pp. 204–207 for explanations, pp. xi–xii for abbreviations.

Comments: GI intolerance decreases over time. Take with food if possible (serum levels increase 15%, fewer GI side effects). Separate dosing from ddI by 2 hours. Refrigerate capsules (not oral solution) if temperature to exceed 78°F. Do not refrigerate oral tablets, they are not heat stable. Tablets are not bioequivalent to capsules and patients may experience more GI side effects when switched to tablet formulation.
Cerebrospinal Fluid Penetration: < 10%

REFERENCES:

Panel on Antiretroviral Guidelines for Adults and Adolescents. Guidelines for the use of antiretroviral agents in HIV-1-infected adults and adolescents, updated July 14, 2016. Department of Health and Human Services; 1–288. Available at https://aidsinfo.nih.gov/contentfiles/lvguidelines/adultandadolescentgl.pdf.

Piliero PJ. Interaction between ritonavir and statins. Am J Med. 2002;112:510–1.

Rathbun RC, Rossi DR. Low-dose ritonavir for protease inhibitor pharmacokinetic enhancement. Ann Pharmacother. 2002;36:702–6.

Product Information: Norvir oral tablet, solution, ritonavir oral tablet, solution. Abbott Laboratories, North Chicago, IL; 2012.

Saquinavir (Invirase) (SQV)

Drug Class: Antiretroviral; protease inhibitor
Usual Dose: Saquinavir 1000 mg (PO) bid with ritonavir 100 mg (PO) bid; take with food
How Supplied: Oral capsule: 200 mg; oral tablet: 500 mg
Pharmacokinetic Parameters:
Peak serum level: 0.07 mcg/mL
Bioavailability: Hard-gel (4%)
Excreted unchanged (urine): 13%
Serum half-life (normal/ESRD): 13 h/no data
Plasma protein binding: 98%

Volume of distribution (V_d): 10 L/kg
Primary Mode of Elimination: Hepatic
Dosage Adjustments*

CrCl 50–80 mL/min	No change
CrCl 10–50 mL/min	No change
CrCl < 10 mL/min	No change
Post-HD dose	None
Post-PD dose	None
CVVH dose	No change
Mild-moderate hepatic insufficiency	Use with caution
Severe hepatic insufficiency	Contraindicated

Antiretroviral Dosage Adjustments

Darunavir	Avoid
Delavirdine	No information
Efavirenz	(SQV 1000 mg + RTV 100 mg) bid
Indinavir	No information
Lopinavir/ritonavir 3 capsules bid	Saquinavir 500 mg bid
Nelfinavir	Saquinavir 1 g bid or 1200 mg bid
Nevirapine	(SQV 1000 mg + RTV 100 mg) bid
Ritonavir	Ritonavir 100 mg bid + saquinavir 1 g bid
Rifampin	Contraindicated
Rifabutin	Avoid

"Usual dose" assumes normal renal/hepatic function. * For renal insufficiency, give usual dose × 1 followed by maintenance dose per CrCl. For dialysis patients, dose the same as for CrCl < 10 mL/min and give supplemental (post-HD/PD dose) immediately after dialysis. CrCl = creatinine clearance; CVVH = continuous venovenous hemofiltration; HD/PD = hemodialysis/peritoneal dialysis. See pp. 204–207 for explanations, pp. xi–xii for abbreviations.

Etravirine	(SQV 1000 mg + RTV 100 mg) bid
Maraviroc	300 mg bid
Raltegravir	No data

Drug Interactions: Antiretrovirals, rifabutin, rifampin (see dose adjustment grid above); astemizole, terfenadine, benzodiazepines, cisapride, ergotamine, statins, St. John's wort (avoid if possible); carbamazepine, phenytoin, phenobarbital, dexamethasone, prednisone (↓ saquinavir levels, ↑ interacting drug levels; monitor anticonvulsant levels); clarithromycin, erythromycin, telithromycin (↑ saquinavir and macrolide levels); grapefruit juice, itraconazole, voriconazole, ketoconazole (↑ saquinavir levels); sildenafil (do not give > 25 mg/48 hrs); tadalafil (max. 10 mg/72 hrs), vardenafil (max. 2.5 mg/72 hrs); rivaroxaban (↑rivaroxaban); warfarin (↑ warfarin, monitor INR).

Adverse Effects: Anorexia, headache, anemia, leukopenia, hyperglycemia (including worsening diabetes, new-onset diabetes, DKA), ↑ cholesterol/triglycerides (evaluate risk for coronary disease/pancreatitis), ↑ SGOT/SGPT, hyperuricemia, fat redistribution, possible increased bleeding in hemophilia. May cause QT interval prolongation when combined with ritonavir.

Allergic Potential: Low
Safety in Pregnancy: B
Comments: Take with food. Avoid garlic supplements, which ↓saquinavir levels ~ 50%.
Cerebrospinal Fluid Penetration: < 1%

REFERENCES:

Borck C. Garlic supplements and saquinavir. Clin Infect Dis. 2002;35:343.

Hsu A, Granneman GR, Cao G, et al. Pharmacokinetic interactions between two human immunodeficiency virus protease inhibitors, ritonavir and saquinavir. Clin Pharmacol Ther. 1998;63:453–64.

Panel on Antiretroviral Guidelines for Adults and Adolescents. Guidelines for the use of antiretroviral agents in HIV-1-infected adults and adolescents, updated July 14, 2016. Department of Health and Human Services. 1–288. Available at https://aidsinfo.nih.gov/contentfiles/lvguidelines/adultandadolescentgl.pdf.

Product Information: Invirase oral capsules, oral tablets, saquinavir mesylate oral capsules, oral tablets. Genentech USA, Inc. (per FDA), South San Francisco, CA; 2016.

Vella S, Floridia M. Saquinavir: Clinical pharmacology and efficacy. Clin Pharmacokinet. 1998;34:189–201.

Simeprevir (Olysio) (SMV)

Drug Class: Anti-hepatitis C agent (NS3/4A protease inhibitor); HCV genotype 1
Usual Dose: 150 mg (PO) once daily with food
How Supplied: Oral capsule, 150 mg
Treatment Duration: 12 or 24 weeks; off-label use listed below based on HCV treatment guidelines (updated September 2016).

Naïve, GT1a without cirrhosis	SMV/SOF	12 weeks
Naïve, GT1a with compensated (Child-Pugh A) cirrhosis and without Q80K polymorphism	SMV/ SOF +/– weight- based RBV	24 weeks
Naïve, GT1b without cirrhosis	SMV/SOF	12 weeks

"Usual dose" assumes normal renal/hepatic function. * For renal insufficiency, give usual dose × 1 followed by maintenance dose per CrCl. For dialysis patients, dose the same as for CrCl < 10 mL/min and give supplemental (post-HD/PD dose) immediately after dialysis. CrCl = creatinine clearance; CVVH = continuous venovenous hemofiltration; HD/PD = hemodialysis/peritoneal dialysis. See pp. 204–207 for explanations, pp. xi–xii for abbreviations.

Naïve, GT1b with compensated (Child-Pugh A) cirrhosis	SMV/ SOF +/– weight-based RBV	24 weeks
Treatment-experienced (failed PegIFN/RBV) GT1a without cirrhosis	SMV/SOF	12 weeks
Treatment-experienced (failed PegIFN/RBV) GT1a with compensated cirrhosis (Child-Pugh A) and without Q80K polymorphism	SMV/ SOF +/– weight-based RBV	24 weeks
Treatment-experienced (failed PegIFN/RBV) GT1b without cirrhosis	SMV/SOF	12 weeks
Treatment-experienced (failed PegIFN/RBV) GT1b with compensated cirrhosis (Child-Pugh A)	SMV/ SOF +/– weight-based RBV	24 weeks

*SMV: simeprevir; SOF: sofosbuvir; PegIFN: pegylated interferon alfa; RBV: ribavirin

Studies of PEG-interferon, ribavirin, and simeprevir in patients with genotype 1a demonstrated that the presence at baseline of the NS3 Q80K polymorphism reduced treatment response. If this polymorphism is detected on pretreatment screening, alternate HCV therapies should be considered.

Pharmacokinetic Parameters:
Excreted unchanged: 91% (feces)

Serum half-life: 10–13 hours in HCV uninfected; 41 hours in HCV infected
Plasma protein binding: 98.9%
Primary Mode of Elimination: Hepatic
Dosage Adjustments for Renal and Hepatic Insufficiency

CrCl 50–80 mL/min	No change
CrCl 30–50 mL/min	No change
CrCl < 30 mL/min	No change
Post-HD dose	Not established
Post-PD dose	Not established
Mild hepatic insufficiency	No change
Moderate-severe hepatic insufficiency	Not established

Drug Interactions: Simeprevir is primarily metabolized by CYP3A. As such, administration of simeprevir with inhibitors of CYP3A will significantly increase plasma concentrations, while inducers will decrease simeprevir levels. As all HIV non-nucleoside inhibitors, protease inhibitors, and the PK booster cobicistat influence CYP3A, they should not be given with simeprevir. Other drugs that are not recommended: carbamazepine, oxacarbazepine, phenobarbital, phenytoin, erythromycin, clarithromycin, telithromycin, itraconazole, ketoconazole, posaconazole, fluconazole, voriconazole, rifampin, rifabutin, rifapentine, dexamethasone, cisapride, milk thistle, St John's wort. Numerous other drugs should be used with caution—see prescribing information for details.
Adverse Effects: Serious photosensitivity reactions have been observed with

"Usual dose" assumes normal renal/hepatic function. * For renal insufficiency, give usual dose × 1 followed by maintenance dose per CrCl. For dialysis patients, dose the same as for CrCl < 10 mL/min and give supplemental (post-HD/PD dose) immediately after dialysis. CrCl = creatinine clearance; CVVH = continuous venovenous hemofiltration; HD/PD = hemodialysis/peritoneal dialysis. See pp. 204–207 for explanations, pp. xi–xii for abbreviations.

simeprevir; patients must use sun protection measures and limit sun exposure. Rash, pruritus, and nausea were also reported more commonly in those receiving simeprevir than placebo. Contraindicated in patients with decompensated cirrhosis Child-Pugh score ≥7, Model for End stage Liver Disease (MELD) ≥15, and/orclinical manifestations of decompensation.

Allergic Potential: Moderate

Safety in Pregnancy: C

If used with ribavirin (contraindicated in pregnancy), pregnancy warnings for ribavirin apply to the combination. See ribavirin prescribing information for details.

REFERENCES:

AASLD-IDSA. Recommendations for testing, managing, and treating hepatitis C. http://www.hcvguidelines.org. Accessed on September 27, 2016.

Kwo P, Gitlin N, Nahass R et al. Simeprevir plus sofosbuvir (12 and 8 weeks) in HCV genotype 1-infected patients without cirrhosis: OPTIMIST-1, a phase 3, randomized study. Hepatology. 2016 Jan 22. doi: 10.1002/hep.28467 [Epub ahead of print].

Lawitz E, Matusow G, DeJesus E et al. Simeprevir plus sofosbuvir in patients with chronic hepatitis C virus genotype 1 infection and cirrhosis: A phase 3 study (OPTIMIST-2). Hepatology. 2015 Dec 24. doi: 10.1002/hep.28422 [Epub ahead of print].

Lawitz E, Sulkowski M, Ghalib R, et al. Simeprevir plus sofosbuvir, with or without ribavirin, to treat chronic infection with hepatitis C virus genotype 1 in non-responders to pegylated interferon and ribavirin and treatment-naïve patients: the COSMOS randomized study. Lancet 2014;384:1756–65.

Product Information: Olysio oral capsules, simeprevir oral capsules. Janssen Products, Titusville, NJ; 2015.

Sofosbuvir (Sovaldi) (SOF)

Drug Class: Anti-hepatitis C agent (NS5B nucleotide polymerase inhibitor); HCV genotypes 1–4

Usual Dose: 400 mg once daily with or without food

How Supplied: Oral tablet, 400 mg

Treatment Duration: 8–24 weeks in combination with simeprevir, ledipasvir, daclatasvir, or velpatasvir with or without ribavirin. See individual drug monographs for complete details on dosing and duration.

Pharmacokinetic Parameters:

Excreted unchanged: 80% (urine), 14% (feces), 2.5% (air)

Serum half-life of the primary circulating metabolite GS-331007: 27 hours

Plasma protein binding: 61–65% for sofosbuvir, minimal for GS-331007

Primary Mode of Elimination: Renal

Dosage Adjustments for Renal and Hepatic Insufficiency

CrCl 50–80 mL/min	No change
CrCl 30–50 mL/min	No change
CrCl < 30 mL/min	Avoid
Post-HD dose	Avoid
Post-PD dose	Avoid
Mild-moderate hepatic insufficiency	No change
Severe hepatic insufficiency	No change

Dosage Adjustments with Antiretroviral Agents: None required.

Drug Interactions: Warning: Amiordarone not recommended due to risk of serious symptomatic bradycardia, particularly when taken in combination with beta blockers or in patients with underlying cardiac disease and/or advanced liver disease.

"Usual dose" assumes normal renal/hepatic function. * For renal insufficiency, give usual dose × 1 followed by maintenance dose per CrCl. For dialysis patients, dose the same as for CrCl < 10 mL/min and give supplemental (post-HD/PD dose) immediately after dialysis. CrCl = creatinine clearance; CVVH = continuous venovenous hemofiltration; HD/PD = hemodialysis/peritoneal dialysis. See pp. 204–207 for explanations, pp. xi–xii for abbreviations.

Concomitant Drug Class: Drug Name	Effect on Concentration[b]	Clinical Comment
Anticonvulsants: carbamazepine phenytoin phenobarbital oxcarbazepine	↓ sofosbuvir ↓ GS-331007	Coadministration of sofosbuvir with carbamazepine, phenytoin, phenobarbital, or oxcarbazepine is expected to decrease the concentration of sofosbuvir, leading to reduced therapeutic effect of sofosbuvir. Coadministration is not recommended.
Antimycobacterials: rifabutin rifampin rifapentine	↓ sofosbuvir ↓ GS-331007	Coadministration of sofosbuvir with rifabutin or rifapentine is expected to decrease the concentration of sofosbuvir, leading to reduced therapeutic effect of sofosbuvir. Coadministration is not recommended. Sofosbuvir should not be used with rifampin, a potent intestinal P-gp inducer.
Herbal Supplements: St. John's wort (Hypericum perforatum)	↓ sofosbuvir ↓ GS-331007	Sofosbuvir should not be used with St. John's wort, a potent intestinal P-gp inducer.
HIV Protease Inhibitors: tipranavir/ritonavir	↓ sofosbuvir ↓ GS-331007	Coadministration of sofosbuvir with tiipranavir/ritonavir is expected to decrease the concentration of sofosbuvir, leading to reduced therapeutic effect of sofosbuvir. Coadministration is not recommended.

[a] This table is not all inclusive. See prescribing information for full details.

[b] ↓ = decrease.

Sofosbuvir is a substrate of P-gp and breast cancer resistance protein (BCRP), while GS-331007 (the primary circulating metabolite) is not. Drugs that are potent P-gp inducers in the intestine (e.g., rifampin or St John's wort) may decrease sofosbuvir's plasma concentration and should not be used. See table above for other potentially significant drug-drug interactions.

Adverse Effects: The most common adverse events (incidence greater than or equal to 20%, all grades) observed with sofosbuvir in combination with ribavirin were fatigue and headache. The most common adverse events observed with sofosbuvir in combination with peginterferon alfa and ribavirin were fatigue, headache, nausea, insomnia, and anemia. These side effects are seen with these agents when not given with sofosbuvir.

Allergic Potential: Low

Safety in Pregnancy: B.

If used with ribavirin (contraindicated in pregnancy), pregnancy warnings for ribavirin apply to the combination. See ribavirin prescribing information for details.

"Usual dose" assumes normal renal/hepatic function. * For renal insufficiency, give usual dose × 1 followed by maintenance dose per CrCl. For dialysis patients, dose the same as for CrCl < 10 mL/min and give supplemental (post-HD/PD dose) immediately after dialysis. CrCl = creatinine clearance; CVVH = continuous venovenous hemofiltration; HD/PD = hemodialysis/peritoneal dialysis. See pp. 204–207 for explanations, pp. xi–xii for abbreviations.

REFERENCES:

AASLD-IDSA. Recommendations for testing, managing, and treating hepatitis C. http://www.hcvguidelines.org. Accessed on September 27, 2016.

Kwo P, Gitlin N, Nahass R et al. Simeprevir plus sofosbuvir (12 and 8 weeks) in HCV genotype 1-infected patients without cirrhosis: OPTIMIST-1, a phase 3, randomized study. Hepatology. 2016 Jan 22. doi: 10.1002/hep.28467 [Epub ahead of print].

Lawitz E, Matusow G, DeJesus E, et al. Simeprevir plus sofosbuvir in patients with chronic hepatitis C virus genotype 1 infection and cirrhosis: A phase 3 study (OPTIMIST-2). Hepatology. 2015 Dec 24. doi: 10.1002/hep.28422 [Epub ahead of print].

Lawitz E, Sulkowski M, Ghalib R, et al. Simeprevir plus sofosbuvir, with or without ribavirin, to treat chronic infection with hepatitis C virus genotype 1 in non-responders to pegylated interferon and ribavirin and treatment-naïve patients: the COSMOS randomized study. Lancet 2014;384:1756–65.

Product Information: Sovaldi oral tablets, sofosbuvir oral tablets. Gilead Sciences, Foster City, CA; 2015.

Sofosbuvir/Velpatasvir (Epclusa) (SOF/VEL)

Drug Class: Anti-hepatitis C agents; sofosbuvir (NS5B nucleotide polymerase inhibitor), velpatasvir (NS5A replication complex inhibitor)

Indication: Hepatitis C virus, genotypes 1–6 with or without cirrhosis

Usual Dose: 1 tablet by mouth daily with or without food

How Supplied: Tablet, containing sofosbuvir 400 mg and velpatasvir 100 mg

Treatment Duration: 12 weeks

Without cirrhosis or compensated cirrhosis (CTP A)	Sofosbuvir/ velpatasvir	12 weeks
With decompensated cirrhosis (CTP B or C)	Sofosbuvir/ velpatasvir + RBV[¶]	12 weeks

RBV: ribavirin.

[¶] In patients eligible to receive ribavirin with decompensated cirrhosis, initiate ribavirin at 600 mg/day and titrate as tolerated up to 1000 mg/day (weight < 75 kg) or 1200 mg/day (weight > 75 kg) in 2 divided doses with food. If unable to tolerate at the initial dose, further dose reductions may be made. See ribavirin prescribing information for more details.

Pharmacokinetic Parameters:
Peak serum level: 567/259 ng/mL
Excreted unchanged: 80% urine, 14% feces (sofosbuvir); 94% feces (velpatasvir)
Serum half-life: 0.5h (sofosbuvir), 27h (GS-331007); 15h (velpatasvir)
Plasma protein binding: 61–65/> 99.5%
Primary Mode of Elimination: Renal/fecal
Dosage Adjustments:

CrCl 50–80 mL/min	No change
CrCl 30–50 mL/min	No change
CrCl < 30 mL/min	Avoid
Post-HD dose	Avoid
Post-PD dose	Avoid
Mild-moderate hepatic insufficiency	No change
Severe hepatic insufficiency	No change

Drug Interactions: Sofosbuvir and velpatasvir are P-gp and BCRP substrates. In addition, velpatasvir inhibits P-gp, BCRP, OATP1B1/3 and 2B1. Slow turnover of

---

velpatasvir by CYP2B6, CYP2C8, and CYP3A4 were observed in vitro. P-gp inducers and moderate-to-potent CYP2B6, CYP2C8, or CYP3A4 inducers may decrease plasma velpatasvir concentrations, leading to reduced effectiveness.

Acid-reducing agents	↓ velpatasvir	Velpatasvir solubility decreases with increased gastric pH.
Antacids		Separate antacids by 4 hours.
H$_2$-receptor antagonists		Administer H$_2$-receptor antagonists simultaneously with velpatasvir or separate by 12 hours.
Proton pump inhibitors		Avoid pump inhibitors (if unavoidable, administer velpatasvir with food and 2 hours before omeprazole 20 mg max).
Digoxin	↑ digoxin	Therapeutic drug monitoring and possible dose adjustment recommended; see prescribing information.
Topotecan	↑ topotecan	Coadministration not recommended.
Anticonvulsants (carbamazepine, phenytoin, phenobarbital, oxcarbazepine)	↓ sofosbuvir ↓ velpatasvir	Coadministration not recommended.
Antimycobacterials (rifampin, rifapentine, rifabutin)	↓ sofosbuvir ↓ velpatasvir	Coadministration not recommended.
Efavirenz	↓ velpatasvir	Coadministration not recommended.
Tenofovir	↑ tenofovir	Close monitoring for renal effects; see tenofovir or tenofovir-containing product information.
Tipranavir/ritonavir	↓ sofosbuvir ↓ velpatasvir	Coadministration not recommended.
St. John's wort	↓ sofosbuvir ↓ velpatasvir	Coadministration not recommended.
HMG-CoA reductase inhibitors (rosuvastatin, atorvastatin)	↑ rosuvastatin ↑ atorvastatin	Close monitoring for myopathy or rhabdomyolysis recommended.

"Usual dose" assumes normal renal/hepatic function. * For renal insufficiency, give usual dose × 1 followed by maintenance dose per CrCl. For dialysis patients, dose the same as for CrCl < 10 mL/min and give supplemental (post-HD/PD dose) immediately after dialysis. CrCl = creatinine clearance; CVVH = continuous venovenous hemofiltration; HD/PD = hemodialysis/peritoneal dialysis. See pp. 204–207 for explanations, pp. xi–xii for abbreviations.

Warning: Amiodarone not recommended due to risk of serious symptomatic bradycardia with SOF. *See SOF monograph for more details.*

Other Significant Interactions:

Adverse Effects:

Common: Nausea (9–15%), diarrhea (10%), headache (11–22%), fatigue (15–32%)

Other: Elevated lipase (2–6%), increased CK (2%), anemia (with ribavirin 26%), insomnia (5–11%), irritability (5%), depression (1%)

Allergic Potential: Low

Safety in Pregnancy: Unknown safety in humans. No observable effects in animal studies; unknown whether velpatasvir/sofosbuvir negatively affects pregnancy outcomes.

If used with ribavirin (contraindicated in pregnancy), pregnancy warnings for ribavirin apply to the combination. See ribavirin prescribing information for details.

REFERENCES:

AASLD-IDSA. Recommendations for testing, managing, and treating hepatitis C. http://www.hcvguidelines.org. Accessed on September 27, 2016.

Feld JJ, Jacobson IM, Hézode C, et al. Sofosbuvir and velpatasvir for HCV genotype 1, 2, 4, 5, and 6 infection. N Engl J Med. 2015 Dec 31;373(27):2599–607.

Product Information: Epclusa oral tablets, sofosbuvir, velpatasvir oral tablets. Gilead Sciences Inc, Foster City, CA; 2016.

Stavudine (Zerit) (d4t)

Drug Class: Antiretroviral NRTI (nucleoside reverse transcriptase inhibitor)

Usual Dose: ≥ 60 kg: 40 mg (PO) bid; < 60 kg: 30 mg (PO) bid with or without food

How Supplied: Oral capsule: 15 mg, 20 mg, 30 mg, 40 mg; oral powder for solution: 1 mg/mL

Pharmacokinetic Parameters:

Peak serum level: 4.2 mcg/mL

Bioavailability: 86%

Excreted unchanged (urine): 40%

Serum half-life (normal/ESRD): 1.0/5.1 hrs

Plasma protein binding: 0%

Volume of distribution (V_d): 0.5 L/kg

Primary Mode of Elimination: Renal

Dosage Adjustments* ≥ 60 kg/(≤ 60 kg)

CrCl 50–80 mL/min	40 mg (PO) bid (30 mg [PO] bid)
CrCl 26–50 mL/min	20 mg (PO) bid (15 mg [PO] bid)
CrCl ~ 10–25 mL/min	20 mg (PO) QD (15 mg [PO] QD)
Post-HD dose	20 mg (PO) (15 mg [PO])
Post-PD dose	No information
CVVH dose	20 mg (PO) QD (15 mg [PO] QD)
Moderate hepatic insufficiency	No recommendation
Severe hepatic insufficiency	No recommendation

Drug Interactions: Ribavirin (↓ stavudine efficacy, ↑ risk of lactic acidosis); zidovudine (↓ stavudine levels); dapsone, INH, other neurotoxic agents (↑ risk of neuropathy), didanosine (↑ risk of neuropathy, lactic acidosis).

Adverse Effects: Drug fever/rash, nausea, vomiting, GI upset, diarrhea, headache, insomnia, dose-dependent peripheral neuropathy, myalgias, pancreatitis, ↑SGOT/SGPT, ↑cholesterol, facial fat pad wasting, lipodystrophy, thrombocytopenia,

leukopenia, lactic acidosis with hepatic steatosis (rare, but potentially life-threatening toxicity with use of NRTIs).
Allergic Potential: Low
Safety in Pregnancy: C
Comments: Pancreatitis may be severe/fatal. Avoid coadministration with AZT. Decrease dose in patients with peripheral neuropathy to 20 mg (PO) bid. Pregnant women may be at increased risk for lactic acidosis/liver damage when stavudine is used with didanosine (ddI).
Cerebrospinal Fluid Penetration: 30%

REFERENCES:
Dudley MN, Graham KK, Kaul S, et al. Pharmacokinetics of stavudine in patients with AIDS and AIDS-related complex. J Infect Dis. 1992;166:480–5.
Lea AP, Faulds D. Stavudine: A review of its pharmacodynamic and pharmacokinetic properties and clinical potential in HIV infection. Drugs. 1996;51:846–64.
Murphy RL, Brun S, Hicks C, et al. ABT-378/ritonavir plus stavudine and lamivudine for the treatment of antiretroviral-naïve adults with HIV-1 infection: 48-week results. AIDS. 2001;15:F1–9.
Panel on Antiretroviral Guidelines for Adults and Adolescents. Guidelines for the use of antiretroviral agents in HIV-1-infected adults and adolescents, updated July 14, 2016. Department of Health and Human Services; 1–288. Available at https://aidsinfo.nih.gov/contentfiles/lvguidelines/adultandadolescentgl.pdf.
Product Information: Zerit oral capsules, oral solution, stavudine oral capsules, oral solution. Bristol-Myers Squibb Company, Princeton, NJ; 2010

Telbivudine (Tyzeka) (LdT)

Drug Class: Anti-hepatitis B agent (nucleoside reverse transcriptase inhibitor)
Usual Dose: 600 mg (PO) daily
How Supplied: Oral tablet: 600 mg; oral solution: 100 mg/5 mL

Pharmacokinetic Parameters:
Peak serum level: 3.69 mcg/mL
Bioavailability: Unknown
Excreted unchanged: 0% (feces), 42% (urine)
Serum half-life (normal/ESRD): 40–49 h/ no data
Plasma protein binding: 3.3%
Volume of distribution (V_d): Not studied
Primary Mode of Elimination: Renal
Dosage Adjustments:

CrCl 50–80 mL/min	No change
CrCl 30–49 mL/min	600 mg q2d
CrCl < 30 mL/min	600 mg q3d
ESRD	600 mg q4d
Post-HD dose	Give dose after HD
Post-PD dose	Not studied
CVVH dose	Not studied
Mild to moderate hepatic insufficiency	No change
Severe hepatic insufficiency	No change

Drug Interactions: Telbivudine use with Peginterferon Alfa-2a: Increased risk of peripheral neuropathy. Telbivudine is not metabolized by the liver and it is not a substrate or inhibitor of the cytochrome P450 enzyme system, and no other drug interactions have been established.
Adverse Effects: Boxed warnings: Lactic acidosis/hepatomegaly, including fatal cases, have been reported with the use of nucleoside analogues alone or in combination with other antiretrovirals. Signs/symptoms of lactic acidosis

---

"Usual dose" assumes normal renal/hepatic function. * For renal insufficiency, give usual dose × 1 followed by maintenance dose per CrCl. For dialysis patients, dose the same as for CrCl < 10 mL/min and give supplemental (post-HD/PD dose) immediately after dialysis. CrCl = creatinine clearance; CVVH = continuous venovenous hemofiltration; HD/PD = hemodialysis/peritoneal dialysis. See pp. 204–207 for explanations, pp. xi–xii for abbreviations.

include: nausea, vomiting, abdominal pain, tachypnea, decreased renal function, or decreased liver function. Severe acute exacerbations of hepatitis B have been reported in patients who have discontinued anti-hepatitis B therapy. Myopathy has also been associated with telbivudine use. Other less serious adverse effects include: abdominal pain, dizziness, headache, nasopharyngitis, malaise, and fatigue.

Allergic Potential: Low

Safety in Pregnancy: B

Comments: May be administered without regard to food. Telbivudine does not exhibit any clinically relevant activity against HIV type 1. The efficacy and safety in patients co-infected with HIV, hepatitis C virus, hepatitis D virus, a history or signs of hepatic decompensation, or a history of alcohol or illicit substance abuse within the preceding 2 years are unknown. Severe, acute exacerbation of hepatitis B may occur upon discontinuation. Monitor liver function several months after stopping treatment; re-initiation of anti-hepatitis B therapy may be required.

REFERENCES:

Chan HL, Heathcote EJ, Marcellin P. Treatment of hepatitis B e antigen positive chronic hepatitis with telbivudine or adefovir: a randomized trial. Ann Intern Med. 2007;147(11):745–54.

Gane E, Lai CL, Liaw YF, et al. Phase III comparison of telbivudine vs lamivudine in HBeAg-positive patients with chronic hepatitis B: efficacy, safety, and predictors of response at 1 year. J Hepatol. 2006;44(suppl 2): S183–S184.

Lai CL, Gane E, Liaw YF, et al. Telbivudine (LdT) vs. lamivudine for chronic hepatitis B: first-year results from the international phase III GLOBE trial. Hepatology. 2005;42(Supp 1):748A.

Lai CL, Gane E, Liaw YF, et al. Telbivudine versus lamivudine in patients with chronic hepatitis B. N Engl J Med. 2007;357(25):2576–88.

Lai CL, Leung N, Teo EK, et al. A 1-year trial of telbivudine, lamivudine, and the combination in patients with hepatitis B e antigen-positive chronic hepatitis B. Gastroenterology. 2005;129(2):528–36.

Product Information: Tyzeka oral tablets, telbivudine oral tablets. Novartis Pharmaceuticals Corporation, East Hanover, NJ; 2006.

Zhou X, Marbury TC, Alcorn HW, et al. Pharmacokinetics of telbivudine in subjects with various degrees of hepatic impairment. Antimicrob Agents Chemother. 2006;50(5):1721–26.

Zhou XJ, Myers M, Chao G, et al. Clinical pharmacokinetics of telbivudine, a potent antiviral for hepatitis B, in subjects with impaired hepatic or renal function. J Hepatol. 2004;40(Suppl 1):452.

Tenofovir disoproxil fumarate (Viread) (TDF)

Drug Class: Antiretroviral; (nucleotide analogue) (HIV) (HBV)

Usual Dose: 300 mg (PO) daily (HIV); 300 mg (PO) daily (HBV) with or without food

How Supplied: Oral tablets: 150 mg, 200 mg, 250mg, 300 mg; oral powder: 40 mg/g

Pharmacokinetic Parameters:

Peak serum level: 0.29 mcg/mL

Bioavailability: 25%/39% (fasting/high-fat meal)

Excreted unchanged (urine): 32%

Serum half-life (normal/ESRD): 17 h/no data

Plasma protein binding: 0.7–7.2%

Volume of distribution (V_d): 1.3 L/kg

Primary Mode of Elimination: Renal

"Usual dose" assumes normal renal/hepatic function. * For renal insufficiency, give usual dose × 1 followed by maintenance dose per CrCl. For dialysis patients, dose the same as for CrCl < 10 mL/min and give supplemental (post-HD/PD dose) immediately after dialysis. CrCl = creatinine clearance; CVVH = continuous venovenous hemofiltration; HD/PD = hemodialysis/peritoneal dialysis. See pp. 204–207 for explanations, pp. xi–xii for abbreviations.

Dosage Adjustments*

CrCl ≥ 50 mL/min	No change
CrCl 30–49 mL/min	300 mg (PO) q2d
CrCl 10–29 mL/min	300 mg (PO) 2×/week
CrCl < 10 mL/min	No information
Post-HD dose	300 mg q7d or after 12 hours on HD
Post-PD dose	No information
CVVH dose	No information
Moderate hepatic insufficiency	No change
Severe hepatic insufficiency	No change

Drug Interactions: Didanosine (avoid concomitant didanosine due to impaired CD4 response and increased risk of virologic failure); valganciclovir (↑ tenofovir levels); atazanavir, lopinavir/ritonavir (↑ tenofovir levels)(↓ atazanavir levels; use atazanavir 300 mg/ritonavir 100 mg with tenofovir); no clinically significant interactions with lamivudine, efavirenz, methadone, oral contraceptives. Not a substrate/inhibitor of cytochrome P-450 enzymes.

Adverse Effects: Mild nausea, vomiting, GI upset, asthenia, headache, diarrhea, lactic acidosis with hepatic steatosis (rare, but potentially life-threatening with NRTIs), renal tubular acidosis, acute renal failure, and Fanconi syndrome have been reported, ↓ bone density.

Allergic Potential: Low
Safety in Pregnancy: B

Comments: Eliminated by glomerular filtration/tubular secretion. May be taken with or without food. If possible, avoid concomitant didanosine (see drug interactions).

Cerebrospinal Fluid Penetration: See emtricitabine/tenofovir monograph for details.

REFERENCES:

Jullien V, Treluyer JM, Rey E, et al. Population pharmacokinetics of tenofovir in human immunodeficiency virus–infected patients taking highly active antiretroviral therapy. Antimicrobial Agents and Chemotherapy. 2005;49:3361–66.

Panel on Antiretroviral Guidelines for Adults and Adolescents. Guidelines for the use of antiretroviral agents in HIV-1-infected adults and adolescents, updated July 14, 2016. Department of Health and Human Services; 1–288. Available at https://aidsinfo.nih.gov/contentfiles/lvguidelines/adultandadolescentgl.pdf.

Product Information: Viread oral tablets, oral powder, tenofovir disoproxil fumarate oral tablets, oral powder. Gilead Sciences, Inc., Foster City, CA; 2012.

Tipranavir (Aptivus) (TPV)

Drug Class: Antiretroviral; protease inhibitor
Usual Dose: 500 mg (PO) with ritonavir 200 mg (PO) bid
How Supplied: Oral capsule, liquid filled: 250 mg, oral solution: 100 mg/mL
Pharmacokinetic Parameters:
Peak serum level: 77–94 mcg/mL
Bioavailability: No data
Excreted unchanged (urine): 44%
Serum half-life (normal/ESRD): 5.5–6 h/no data
Plasma protein binding: 99.9%
Volume of distribution (V_d): 7–10 L/kg

"Usual dose" assumes normal renal/hepatic function. * For renal insufficiency, give usual dose × 1 followed by maintenance dose per CrCl. For dialysis patients, dose the same as for CrCl < 10 mL/min and give supplemental (post-HD/PD dose) immediately after dialysis. CrCl = creatinine clearance; CVVH = continuous venovenous hemofiltration; HD/PD = hemodialysis/peritoneal dialysis. See pp. 204–207 for explanations, pp. xi–xii for abbreviations.

Primary Mode of Elimination: Hepatic

Dosage Adjustments*

CrCl 50–80 mL/min	No change
CrCl 10–50 mL/min	No change
CrCl < 10 mL/min	No change
Post-HD dose	No change
Post-PD dose	No change
CVVH dose	No change
Mild hepatic insufficiency	No change; use caution
Moderate or severe hepatic insufficiency	Avoid

Drug Interactions: Rifabutin (↑ levels), clarithromycin (↑ levels), loperamide (↓ levels), statins (↑ risk of myopathy); abacavir, saquinavir, tenofovir, zidovudine, amprenavir/RTV, lopinavir/RTV (↓ levels). Aluminum/magnesium antacids (↓ absorption 25–30%). Ritonavir (↑ risk of hepatitis). St. John's wort (↓ tipranavir levels). Maraviroc (dose maraviroc 300 mg bid). Rivaroxaban (↑ rivaroxaban), warfarin (↑ warfarin, monitor INR)

Adverse Effects: Contraindicated in moderate/severe hepatic insufficiency. ↑risk of hepatotoxicity in HIV patients co-infected with HBV/HCV. Case reports of intracerebral hemorrhage—use with caution in patients with coagulopathies.

Allergic Potential: High. Tipranavir has a sulfonamide moiety; use with caution in patients with sulfonamide allergies.

Safety in Pregnancy: C

Comments: Should be taken with food. Increased bioavailability when taken with meals. Must be coadministered with 200 mg ritonavir. Tipranavir contains a sulfonamide moiety (as do darunavir and fosamprenavir). Refrigerate capsules; can be stored at temperature for up to 60 days. Store oral solution at room temperature; use within 60 days after opening.

Cerebrospinal Fluid Penetration: No data

REFERENCES:

Hicks CB, Cahn P, Cooper DA, et al. Durable efficacy of tipranavir-ritonavir in combination with an optimised background regimen of antiretroviral drugs for treatment-experienced HIV-1-infected patients at 48 weeks in the Randomized Evaluation of Strategic Intervention in multi-drug resistant patients with tipranavir (RESIST) studies: an analysis of combined data from two randomized open-label trials. Lancet. 2006; 368:466–75.

Kandula VR, Khanlou H, Farthing C. Tipranavir: a novel second-generation nonpeptidic protease inhibitor. Expert Rev Anti Infect Ther. 2005;3:9–21.

Kashuba AD. Drug-drug interactions and the pharmacotherapy of HIV infection. Top HIV Med. 2005;13:64–9.

Panel on Antiretroviral Guidelines for Adults and Adolescents. Guidelines for the use of antiretroviral agents in HIV-1-infected adults and adolescents, updated July 14, 2016. Department of Health and Human Services; 1–288. Available at https://aidsinfo.nih.gov/contentfiles/lvguidelines/adultandadolescentgl.pdf.

Plosker GL, Figgitt DP. Tipranavir. Drugs. 2003;63: 1611–8.

Product Information: Aptivus oral capsules, solution, tipranavir oral capsules, solution. Boehringer Ingelheim Pharmaceuticals, Inc, Ridgefield, CT; 2011.

Zidovudine (Retrovir) (ZDV)

Drug Class: Antiretroviral; NRTI (nucleoside reverse transcriptase inhibitor)

Usual Dose: 300 mg (PO) bid (see comments). IV solution 10 mg/mL (dose 1 mg/kg 5–6×/day)

"Usual dose" assumes normal renal/hepatic function. * For renal insufficiency, give usual dose × 1 followed by maintenance dose per CrCl. For dialysis patients, dose the same as for CrCl < 10 mL/min and give supplemental (post-HD/PD dose) immediately after dialysis. CrCl = creatinine clearance; CVVH = continuous venovenous hemofiltration; HD/PD = hemodialysis/peritoneal dialysis. See pp. 204–207 for explanations, pp. xi–xii for abbreviations.

How Supplied: Oral capsule: 100 mg; oral tablet: 300 mg; oral syrup: 50 mg/5 mL; intravenous solution: 10 mg/mL

Pharmacokinetic Parameters:
Peak serum level: 1.2 mcg/mL
Bioavailability: 64%
Excreted unchanged (urine): 16%
Serum half-life (normal/ESRD): 1.1/1.4 h
Plasma protein binding: < 38%
Volume of distribution (V_d): 1.6 L/kg

Primary Mode of Elimination: Hepatic
Dosage Adjustments*

CrCl 50–80 mL/min	No change
CrCl 15–450 mL/min	No change
CrCl < 15 mL/min	300 mg (PO) QD
HD/PD	100 mg (PO) q6–8h
Post-HD/PD dose	None
CVVH dose	300 mg (PO) QD
Moderate or severe hepatic insufficiency	No information

Drug Interactions: Acetaminophen, atovaquone, fluconazole, methadone, probenecid, valproic acid (↑ zidovudine levels); clarithromycin, nelfinavir, rifampin, rifabutin (↓ zidovudine levels); dapsone, flucytosine, ganciclovir, interferon alpha, bone marrow suppressive/cytotoxic agents (↑ risk of hematologic toxicity); indomethacin (↑ levels of zidovudine toxic metabolite); phenytoin (↑ zidovudine levels; ↑ or ↓ phenytoin levels); ribavirin (↓ zidovudine effect; avoid).

Adverse Effects: Nausea, vomiting, GI upset, diarrhea, malaise, anorexia, leukopenia, severe anemia, macrocytosis, thrombocytopenia, headaches, ↑ SGOT/SGPT, hepatotoxicity, myalgias, myositis, symptomatic myopathy, insomnia, blue/black nail discoloration, asthenia, lactic acidosis with hepatic steatosis (rare, but potentially life-threatening toxicity with use of NRTIs).

Allergic Potential: Low
Safety in Pregnancy: C
Comments: Antagonized by ganciclovir or ribavirin. Also a component of Combivir and Trizivir. Patients on IV therapy should be switched to PO as soon as able to take oral medication. For IV administration, dilute in D5W to a concentration no greater than 4 mg/mL and infuse over 1 hour.
Cerebrospinal Fluid Penetration: 60%

REFERENCES:

Barry M, Mulcahy F, Merry C, et al. Pharmacokinetics and potential interactions amongst antiretroviral agents used to treat patients with HIV infection. Clin Pharmacol. 1999;36:289–304.

McDowell JA, Lou Y, Symonds WS, et al. Multiple-dose pharmacokinetics and pharmacodynamics of abacavir alone and in combination with zidovudine in human immunodeficiency virus-infected adults. Antimicrob Agents Chemother. 2000;44:2061–7.

Panel on Antiretroviral Guidelines for Adults and Adolescents. Guidelines for the use of antiretroviral agents in HIV-1-infected adults and adolescents, updated July 14, 2016. Department of Health and Human Services; 1–288. Available at https://aidsinfo.nih.gov/contentfiles/lvguidelines/adultandadolescentgl.pdf.

Piscitelli SC, Gallicano KD. Interactions among drugs for HIV and opportunistic infections. N Engl J Med. 2001; 344:984–996.

Simpson DM. Human immunodeficiency virus-associated dementia: A review of pathogenesis, prophylaxis, and treatment studies of zidovudine therapy. Clin Infect Dis. 1999;29:19–34.

Appendix 1*

*   Reprinted with permission and updates from the International Antiviral Society–USA. Wensing AM,
    Calvez V, Günthard HF, et al. 2017 Update of the drug resistance mutations in HIV-1. *Topics in Antiviral
    Medicine*. December 2016/January 2017; 24(4): 2017 Resistance Mutations Update. © 2017 IAS–USA.
    Updated information and User Notes are available at www.iasusa.org.

MUTATIONS IN THE REVERSE TRANSCRIPTASE GENE ASSOCIATED WITH RESISTANCE TO REVERSE TRANSCRIPTASE INHIBITORS

Nucleoside and Nucleotide Analogue Reverse Transcriptase Inhibitors (nRTIs)[a]

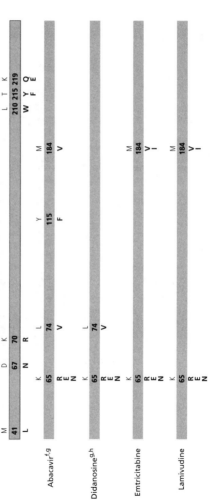

Multi-nRTI Resistance: 69 Insertion Complex[b] (affects all nRTIs currently approved by the US FDA)

Multi-nRTI Resistance: 151 Complex[c] (affects all nRTIs currently approved by the US FDA except tenofovir)

Multi-nRTI Resistance: Thymidine Analogue-Associated Mutations[d,e] (TAMs; affect all nRTIs currently approved by the US FDA other than emtricitabine and lamivudine)

Abacavir[f,g]

Didanosine[g,h]

Emtricitabine

Lamivudine

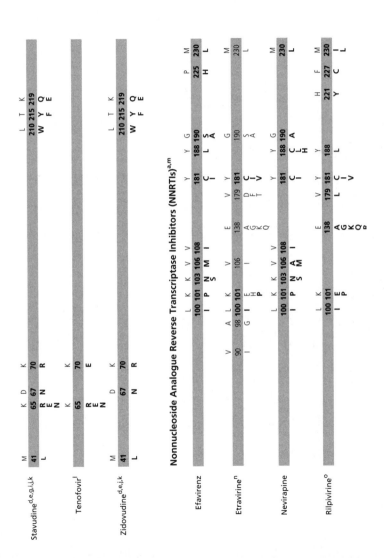

Nonnucleoside Analogue Reverse Transcriptase Inhibitors (NNRTIs)[a,m]

MUTATIONS IN THE PROTEASE GENE ASSOCIATED WITH RESISTANCE TO PROTEASE INHIBITORS[p,q,r]

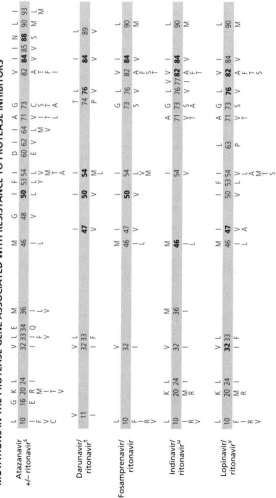

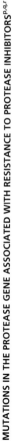

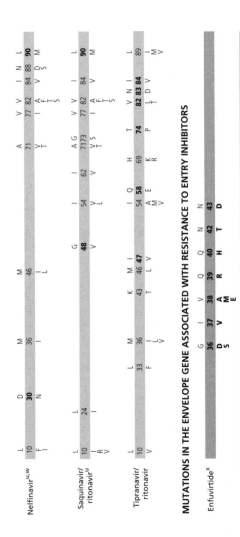

MUTATIONS IN THE ENVELOPE GENE ASSOCIATED WITH RESISTANCE TO ENTRY INHIBITORS

MUTATIONS IN THE INTEGRASE GENE ASSOCIATED WITH RESISTANCE TO INTEGRASE INHIBITORS[z]

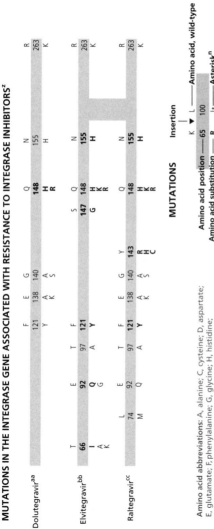

Dolutegravir[aa]

	T		E	T		F		E	G			Q		N		R
	66		92	97		121		138	140			148		155		263
	I		Q	A		Y		A	A			H		H		K
	A		G					K	S			R				
	K															

Elvitegravir[bb]

			E	T		F		E	G		S	Q		N		R
			92	97		121		138	140		147	148		155		263
			Q	A		Y		A	A		G	H		H		K
			G					K	S			K				
												R				

Raltegravir[cc]

	L		E	T		F		E	G	Y		Q		N		R
	74		92	97		121		138	140	143		148		155		263
	M		Q	A		Y		A	A	R		H		H		K
								K	S	H		K				
										C		R				

MUTATIONS

Insertion

K ▶ L ——— Amino acid, wild-type

Amino acid position ——— 65 100

Amino acid substitution ——— R I* ——— Asterisk[n]
conferring resistance

Amino acid abbreviations: A, alanine; C, cysteine; D, aspartate;
E, glutamate; F, phenylalanine; G, glycine; H, histidine;
I, isoleucine; K, lysine; L, leucine; M, methionine; N, asparagine;
P, proline; Q, glutamine; R, arginine; S, serine; T, threonine;
V, valine; W, tryptophan; Y, tyrosine.

IAS–USA DRUG RESISTANCE MUTATIONS IN HIV-1: January 2017

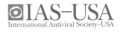

International Antiviral Society–USA

The IAS–USA Drug Resistance Mutations Group reviews new data on HIV-1 drug resistance that have been published or presented at scientific conferences to maintain a current list of mutations associated with antiretroviral drug resistance. The compilation includes mutations that may contribute to a reduced virologic response to a drug. It should not be assumed that the list presented here is exhaustive. Drugs that have been approved by the US Food and Drug Administration (FDA), as well as any drugs available in expanded access programs, are included and listed in alphabetic order within each drug class.

The mutations listed have been identified by one or more of the following criteria: (1) in vitro passage experiments or validation of contribution to resistance by using site-directed mutagenesis, (2) susceptibility testing of laboratory or clinical isolates, (3) nucleotide sequencing of viruses from patients in whom the drug is failing, (4) correlation studies between genotype at baseline and virologic response in patients exposed to a drug. The availability of more recently approved drugs that cannot be tested as monotherapy precludes assessment of the impact of resistance on antiretroviral activity that is not seriously confounded by activity of other drug components in the background regimen. Readers are encouraged to consult the literature and experts in the field for clarification or more information about specific mutations and their clinical impact. Polymorphisms associated with impaired treatment responses that occur in wild-type viruses should not be used *in epidemiologic analyses to identify transmitted HIV-1 drug resistance. For more in-depth reading and an extensive reference list, see the 2008 IAS–USA panel recommendations for resistance testing (Hirsch MS, Günthard HF, Schapiro JM, et al, Clin Infect Dis. 2008;47:266–285) and 2014 IAS-USA panel recommendations for antiretroviral therapy (Günthard HF, Aberg JA, Eron JJ, et al. JAMA. 2014; 312(4): 410–425).*

Updates and reference list are posted at www.iasusa.org EOS.

USER NOTES

a. Some nucleoside (or nucleotide) analogue reverse transcriptase inhibitor (nRTI) mutations, like T215Y and H208Y,[1] may lead to viral hypersusceptibility to the nonnucleoside analogue reverse transcriptase inhibitors (NNRTIs), including etravirine,[2] in nRTI-treated individuals. The presence of these mutations may improve subsequent virologic response to NNRTI-containing regimens (nevirapine or efavirenz) in NNRTI-naive individuals,[3-7] although no clinical data exist for improved response to etravirine in NNRTI-experienced individuals. Mutations at the C-terminal reverse transcriptase domains (amino acids 293–560) outside of regions depicted on the figure bars may prove to be important for nRTI and NNRTI HIV-1 drug resistance. The clinical relevance of these connection domain mutations arises mostly in conjunction with thymidine analogue-associated mutations (TAMs) and M184V and have not been associated with increased rates of virologic failure of etravirine or rilpivirine in clinical trials.[8-10]

K65E/N variants are increasingly reported in patients experiencing treatment failure with tenofovir, stavudine, or didanosine. K65E usually occurs in mixtures with wild type. K65N gives an approximately 4-fold decrease in susceptibility. Patient-derived viruses with K65E and site-directed mutations replicate very poorly in vitro; as such, no susceptibility testing can be performed.[11,12]

b. The 69 insertion complex consists of a substitution at codon 69 (typically T69S) and an insertion of two or more amino acids (S-S, S-A, S-G, or others). The 69 insertion complex is associated with resistance to all nRTIs currently approved by the US Food and Drug Administration (FDA) when present with one or more thymidine analogue–associated mutations (TAMs) at codons 41, 210, or 215.[13] Some other amino acid changes from the wild-type T at codon 69 without the insertion may be associated with broad nRTI resistance.

c. Tenofovir retains activity against the Q151M complex of mutations.[13] Q151M is the most important mutation in the complex (i.e., the other mutations in the complex [A62V, V75I, F77L, and F116Y] in isolation may not reflect multidrug resistance).

d. Mutations known to be selected by TAMs (M41L, D67N, K70R, L210W, T215Y/F, and K219Q/E) also confer reduced susceptibility to all approved nRTIs,[14] except emtricitabine and lamivudine, which in fact reverse the magnitude of resistance and are recommended with tenofovir or zidovudine in the presence of TAMS. The degree to which cross-resistance is observed depends on the specific mutations and number of mutations involed.[15–18]

e. Although reverse transcriptase changes associated with the E44D and V118I mutations may have an accessory role in increased resistance to nRTIs in the presence of TAMs, their clinical relevance is very limited.[19–21]

f. The M184V mutation alone does not appear to be associated with a reduced virologic response to abacavir in vivo. When associated with TAMs, M184V increases abacavir resistance.[22,23]

g. As with tenofovir, the K65R mutation may be selected by didanosine, abacavir, or stavudine (particularly in patients with nonsubtype-B clades) and is associated with decreased viral susceptibility to these drugs.[22,24,25] Data are lacking on the potential negative impact of K65R on clinical response to didanosine.

h. The presence of three of the following mutations—M41L, D67N, L210W, T215Y/F, K219Q/E—is associated with resistance to didanosine.[26] The presence of K70R or M184V alone does not decrease virologic response to didanosine.[27]

i. K65R is selected frequently (4%–11%) in patients with nonsubtype-B clades for whom stavudine-containing regimens are failing in the absence of tenofovir.[28,29]

j. The presence of M184V appears to delay or prevent emergence of TAMs.[30] This effect may be overcome by an accumulation of TAMs or other mutations.

k. The T215A/C/D/E/G/H/I/L/N/S/V substitutions are revertant mutations at codon 215 that confer increased risk of virologic failure of zidovudine or stavudine in antiretroviral-naive patients.[31,32] The T215Y mutant may emerge quickly from one of these mutations in the presence of zidovudine or stavudine.[33]

l. The presence of K65R is associated with a reduced virologic response to tenofovir.[13] A reduced response also occurs in the presence of three or more TAMs inclusive of either M41L or L210W.[13] The presence of TAMs or combined treatment with zidovudine prevents the emergence of K65R in the presence of tenofovir.[34–36] There are no data to indicate differences in resistance patterns between tenofovir disoproxil fumarate and tenofovir alafenamide because the active drug component in both formulations is tenofovir.

m. There is no evidence for the utility of efavirenz, nevirapine, or rilpivirine in patients with NNRTI resistance.[37]

n. Resistance to etravirine has been extensively studied only in the context of coadministration with ritonavir-booster darunavir. In this context, mutations associated with virologic outcome have been assessed and their relative weights (or magnitudes of impact) assigned. In addition, phenotypic cutoff values have been calculated, and assessment of genotype-phenotype correlations from a large clinical database have determined relative importance of the various mutations. These two approaches are in agreement for many, but not all, mutations and weights.[38-40] The single mutations L100I, K101P, and Y181C*/I*/V have a high relative weight with regard to reduced susceptibility and reduced clinical response compared with other mutations. The presence of K103N alone does not affect etravirine response.[41,42] Accumulation of several mutations results in greater reductions in susceptibility and virologic response than do single mutations.[43-45]

o. Fifteen mutations have been associated with decreased rilpivirine susceptibility (K101E/P, E138A/G/K/Q/R, V179L, Y181C/I/V, H221Y, F227C, and M230I/L).[46-48] A 16th mutation, Y188L, reduces rilpivirine susceptibility 6 fold.[49] K101P and Y181I/V reduce rilpivirine susceptibility approximately 50 fold and 15 fold, respectively, but are uncommonly observed in patients receiving rilpivirine.[49-51] Mutations at position 138 (most notably 138A) may occur as natural polymorphisms, especially in non-B subtypes.[52] K101E, E138K, and Y181C, each of which reduces rilpivirine susceptibility 2.5 fold to 3 fold, occur commonly in patients receiving rilpivirine. E138K, and to a lesser extent K101E, usually occur in combination with the nRTI resistance mutation M184I, which alone does not reduce rilpivirine susceptibility. When M184I is combined with E138K or K101E, rilpivirine susceptibility is reduced approximately 7 fold and 4.5 fold, respectively.[51,53-55] The combinations of reverse transcriptase–associated mutations L100I plus K103N/S and L100I plus K103R plus V179D were strongly associated with reduced susceptibility to rilpivirine. However, for isolates harboring the K103N/R/S or V179D as single mutations, no reduction in susceptibility was detected.[48,56]

p. Often, numerous mutations are necessary to substantially impact virologic response to a ritonavir-boosted protease inhibitor (PI).[57] In some specific circumstances, atazanavir might be used unboosted. In such cases, the mutations that are selected are the same as with ritonavir-boosted atazanavir, but the relative frequency of mutations may differ.

q. Resistance mutations in the protease gene are classified as "major" or "minor."

Major mutations in the protease gene (positions in **bold** type) are defined as those selected first in the presence of the drug or those substantially reducing drug susceptibility. These mutations tend to be the primary contact residues for drug binding, and may also be associated with reductions in virologic responses to therapy

Minor mutations generally emerge later than major mutations and by themselves do not have a substantial effect on phenotype. They may improve replication of viruses containing major mutations. Some minor mutations are present as common polymorphic changes in HIV-1 nonsubtype-B clades.

Mutations in *gag* cleavage sites may confer resistance to all PIs and may emerge before mutations in protease. A large proportion of virus samples from patients with confirmed virologic failure on a PI-containing regimen is not found to have PI resistance–associated mutations. Preliminary data from recent studies suggest that several mutations in the Gag protein[58] may be responsible for reduced PI susceptibility in a subset of these patients.

r. Ritonavir is not listed separately, as it is currently used only at low dose as a pharmacologic booster of other PIs.

s. Many mutations are associated with atazanavir resistance. Their impacts differ, with I50L, I84V, and N88S having the greatest effect. Higher atazanavir levels obtained with ritonavir boosting increase the number of mutations required for loss of activity. The presence of M46I plus L76V might increase susceptibility to atazanavir when no other related mutations are present.[59]

t. HIV-1 RNA response to ritonavir-boosted darunavir correlates with baseline susceptibility and the presence of several specific PI resistance-associated mutations. Reductions in response are associated with increasing numbers of the mutations indicated in the figure bar. The negative impact of the protease mutations I47V, I54M, T74P, and I84V and the positive impact of the protease mutation V82A on virologic response to ritonavir-boosted darunavir were shown in two data sets independently.[60,61] Some of these mutations appear to have a greater effect on susceptibility than others (e.g., I50V vs. V11I). The presence at baseline of two or more of the substitutions V11I, V32I, L33F, I47V, I50V, I54L or M, T74P, L76V, I84V, or L89V was associated with a decreased virologic response to ritonavir-boosted darunavir.[62]

u. The mutations depicted on the figure bar cannot be considered comprehensive because little relevant research has been reported in recent years to update the resistance and cross-resistance patterns for this drug.

v. In PI-experienced patients, the accumulation of six or more of the mutations indicated on the figure bar is associated with a reduced virologic response to ritonavir-booster lopinavir.[63, 64] The product information states that accumulation of seven or eight mutations confers resistance to the drug.[65] However, there is emerging evidence that specific mutations, most notably I47A (and possibly I47V) and V32I, are associated with high-level resistance.[66–68] The addition of L76V to three PI resistance–associated mutations substantially increases resistance to ritonavir-boosted lopinavir.[59]

w. In some nonsubtype-B HIV-1, D30N is selected less frequently than are other PI resistance-associated mutations.[69]

x. Resistance to enfuvirtide is associated primarily with mutations in the first heptad repeat (HR1) region of the gp41 envelope gene. However, mutations or polymorphisms in other regions of the envelope (e.g., the HR2 region or those yet to be identified) as well as coreceptor usage and density may affect susceptibility to enfuvirtide.[70–72]

y. The activity of CC chemokine receptor 5 (CCR5) antagonists is limited to patients with virus that uses only CCR5 for entry (R5 virus). Viruses that use both CCR5 and CXC chemokine receptor 4 (CXCR4; termed dual/mixed [D/M] virus) or only CXCR4 (X4 virus) do not respond to treatment with CCR5 antagonists. Virologic failure of these drugs frequently is associated with outgrowth of D/M or X4 virus from a preexisting minority population present at levels below the limit of assay detection. Mutations in HIV-1 gp120 that allow the virus to bind to the drug-bound form of CCR5 have been described in viruses from some patients whose virus remained R5 after virologic failure of a CCR5 antagonist. Most of these mutations are found in the V3 loop, the major determinant of viral tropism.[73] There is as yet no consensus on specific signature mutations for CCR5 antagonist resistance, so they are not depicted in the figure. Some CCR5 antagonist-resistant viruses selected in vitro have shown mutations in gp41 without mutations in V3;[74] the clinical significance of such mutations is not yet known.

z. In site-directed mutants and clinical isolates, the mutation F121Y has a profound effect on susceptibility to elvitegravir and raltegravir and to a lesser extent to dolutegravir. Mutation R263K can be selected in vivo during treatment with dolutegravir and raltegravir and results in a 2- to 5-fold reduction in susceptibility to dolutegravir, elvitegravir, and raltegravir.[75–80]

aa. Several mutations are required in HIV integrase to confer high-level resistance to dolutegravir.[81] Cross-resistance studies with raltegravir- and elvitegravir-resistant viruses in vitro indicate that Q148H/R and G140S in combination with mutations L74I/M, E92Q, T97A, E138A/K, G140A, or N155H are associated with 5-fold to 20-fold reduced dolutegravir susceptibility[82] and reduced virologic suppression in patients.[83–86]

bb. Seven elvitegravir codon mutations have been observed in integrase strand transfer inhibitor treatment-naive and -experienced patients in whom therapy is failing.[87–93] T97A results in only a 2-fold change in elvitegravir susceptibility and may require additional mutations for resistance.[92,93] The sequential use of elvitegravir and raltegravir (in either order) is not recommended because of cross-resistance between these drugs.[92]

cc. Raltegravir failure is associated with integrase mutations in at least three distinct genetic pathways defined by two or more mutations including (1) a signature (major) mutation at Q148H/K/R, N155H, or Y143R/H/C; and (2) one or more additional minor mutations. Minor mutations described in the Q148H/K/R pathway include L74M plus E138A, E138K, or G140S. The most common mutational pattern in this pathway is Q148H plus G140S, which also confers the greatest loss of drug susceptibility. Mutations described in the N155H pathway include this major mutation plus either L74M, E92Q, T97A, E92Q plus T97A, Y143H, G163K/R, V151I, or D232N.[95] The Y143R/H/C mutation is uncommon.[96–100] E92Q alone reduces susceptibility to elvitegravir more than 20 fold and causes limited (< 5 fold) cross-resistance to raltegravir.[101–103] N155H mutants tend to predominate early in the course of raltegravir failure but are gradually replaced by viruses with higher resistance, often bearing mutations G140S plus Q148H/R/K, with continuing raltegravir treatment.[96]

REFERENCES TO THE USER NOTES

1. Clark SA, Shulman NS, Bosch RJ, Mellors JW. Reverse transcriptase mutations 118I, 208Y, and 215Y cause HIV-1 hypersusceptibility to non-nucleoside reverse transcriptase inhibitors. AIDS. 2006;20(7):981–984.

2. Picchio G, Vingerhoets J, Parkin N, Azijn H, de Bethune MP. Nucleoside-associated mutations cause hypersusceptibility to etravirine. Antivir Ther. 2008;13(Suppl 3):A25.

3. Shulman NS, Bosch RJ, Mellors JW, Albrecht MA, Katzenstein DA. Genetic correlates of efavirenz hypersusceptibility. AIDS. 2004;18(13):1781–1785.

4. Demeter LM, DeGruttola V, Lustgarten S, et al. Association of efavirenz hypersusceptibility with virologic response in ACTG 368, a randomized trial of abacavir (ABC) in combination with efavirenz (EFV) and indinavir (IDV) in HIV-infected subjects with prior nucleoside analog experience. HIV Clin Trials. 2008;9(1):11–25.

5. Haubrich RH, Kemper CA, Hellmann NS, et al. The clinical relevance of non-nucleoside reverse transcriptase inhibitor hypersusceptibility: a prospective cohort analysis. AIDS. 2002;16(15):F33–F40.

6. Tozzi V, Zaccarelli M, Narciso P, et al. Mutations in HIV-1 reverse transcriptase potentially associated with hypersusceptibility to nonnucleoside reverse-transcriptase inhibitors: effect on response to efavirenz-based therapy in an urban observational cohort. J Infect Dis. 2004;189(9):1688–1695.

7. Katzenstein DA, Bosch RJ, Hellmann N, et al. Phenotypic susceptibility and virological outcome in nucleoside-experienced patients receiving three or four antiretroviral drugs. AIDS. 2003;17(6):821–830.

8. von Wyl V, Ehteshami M, Demeter LM, et al. HIV-1 reverse transcriptase connection domain mutations: dynamics of emergence and implications for success of combination antiretroviral therapy. Clin Infect Dis. 2010;51(5):620–628.

9. Gupta S, Vingerhoets J, Fransen S, et al. Connection domain mutations in HIV-1 reverse transcriptase do not impact etravirine susceptibility and virologic responses to etravirine-containing regimens. Antimicrob Agents Chemother. 2011; 55(6):2872–2879.

10. Rimsky L, Van Eygen V, Vingerhoets J, Leijskens E, Picchio G. Reverse transcriptase connection domain mutations were not associated with virological failure or phenotypic resistance in rilpivirine-treated patients from the ECHO and THRIVE Phase III trials (week 96 analysis). Antivir Ther. 2012;17(Suppl 1):A36.

11. Fourati S, Visseaux B, Armenia D, et al. Identification of a rare mutation at reverse transcriptase Lys65 (K65E) in HIV-1-infected patients failing on nucleos(t)ide reverse transcriptase inhibitors. J Antimicrob Chemother. 2013;68(10):2199–2204.

12. Chunduri H, Crumpacker C, Sharma PL. Reverse transcriptase mutation K65N confers a decreased

replication capacity to HIV-1 in comparison to K65R due to a decreased RT processivity. *Virology*. 2011; 414(1):34–41.

13. Miller MD, Margot N, Lu B, et al. Genotypic and phenotypic predictors of the magnitude of response to tenofovir disoproxil fumarate treatment in antiretroviral-experienced patients. *J Infect Dis*. 2004; 189(5):837–846.

14. Whitcomb JM, Parkin NT, Chappey C, Hellman NS, Petropoulos CJ. Broad nucleoside reverse-transcriptase inhibitor cross-resistance in human immunodeficiency virus type 1 clinical isolates. *J Infect Dis*. 2003;188(7):992–1000.

15. Larder BA, Kemp SD. Multiple mutations in HIV-1 reverse transcriptase confer high-level resistance to zidovudine (AZT). *Science*. 1989; 246(4934): 1155–1158.

16. Kellam P, Boucher CA, Larder BA. Fifth mutation in human immunodeficiency virus type 1 reverse transcriptase contributes to the development of high-level resistance to zidovudine. *Proc Natl Acad Sci USA*. 1992;89(5):1934–1938.

17. Calvez V, Costagliola D, Descamps D, et al. Impact of stavudine phenotype and thymidine analogues mutations on viral response to stavudine plus lamivudine in ALTIS 2 ANRS trial. *Antivir Ther*. 2002; 7(3):211–218.

18. Kuritzkes DR, Bassett RL, Hazelwood JD, et al. Rate of thymidine analogue resistance mutation accumulation with zidovudine- or stavudine-based regimens. *JAIDS*. 2004;36(1):600–603.

19. Romano L, Venturi G, Bloor S, et al. Broad nucleoside-analogue resistance implications for human immunodeficiency virus type 1 reverse-transcriptase mutations at codons 44 and 118. *J Infect Dis*. 2002;185(7):898–904.

20. Walter H, Schmidt B, Werwein M, Schwingel E, Korn K. Prediction of abacavir resistance from genotypic data: impact of zidovudine and lamivudine resistance in vitro and in vivo. *Antimicrob Agents Chemother*. 2002;46(1):89–94.

21. Mihailidis C, Dunn D, Pillay D, Pozniak A. Effect of isolated V118I mutation in reverse transcriptase on response to first-line antiretroviral therapy. *AIDS*. 2008;22(3):427–430.

22. Harrigan PR, Stone C, Griffin P, et al. Resistance profile of the human immunodeficiency virus type 1 reverse transcriptase inhibitor abacavir (1592U89) after monotherapy and combination therapy. CNA2001 Investigative Group. *J Infect Dis*. 2000;181(3):912–920.

23. Lanier ER, Ait-Khaled M, Scott J, et al. Antiviral efficacy of abacavir in antiretroviral therapy-experienced adults harbouring HIV-1 with specific patterns of resistance to nucleoside reverse transcriptase inhibitors. *Antivir Ther*. 2004;9(1):37–45.

24. Winters MA, Shafer RW, Jellinger RA, Mamtora G, Gingeras T, Merigan TC. Human immunodeficiency virus type 1 reverse transcriptase genotype and drug susceptibility changes in infected individuals receiving dideoxyinosine monotherapy for 1 to 2 years. *Antimicrob Agents Chemother*. 1997;41(4):757–762.

25. Svarovskaia ES, Margot NA, Bae AS, et al. Low-level K65R mutation in HIV-1 reverse transcriptase of treatment-experienced patients exposed to abacavir or didanosine. *JAIDS*. 2007;46(2):174–180.

26. Marcelin AG, Flandre P, Pavie J, et al. Clinically relevant genotype interpretation of resistance to didanosine. *Antimicrob Agents Chemother*. 2005;49(5): 1739–1744.

27. Molina JM, Marcelin AG, Pavie J, et al. Didanosine in HIV-1-infected patients experiencing failure of antiretroviral therapy: a randomized placebo-controlled trial. *J Infect Dis*. 2005;191(6):840–847.

28. Hawkins CA, Chaplin B, Idoko J, et al. Clinical and genotypic findings in HIV-infected patients with the K65R mutation failing first-line antiretroviral therapy in Nigeria. *JAIDS*. 2009;52(2):228–234.

29. Wallis CL, Mellors JW, Venter WD, Sanne I, Stevens W. Varied patterns of HIV-1 drug resistance on failing first-line antiretroviral therapy in South Africa. *JAIDS*. 2010;53(4):480–484.

30. Kuritzkes DR, Quinn JB, Benoit SL, et al. Drug resistance and virologic response in NUCA 3001, a randomized trial of lamivudine (3TC) versus zidovudine (ZDV) versus ZDV plus 3TC in previously untreated patients. *AIDS*. 1996;10(9):975–981.

31. Violin M, Cozzi-Lepri A, Velleca R, et al. Risk of failure in patients with 215 HIV-1 revertants starting their first thymidine analog-containing highly active antiretroviral therapy. *AIDS*. 2004;18(2):227–235.

32. Chappey C, Wrin T, Deeks S, Petropoulos CJ. Evolution of amino acid 215 in HIV-1 reverse transcriptase in response to intermittent drug selection. *Antivir Ther*. 2003;8:S37.

33. Garcia-Lerma JG, MacInnes H, Bennett D, Weinstock H, Heneine W. Transmitted human immunodeficiency virus type 1 carrying the D67N or K219Q/E mutation evolves rapidly to zidovudine resistance in vitro and shows a high replicative fitness in the presence of zidovudine. *J Virol*. 2004;78(14):7545–7552.

34. Parikh UM, Zelina S, Sluis-Cremer N, Mellors JW. Molecular mechanisms of bidirectional antagonism between K65R and thymidine analog mutations in HIV-1 reverse transcriptase. *AIDS*. 2007;21(11):1405–1414.

35. Parikh UM, Barnas DC, Faruki H, Mellors JW. Antagonism between the HIV-1 reverse-transcriptase mutation K65R and thymidine-analogue mutations at the genomic level. *J Infect Dis*. 2006;194(5):651–660.

36. von Wyl V, Yerly S, Böni J, et al. Factors associated with the emergence of K65R in patients with HIV-1 infection treated with combination antiretroviral therapy containing tenofovir. *Clin Infect Dis*. 2008;46(8):1299–1309.

37. Antinori A, Zaccarelli M, Cingolani A, et al. Cross-resistance among nonnucleoside reverse transcriptase inhibitors limits recycling efavirenz after nevirapine failure. *AIDS Res Hum Retroviruses*. 2002; 18(12):835–838.

38. Benhamida J, Chappey C, Coakley E, Parkin NT. HIV-1 genotype algorithms for prediction of etravirine susceptibility: novel mutations and weighting factors identified through correlations to phenotype. *Antivir Ther*. 2008;13(Suppl 3):A142.

39. Coakley E, Chappey C, Benhamida J, et al. Biological and clinical cut-off analyses for etravirine in the PhenoSense HIV assay. *Antivir Ther*. 2008;13(Suppl 3):A134.

40. Vingerhoets J, Tambuyzer L, Azijn H, et al. Resistance profile of etravirine: combined analysis of baseline genotypic and phenotypic data from the randomized, controlled Phase III clinical studies. *AIDS*. 2010;24(4):503–514.

41. Haddad M, Stawiski E, Benhamida J, Coakley E. Improved genotypic algorithm for predicting etravirine susceptibility: comprehensive list of mutations identified through correlation with matched phenotype. 17th Conference on Retroviruses and Opportunistic Infections (CROI). February 16–19, 2010; San Francisco, California.

42. Etravirine [prescribing information]. 2013. Titusville, NJ, Janssen Therapeutics.

43. Scherrer AU, Hasse B, Von Wyl V, et al. Prevalence of etravirine mutations and impact on response to treatment in routine clinical care: the Swiss HIV Cohort Study (SHCS). *HIV Med*. 2009;10(10):647–656.

44. Tambuyzer L, Nijs S, Daems B, Picchio G, Vingerhoets J. Effect of mutations at position E138 in HIV-1 reverse transcriptase on phenotypic susceptibility and virologic response to etravirine. *JAIDS*. 2011; 58(1):18–22.

45. Tudor-Williams G, Cahn P, Chokephaibulkit K, et al. Etravirine in treatment-experienced, HIV-1-infected children and adolescents: 48-week safety, efficacy and resistance analysis of the phase II PIANO study. *HIV Med*. 2014;15(9):513–524.

46. Rilpivirine [prescribing information]. 2015. Titusville, NJ, Janssen Therapeutics.

47. Azijn H, Tirry I, Vingerhoets J, et al. TMC278, a next-generation nonnucleoside reverse transcriptase inhibitor (NNRTI), active against wild-type and NNRTI-resistant HIV-1. *Antimicrob Agents Chemother*. 2010;54(2):718–727.

48. Picchio GR, Rimsky LT, Van Eygen V, Haddad M, Napolitano LA, Vingerhoets J. Prevalence in the USA of rilpivirine resistance-associated mutations in clinical samples and effects on phenotypic susceptibility to rilpivirine and etravirine. *Antivir Ther*. 2014;19(8):819–823.

49. Cohen CJ, Andrade-Villanueva J, Clotet B, et al. Rilpivirine versus efavirenz with two background nucleoside or nucleotide reverse transcriptase inhibitors in treatment-naive adults infected with HIV-1 (THRIVE): a phase 3, randomised, non-inferiority trial. *Lancet*. 2011; 378(9787):229–237.

50. Molina JM, Cahn P, Grinsztejn B, et al. Rilpivirine versus efavirenz with tenofovir and emtricitabine in treatment-naive adults infected with HIV-1 (ECHO): a phase 3 randomised double-blind active-controlled trial. *Lancet*. 2011;378(9787):238–246.

51. Rimsky L, Vingerhoets J, Van Eygen V, et al. Genotypic and phenotypic characterization of HIV-1 isolates obtained from patients on rilpivirine therapy experiencing virologic failure in the phase 3 ECHO and THRIVE studies: 48-week analysis. *JAIDS*. 2012;59(1):39–46.

52. Hofstra M, Sauvageot N, Albert J, et al. Transmission of HIV drug resistance and the predicted effect on current first-line regimens in Europe. *Clin Infect Dis*. 2016;62(5):655–663.

53. Kulkarni R, Babaoglu K, Lansdon EB, et al. The HIV-1 reverse transcriptase M184I mutation enhances the E138K-associated resistance to rilpivirine and decreases viral fitness. *JAIDS*. 2012;59(1):47–54.

54. Hu Z, Kuritzkes DR. Interaction of reverse transcriptase (RT) mutations conferring resistance to lamivudine and etravirine: effects on fitness and RT activity of human immunodeficiency virus type 1. *J Virol*. 2011;85(21):11309–11314.

55. Xu HT, Asahchop EL, Oliveira M, et al. Compensation by the E138K mutation in HIV-1 reverse transcriptase for deficits in viral replication capacity and enzyme processivity associated with the M184I/V mutations. *J Virol.* 2011;85(21):11300–11308.

56. Haddad M, Napolitano LA, Frantzell A, et al. Combinations of HIV-1 reverse transcriptase mutations L100I+K103N/S and L100I +K103R+V179D reduce susceptibility to rilpivirine [Abstract H-677]. 53rd Interscience Conference on Antimicrobial Agents and Chemotherapy (ICAAC). September 10–13, 2013; Denver, Colorado.

57. Hirsch MS, Günthard HF, Schapiro JM, et al. Antiretroviral drug resistance testing in adult HIV-1 infection: 2008 recommendations of an International AIDS Society–USA panel. *Clin Infect Dis.* 2008;47(2):266–285.

58. Fun A, Wensing AM, Verheyen J, Nijhuis M. Human immunodeficiency virus Gag and protease: partners in resistance. *Retrovirology.* 2012;9:63.

59. Young TP, Parkin NT, Stawiski E, et al. Prevalence, mutation patterns, and effects on protease inhibitor susceptibility of the L76V mutation in HIV-1 protease. *Antimicrob Agents Chemother.* 2010;54(11):4903–4906.

60. De Meyer S, Descamps D, Van Baelen B, et al. Confirmation of the negative impact of protease mutations I47V, I54M, T74P and I84V and the positive impact of protease mutation V82A on virological response to darunavir/ritonavir. *Antivir Ther.* 2009;14(Suppl 1):A147.

61. Descamps D, Lambert-Niclot S, Marcelin AG, et al. Mutations associated with virological response to darunavir/ritonavir in HIV-1-infected protease inhibitor-experienced patients. *J Antimicrob Chemother.* 2009; 63(3):585–592.

62. Darunavir [prescribing information]. 2015. Titusville, NJ, Janssen Therapeutics.

63. Masquelier B, Breilh D, Neau D, et al. Human immunodeficiency virus type 1 genotypic and pharmacokinetic determinants of the virological response to lopinavir-ritonavir-containing therapy in protease inhibitor-experienced patients. *Antimicrob Agents Chemother.* 2002; 46(9):2926–2932.

64. Kempf DJ, Isaacson JD, King MS, et al. Identification of genotypic changes in human immunodeficiency virus protease that correlate with reduced susceptibility to the protease inhibitor lopinavir among viral isolates from protease inhibitor-experienced patients. *J Virol.* 2001;75(16):7462–7469.

65. Lopinavir/ritonavir [prescribing information]. 2015. Abbott Park, IL, AbbVie Inc.

66. Mo H, King MS, King K, Molla A, Brun S, Kempf DJ. Selection of resistance in protease inhibitor-experienced, human immunodeficiency virus type 1-infected subjects failing lopinavir- and ritonavir-based therapy: mutation patterns and baseline correlates. *J Virol.* 2005; 79(6):3329–3338.

67. Friend J, Parkin N, Liegler T, Martin JN, Deeks SG. Isolated lopinavir resistance after virological rebound of a ritonavir/lopinavir-based regimen. *AIDS.* 2004;18(14):1965–1966.

68. Kagan RM, Shenderovich M, Heseltine PN, Ramnarayan K. Structural analysis of an HIV-1 protease I47A mutant resistant to the protease inhibitor lopinavir. *Protein Sci.* 2005;14(7):1870–1878.

69. Gonzalez LM, Brindeiro RM, Aguiar RS, et al. Impact of nelfinavir resistance mutations on in vitro phenotype, fitness, and replication capacity of human immunodeficiency virus type 1 with subtype B and C proteases. *Antimicrob Agents Chemother.* 2004;48(9):3552–3555.

70. Reeves JD, Gallo SA, Ahmad N, et al. Sensitivity of HIV-1 to entry inhibitors correlates with envelope/coreceptor affinity, receptor density, and fusion kinetics. *Proc Natl Acad Sci USA.* 2002;99(25):16249–16254.

71. Reeves JD, Miamidian JL, Biscone MJ, et al. Impact of mutations in the coreceptor binding site on human immunodeficiency virus type 1 fusion, infection, and entry inhibitor sensitivity. *J Virol.* 2004;78(10):5476–5485.

72. Xu L, Pozniak A, Wildfire A, et al. Emergence and evolution of enfuvirtide resistance following long-term therapy involves heptad repeat 2 mutations within gp41. *Antimicrob Agents Chemother.* 2005; 49(3):1113–1119.

73. Maraviroc [prescribing information]. 2015. Research Triangle Park, NC, ViiV Healthcare.

74. Anastassopoulou CG, Ketas TJ, Sanders RW, Klasse PJ, Moore JP. Effects of sequence changes in the HIV-1 gp41 fusion peptide on CCR5 inhibitor resistance. *Virology.* 2012;428(2):86–97.

75. Malet I, Gimferrer AL, Artese A, et al. New raltegravir resistance pathways induce broad cross-resistance to all currently used integrase inhibitors. *J Antimicrob Chemother.* 2014;69(8):2118–2122.

76. Cahn P, Pozniak AL, Mingrone H, et al. Dolutegravir versus raltegravir in antiretroviral-experienced, integrase-inhibitor-naive adults with HIV: week 48 results

from the randomised, double-blind, non-inferiority SAILING study. *Lancet.* 2013;382(9893):700–708.

77. Quashie PK, Mesplede T, Han YS, et al. Characterization of the R263K mutation in HIV-1 integrase that confers low-level resistance to the second-generation integrase strand transfer inhibitor dolutegravir. *J Virol.* 2012;86(5):2696–2705.

78. Souza Cavalcanti J, Minhoto LA, de Paula Ferreira JL, da Eira M, de Souza Dantas DS, de Macedo Brigido LF. In-vivo selection of the mutation F121Y in a patient failing raltegravir containing salvage regimen. *Antiviral Res.* 2012;95(1):9–11.

79. Margot NA, Hluhanich RM, Jones GS, et al. In vitro resistance selections using elvitegravir, raltegravir, and two metabolites of elvitegravir M1 and M4. *Antiviral Res.* 2012;93(2):288–296.

80. Brenner BG, Lowe M, Moisi D, et al. Subtype diversity associated with the development of HIV-1 resistance to integrase inhibitors. *J Med Virol.* 2011;83(5):751–759.

81. Frantzell A, Petropoulos C, Huang W. Dolutegravir resistance requires multiple primary mutations in HIV-1 integrase [CROI Abstract 121]. In Special Issue: Abstracts from the 2015 Conference on Retroviruses and Opportunistic Infections. *Top Antivir Med.* 2015; 23(e-1):51.

82. Kobayashi M, Yoshinaga T, Seki T, et al. In vitro antiretroviral properties of S/GSK1349572, a next-generation HIV integrase inhibitor. *Antimicrob Agents Chemother.* 2011;55(2):813–821.

83. Raffi F, Rachlis A, Stellbrink HJ, et al. Once-daily dolutegravir versus raltegravir in antiretroviral-naive adults with HIV-1 infection: 48 week results from the randomised, double-blind, non-inferiority SPRING-2 study. *Lancet.* 2013;381(9868):735–743.

84. Eron JJ, Clotet B, Durant J, et al. Safety and efficacy of dolutegravir in treatment-experienced subjects with raltegravir-resistant HIV type 1 infection: 24-week results of the VIKING Study. *J Infect Dis.* 2013; 207(5):740–748.

85. Seki T, Suyama-Kagitani A, Kawauchi-Miki S, et al. Effects of raltegravir or elvitegravir resistance signature mutations on the barrier to dolutegravir resistance in vitro. *Antimicrob Agents Chemother.* 2015; 59(5):2596–2606.

86. DeAnda F, Hightower KE, Nolte RT, et al. Dolutegravir interactions with HIV-1 integrase-DNA: structural rationale for drug resistance and dissociation kinetics. *PLoS One.* 2013;8(10):e77448.

87. Goodman D, Hluhanich R, Waters J, et al. Integrase inhibitor resistance involves complex interactions among primary and second resistance mutations: a novel mutation L68V/I associates with E92Q and increases resistance. *Antivir Ther.* 2008;13(Suppl 3):A15.

88. Waters J, Margot N, Hluhanich R, et al. Evolution of resistance to the HIV integrase inhibitor (INI) elvitegravir can involve genotypic switching among primary INI resistance patterns. Fort Myers, FL. *Antivir Ther.* 2009;14(Supp 1):A137.

89. Doyle T, Dunn DT, Ceccherini-Silberstein F, et al. Integrase inhibitor (INI) genotypic resistance in treatment-naive and raltegravir-experienced patients infected with diverse HIV-1 clades. *J Antimicrob Chemother.* 2015;70(11):3080–3086.

90. Sax PE, DeJesus E, Mills A, et al. Co-formulated elvitegravir, cobicistat, emtricitabine, and tenofovir versus co-formulated efavirenz, emtricitabine, and tenofovir for initial treatment of HIV-1 infection: a randomised, double-blind, phase 3 trial, analysis of results after 48 weeks. *Lancet.* 2012;379(9835):2439–2448.

91. DeJesus E, Rockstroh J, Henry K, et al. Co-formulated elvitegravir, cobicistat, emtricitabine, and tenofovir disoproxil fumarate versus ritonavir-boosted atazanavir plus co-formulated emtricitabine and tenofovir disoproxil fumarate for initial treatment of HIV-1 infection: a randomised, double-blind, phase 3, non-inferiority trial. *Lancet.* 2012; 379(9835):2429–2438.

92. Abram ME, Hluhanich RM, Goodman DD, et al. Impact of primary elvitegravir resistance-associated mutations in HIV-1 integrase on drug susceptibility and viral replication fitness. *Antimicrob Agents Chemother.* 2013;57(6):2654–2663.

93. White K, Kulkarni R, Miller MD. Analysis of early resistance development at the rst failure timepoint in elvitegravir/cobicistat/emtricitabine/tenofovir disoproxil fumarate-treated patients. *J Antimicrob Chemother.* 2015;70(9):2632–2638.

94. Scherrer AU, Yang WL, Kouyos RD, et al. Successful prevention of transmission of integrase resistance in the Swiss HIV Cohort Study. *J Infect Dis.* 2016;214(3):399–402.

95. Hazuda DF, Miller MD, Nguyen BY, Zhao J, for the P005 Study Team. Resistance to the HIV-integrase inhibitor raltegravir: analysis of protocol 005, a phase II study in patients with triple-class resistant HIV-1 infection. *Antivir Ther.* 2007;12:S10.

96. Gatell JM, Katlama C, Grinsztejn B, et al. Long-term efficacy and safety of the HIV integrase inhibitor raltegravir in patients with limited treatment options in a Phase II study. *JAIDS.* 2010;53(4):456–463.

97. Fransen S, Gupta S, Danovich R, et al. Loss of raltegravir susceptibility by human immunodeficiency virus type 1 is conferred via multiple nonoverlapping genetic pathways. *J Virol.* 2009;83(22):11440–11446.

98. Hatano H, Lampiris H, Fransen S, et al. Evolution of integrase resistance during failure of integrase inhibitor-based antiretroviral therapy. *J Acquir Immune De c Syndr.* 2010;54(4):389–393.

99. Wittkop L, Breilh D, Da Silva D, et al. Virological and immunological response in HIV-1-infected patients with multiple treatment failures receiving raltegravir and optimized background therapy, ANRS CO3 Aquitaine Cohort. *J Antimicrob Chemother.* 2009;63(6):1251–1255.

100. Armenia D, Vandenbroucke I, Fabeni L, et al. Study of genotypic and phenotypic HIV-1 dynamics of integrase mutations during raltegravir treatment: a refined analysis by ultra-deep 454 pyrosequencing. *J Infect Dis.* 2012;205(4):557–567.

101. Cooper DA, Steigbigel RT, Gatell JM, et al. Subgroup and resistance analyses of raltegravir for resistant HIV-1 infection. *N Engl J Med.* 2008;359(4):355–365.

102. Malet I, Delelis O, Valantin MA, et al. Mutations associated with failure of raltegravir treatment affect integrase sensitivity to the inhibitor in vitro. *Antimicrob Agents Chemother.* 2008;52(4):1351–1358.

103. Blanco JL, Varghese V, Rhee SY, Gatell JM, Shafer RW. HIV-1 integrase inhibitor resistance and its clinical implications. *J Infect Dis.* 2011;203(9):1204–1214.

These updated figures and additional information about the IAS–USA Drug Resistance Mutations Group are also available on the IAS–USA Web site (www.iasusa.org). To purchase copies of this card, call (415) 544-9400, e-mail the request to info2017@iasusa.org, or write to IAS–USA, 425 California Street, Suite 1450, San Francisco, CA 94104-2120. For permission to reprint or adapt the figures, please contact the IAS–USA.

Reprinted with permission and updates from the International Antiviral Society–USA. Wensing AM, Calvez V, Günthard HF, et al. 2017 Update of the drug resistance mutations in HIV-1. *Topics in Antiviral Medicine.* December 2016/January 2017; 24(4): 2017 Resistance Mutations Update. © 2017 IAS–USA. Updated information and User Notes are available at www.iasusa.org.

Appendix 2

SELECTED KEY INTERNET RESOURCES

- AIDSinfo—A Service of the Department of Health and Human Services (www.aidsinfo.nih.gov)
- Centers for Disease Control HIV (www.cdc.gov/hiv/)
- Clinical Care Options (www.clinicaloptions.com/HIV.aspx)
- Comprehensive HIV/AIDS Resource (www.thebody.com)
- Hepatitis C Treatment Guidelines (hcvguidelines.org)
- HIV Drug Interactions (www.HIV-druginteractions.org)
- HCV Drug Interactions (www.hep-druginteractions.org)
- HIV and Hepatitis.com (www.hivandhepatitis.com)
- HIV and Observations (blogs.jwatch.org/hiv-id-observations/)
- International Antiviral Society—USA (www.iasusa.org)
- Journal Watch: Infectious Diseases (www.jwatch.org/infectious-diseases)
- Medscape HIV/AIDS (www.medscape.com/hiv)
- National AIDS Treatment Advocacy Project (www.natap.org)
- National Clinicians' Post-exposure Prophylaxis Hotline (www.ucsf.edu/hivcntr/Hotlines/PEPline.html)
- National HIV/AIDS Clinicians' Consultation Center (www.nccc.ucsf.edu/)
- National Institute of Allergy and Infectious Diseases (www3.niaid.nih.gov/)
- National Library of Medicine—AIDS Portal (sis.nlm.nih.gov/hiv.html)
- National Library of Medicine—MedlinePlus AIDS page (www.nlm.nih.gov/medlineplus/)
- New York State HIV Guidelines (www.hivguidelines.org)

INDEX